Maximize Your Rotations

ASHP's Student Guide to IPPEs, APPEs, and Beyond

Mate M. Soric

American Society of Health-System Pharmacists®

Bethesda, Maryland

Any correspondence regarding this publication should be sent to the publisher, American Society of Health-System Pharmacists, 7272 Wisconsin Avenue, Bethesda, MD 20814, attention: Special Publishing.

The information presented herein reflects the opinions of the contributors and advisors. It should not be interpreted as an official policy of ASHP or as an endorsement of any product.

Because of ongoing research and improvements in technology, the information and its applications contained in this text are constantly evolving and are subject to the professional judgment and interpretation of the practitioner due to the uniqueness of a clinical situation. The editors, contributors, and ASHP have made reasonable efforts to ensure the accuracy and appropriateness of the information presented in this document. However, any user of this information is advised that the editors, contributors, advisors, and ASHP are not responsible for the continued currency of the information, for any errors or omissions, and/or for any consequences arising from the use of the information in the document in any and all practice settings. Any reader of this document is cautioned that ASHP makes no representation, guarantee, or warranty, express or implied, as to the accuracy and appropriateness of the information contained in this document and specifically disclaims any liability to any party for the accuracy and/or completeness of the material or for any damages arising out of the use or non-use of any of the information contained in this document.

Director, Special Publishing: Jack Bruggeman

Acquisitions Editor: Robin Coleman

Editorial Project Manager: Ruth Bloom

Production Editor: Johnna Hershey

Design: David Wade

Library of Congress Cataloging-in-Publication Data

Maximize your rotations : ASHP's guide to IPPEs, APPEs, and beyond / editor, Mate M. Soric.
    p.; cm.
ASHP's guide to IPPEs, APPEs, and beyond
Includes bibliographical references and index.
ISBN 978-1-58528-354-5
I. Soric, Mate M. II. American Society of Health-System Pharmacists. III. Title: ASHP's guide to IPPEs, APPEs, and beyond.
[DNLM: 1. Education, Pharmacy. 2. Pharmacists. 3. Professional Competence. QV 18]

615.1071--dc23
                    2012046173

ISBN 978-1-58528-354-5

First, to my wife and family for supporting me through the many nights and weekends of writing and editing.

Second, to my students for keeping me on my toes.

Lastly, to all of my preceptors for putting up with me when I was a student.

Table of Contents

PART III: LIFE AFTER ROTATIONS

After countless hours dedicated to lectures, study sessions, and exams, it is finally time to put your skills to the test in the real world. Regardless of the number of simulated patient experiences or multiple-choice questions you have successfully completed, no classroom activity can be a substitute for the hands-on training that the introductory and advanced pharmacy practice experiences (IPPEs and APPEs) can provide. Your rotations will likely be one of the first times you can use what you have learned in pharmacy school to make a significant impact on your patient's health. Often, this transition comes with some degree of difficulty. You will be required to make the leap from hypothetical situations and abstract concepts to addressing real drug-related problems in situations much more complex than anything you can find in a textbook.

Although rotations are vital to the development of the skills needed to practice pharmacy, there is little guidance available to pharmacy students to describe the best way to prepare, let alone how to make the most of these crucial experiences. The purpose of this text is to give pharmacy students a place to turn for all things experiential. It provides you with a glimpse of the general expectations and typical activities of your rotations before they begin, allowing for better preparation and performance. Part I, The Essentials, covers the broad skills needed to succeed on any type of rotation such as professionalism, literature evaluation, and case presentation skills. Part II, The Particulars, delves into the unique skills required to excel in each major type of rotation and is organized by rotation type. Part III, Life After Rotations, deals with the transition from student to pharmacist, with a focus on lifelong learning, getting your first job, and becoming a preceptor yourself.

To ensure that you are getting the best resource possible, an incredible team of pharmacy preceptors from across the country has come together to lend their expertise to the creation of this book. They have included cases that illustrate the common pitfalls that pharmacy students encounter, quotes from students and preceptors that provide first-hand perspectives, and the essential information that will get you the best results from your rotations.

In addition to all of these excellent pharmacy role models, I would like to thank Robin Coleman, Ruth Bloom, Johnna Hershey, and all of the other members of the American Society of Health-System Pharmacists publishing team that provided invaluable guidance as we created this resource for pharmacy students. We all hope that you use the material we have provided to maximize your rotations and start your career off on the right foot.

CONTRIBUTORS

ROBERT D. BECKETT, PharmD, BCPS

Clinical Assistant Professor
Drug Information Specialist
Manchester University
Fort Wayne, Indiana

CARLA BOUWMEESTER, MS, PharmD, BCPS

Assistant Clinical Professor
Bouvé College of Health Sciences
and
Geriatric Clinical Pharmacist
Northeastern University
Boston, Massachusetts

MICHAEL R. BRODEUR, PharmD, CGP, FASCP

Associate Professor
Albany College of Pharmacy and Health Sciences
Albany, New York

SUSAN P. BRUCE, PharmD, BCPS

Chair and Associate Professor
Northeast Ohio Medical University
Rootstown, Ohio

KATHERINE M. COCHRAN, PharmD

Assistant Director of Experiential Education
University of Findlay
Findlay, Ohio

JEAN CUNNINGHAM, PharmD, BCPS

Clinical Content Specialist
Truven Health Analytics
Findlay, Ohio

LINDSAY DAVISON, PharmD

Consumer Safety Officer
Division of Drug Information
Center for Drug Evaluation and Research
Food and Drug Administration
Silver Spring, Maryland

DALE E. ENGLISH II, PharmD, FASHP

Director, Instructional Labs and Professional
  Relations
Associate Professor of Pharmacy Practice
Associate Professor of Pharmaceutical Sciences
Northeast Ohio Medical University
Rootstown, Ohio

LORI ERNSTHAUSEN, PharmD, BCPS

Assistant Professor
University of Findlay
Findlay, Ohio

LAWRENCE A. FRAZEE, PharmD, BCPS

Pharmacotherapy Specialist
Akron General Medical Center
Akron, Ohio

JASON GLOWCZEWSKI, PharmD, MBA

Manager, Pharmacy and Oncology Services
University Hospitals Geauga Medical Center
Chardon, Ohio

MEGAN KAUN, PharmD, BCPS, BCACP

Director of Experiential Education
University of Toledo
Toledo, Ohio

DANIEL KRINSKY, MS, RPh

Associate Professor of Pharmacy Practice
Northeast Ohio Medical University
Rootstown, Ohio

JANIS J. MACKICHAN, PharmD, FAPhA

Vice Chair and Professor
Northeast Ohio Medical University
Rootstown, Ohio

BRANDON MOTTICE, PharmD

Clinical Specialist and PGY1 Residency Coordinator
Medina Hospital
Medina, Ohio

JOHN E. MURPHY, PharmD, FCCP, FASHP
Professor and Associate Dean
University of Arizona College of Pharmacy
Tucson, Arizona

LAURA A. PERRY, PharmD, BCPS
Assistant Professor of Pharmacy Practice
University of Findlay
Findlay, Ohio

STACEY SCHNEIDER, PharmD
Assistant Professor
Northeast Ohio Medical University
Rootstown, Ohio

MICHELLE SERRES, PharmD, BC-ADM, BCACP
Clinical Assistant Professor
University of Toledo
Toledo, Ohio

STEVEN R. SMITH, MS, RPh, BCACP
Clinical Pharmacist, Family Medicine
Toledo Hospital Family Medicine Residency
Toledo, Ohio

MATE M. SORIC, PharmD, BCPS
Clinical Pharmacist
University Hospitals Geauga Medical Center
Chardon, Ohio
and
Assistant Professor
Northeast Ohio Medical University
Rootstown, Ohio

TIMOTHY R. ULBRICH, PharmD
Director of Pharmacy Resident Education
Assistant Professor of Pharmacy Practice
Northeast Ohio Medical University
Rootstown, Ohio

S. SCOTT WISNESKI, PharmD, MBA
Director of Experiential Education
Northeast Ohio Medical University
Rootstown, Ohio

Part I: The Essentials

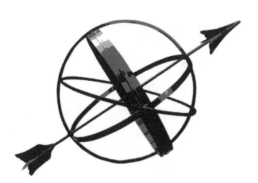

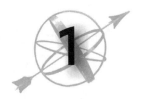

PROFESSIONALISM

S. Scott Wisneski, PharmD, MBA, and Mate M. Soric, PharmD, BCPS

CASE

M.B. is a pharmacy student currently completing her ambulatory care APPE rotation. During the midpoint evaluation, her preceptor expresses concern regarding certain behaviors that she had displayed during the rotation. M.B. arrived late on three separate occasions and did not complete a recent patient case exercise by the assigned due date. The preceptor is also extremely concerned about a comment that M.B. made to a fellow pharmacy student, in which she stated, "I don't like working with the diabetic patients at this clinic; they are all noncompliant and don't follow recommendations for their diet and blood sugar checks. I just want to get through this rotation so I can graduate and start working as a hospital pharmacist." The preceptor informs M.B. that if her professional behavior does not improve over the remaining weeks of the rotation, she will likely receive a failing grade. M.B. is surprised with the evaluation and believes her tardiness was not excessive and that her lateness in completing the assignment should be excused due to the high demands of the rotation. She admits to the comment regarding the clinic patients but states, "I was just joking, and I really care about the patients. I am always professional." She asks to have fewer patients to follow so she can spend more time increasing her drug knowledge. M.B.'s preceptor denies this request; he indicates that he wants her to spend more time counseling patients. He also states that he will not tolerate any further occurrences of tardiness or delays in completing assignments.

WHY IT'S ESSENTIAL

Over the course of the didactic curriculum, you likely heard the term *professionalism* mentioned many times. Although the many definitions of the word may not be easily recited, most students can describe its characteristics and identify its importance to the profession. Faculty and preceptors expect their students to act professionally. Beyond the academic setting, employers, staff, healthcare providers, peers, and patients will all presume a high degree of professionalism from you as well. Professionalism is the essential element of the profession of pharmacy.

To care for patients, you must not only acquire the vital clinical knowledge and practice-related skills but also develop the values, attitudes, and behaviors of a healthcare professional. Without these elements, clinical knowledge cannot be effectively parlayed into improved patient outcomes. Luckily, before your formal training begins, you already possess some of the key values and attitudes of a pharmacist. For example, applicants to a pharmacy school often indicate that wanting to "care for patients" is their prime reason for pursuing a career as a pharmacist. Once in the classroom, students learn the definition of professionalism and its associated behaviors. You may participate in a white coat ceremony, recite a code of ethics, sign a statement of professionalism, and join professional organizations, all of which aid in your professional development.

The IPPEs provide an opportunity to observe preceptors and further develop the attributes and behaviors of professionalism. You will develop professional communication skills through your interactions with practice site staff, healthcare professionals, and patients. Throughout the IPPEs, you are assessed not only on your practice-related skills and knowledge but also your professionalism. Preceptors and experiential program staff will provide feedback and, if needed, counseling on how you can improve your professional behavior. Positive feedback includes statements such as the following:

"The student displays a high level of professionalism and will be an excellent pharmacist."

"The student dressed professionally and was always either on time or early for rotation activities."

"Remarkable student — I would like him to be my partner pharmacist in the future."

When a student has displayed unprofessional behavior, examples of comments from a preceptor may include:

"The student was continually 5 to 10 minutes late to the site and needs to improve if she wants to become a pharmacist."

"The student shows no initiative to want to learn and ask questions."

"Needs to be more aware of his appearance and how he presents himself to my customers."

By the time you begin your APPEs, you should have had ample opportunity to develop appropriate professional behavior. The APPEs bring their own unique circumstances to test one's professionalism. You will be spending more time on rotations, interacting with healthcare providers, and caring for a greater number of patients. There are additional assignments and increased demands placed on you by your preceptors. Being on time for daily activities, maintaining a professional appearance, and interacting properly with others will be more challenging compared to the IPPEs. You need to be aware of this in order to avoid any erosion of your professionalism. By the end of the APPEs, you should have developed your professionalism to a level where you are prepared to begin a career as a pharmacist.

PROFESSIONALISM DEFINED

Many definitions of *professionalism* have been published in the healthcare literature.[1-3] In pharmacy, we often focus on the behavioral attributes of professionalism, including appearance, timeliness, politeness, initiative, and life-long learning. Chalmers described professionalism in the following way:

Professionalism is displayed in the way pharmacists conduct themselves in professional situations. This definition implies a demeanor that is created through a combination of behaviors which include courtesy and politeness when dealing with patients, peers, and other healthcare professionals. Pharmacists should consistently display respect for others and maintain appropriate boundaries of privacy and discretion. Whether dealing with patients or interacting with others on a healthcare team, it is important to possess and display an empathetic manner.[2]

QUICK TIP

Take a moment to reflect on the personal attitudes you have regarding the profession of pharmacy. Have your attitudes changed since you entered pharmacy school? Who or what has influenced those attitudes? How does your professional behavior stem from your attitudes and beliefs about the profession?

The American College of Clinical Pharmacy National StuNet Advisory Committee developed the Tenets of Professionalism for Pharmacy Students, which outlined the key attitudes and behaviors that exemplify professionalism and that should be developed and practiced by all students.[4] These tenets and associated behavioral attributes include the following:

Altruism

- Commit to serve the best interest of the patient above one's own
- Make the patient the top priority in all healthcare decisions
- Place patient care before ability to pay, managerial opinions, or self-interests
- Actively listen; be patient and compassionate when interacting with the patient

Honesty and Integrity

- Display honor and trustworthiness
- Preserve patient and business confidentiality
- Maintain academic honesty in the classroom and on experiential rotations
- Avoid plagiarism

Respect for Others

- Treat others as you would want to be treated
- Show respect for patients, preceptors, faculty, and healthcare providers
- Demonstrate empathy
- Demonstrate effective listening skills
- Display cultural sensitivity and tolerance
- Exhibit self-control in interactions with others
- Value the opinions and recommendations of others in practice

Professional Presence

- Conduct yourself in a professional manner in both professional and personal settings
- Maintain proper professional dress, proper hygiene, grooming, and overall appearance
- Maintain a professional, organized portfolio
- Carry yourself in a way that will instill confidence and trust with patients and colleagues
- Display an enthusiastic attitude and personal commitment to the profession

Professional Stewardship

- Actively participate in professional organizations
- Volunteer for service-oriented activities
- Be a role model for those in the profession and other healthcare fields
- Inform the community about the profession

Dedication and Commitment to Excellence

- Accept responsibility for your own learning and self-development
- Be self-directed and demonstrate accountability in completing tasks
- Demonstrate timeliness and appropriate time-management skills
- Aspire to be a life-long learner
- Stay current with changes in the profession, practice guidelines, new drug therapies, emerging technology, and state and federal legislation

- Proactively seek guidance to achieve the goal of excellence
- Exceed the expectations of others

These tenets are similar to those that have been published elsewhere[1,3,5-8] but are unique by focusing primarily on student professionalism. Throughout the APPEs, you should strive to follow and practice according to these tenets. This will help you to fully incorporate the lifelong attitudes and behaviors expected by members of the pharmacy profession and the patients you will serve.

CASE QUESTION

Which of the tenets of student professionalism is M.B. failing to exhibit? Describe one way that M.B. can improve her behavior based on the tenets of student professionalism described above.

QUICK TIP

Identify whether each tenet of student professionalism can be categorized as challenging or simple to incorporate into your professional practice. For each one that is challenging, develop a plan to bring your behaviors into alignment with professional expectations.

Professionalism in Pharmacy Practice

Historically, pharmacists have been regarded by the public as professionals with a high level of integrity and ethics. A 2009 Gallup poll ranked pharmacists the highest in honesty and moral standards among all professions.[9] In pharmacy practice, the relationship between a pharmacist and a patient is not commercial but covenantal, or fiducial. *Fiducial* is derived from the Latin *fides*, meaning faith, clearly affirming that faith and trust underlie professional interactions.[10] Pharmacists have the knowledge and skills critical to help maintain the well-being of their patients. Because patients do not fully understand the knowledge and skills provided, they entrust the pharmacist with their well-being. As a result, the pharmacist, as a professional, must always act in the best interest of the patient. If the profession is to maintain its prestige, pharmacists and students must keep the covenantal relationship as the core element of their practice. It demands that one be altruistic, maintain a high standard of integrity and competence, and provide expertise on matters of appropriate medication use and health.

In 1990, Hepler and Strand introduced the concept of pharmaceutical care.[11] *Pharmaceutical care* involves the pharmacist assuming responsibility for drug therapy outcomes in addition to the safe, accurate, and efficient distribution of pharmaceutical products. It moved the profession from a product focus to more of a patient focus. This shift in practice brings an expanded sense of professionalism among pharmacists committed to achieving optimal therapeutic outcomes in their patients.[1] Many in the profession have embraced and implemented pharmaceutical care to make a difference in the health and lives of patients. Services such as medication therapy management, collaborative practice, medication reconciliation, and administration of immunizations are just a few examples of pharmacists incorporating pharmaceutical care into practice. As these services become more prevalent, the commitment to professionalism will continue to expand. You need only to refer to the Pledge of Professionalism adopted by the APhA-ASP/AACP Council of Deans Task Force on Professionalism to understand how professionalism is implemented in everyday practice (see **Figure 1-1**).

Figure 1-1. Pledge of Professionalism

As a student of pharmacy, I believe there is a need to build and reinforce a professional identity founded on integrity, ethical behavior, and honor. This development, a vital process in my education, will help to ensure that I am true to the professional relationship I establish between myself and society as I become a member of the pharmacy community. Integrity will be an essential part of my everyday life and I will pursue all academic and professional endeavors with honesty and commitment to service.

To accomplish this goal of professional development, as a student of pharmacy I will:

A.   DEVELOP a sense of loyalty and duty to the profession by contributing to the well-being of others and by enthusiastically accepting responsibility and accountability for membership in the profession.

B.   FOSTER professional competency through lifelong learning. I will strive for high ideals, teamwork, and unity within the profession in order to provide optimal patient care.

C.   SUPPORT my colleagues by actively encouraging personal commitment to the Oath of a Pharmacist and the Code of Ethics for Pharmacists as set forth by the profession.

D.   DEDICATE my life and practice to excellence. This will require an ongoing reassessment of personal and professional values.

E.   MAINTAIN the highest ideals and professional attributes to ensure and facilitate the covenantal relationship required of the pharmaceutical caregiver.

The profession of pharmacy is one that demands adherence to a set of ethical principles. These high ideals are necessary to ensure the quality of care extended to the patients I serve. As a student of pharmacy, I believe this does not start with graduation; rather, it begins with my membership in this professional college community. Therefore, I will strive to uphold this pledge as I advance toward full membership in the profession.

I voluntarily make this pledge of professionalism.

Adapted from the University of Illinois College of Pharmacy's Pledge of Professionalism, 1993.

Developed and adopted by the American Pharmaceutical Association Academy of Students of Pharmacy and the American Association of Colleges of Deans Task Force on Professionalism on June 26, 1994.

Source: Reprinted by permission of APhA. Copyright American Pharmacists Association (APhA). APhA-ASP/AACP-COD Task Force on Professionalism. White paper on pharmacy student professionalism. J Am Pharm Assoc. 2000;40:96-102.

FIRST IMPRESSIONS

At the start of the APPEs, preceptors expect that you already possess a high level of professionalism. You can live up to this standard by displaying a positive first impression when you start a rotation. The following are suggestions for you to consider in making a good first impression:

- Review the guidelines (e.g., APPE Student Manual) provided by the college regarding the APPEs, including rotation objectives and assessment standards.
- Contact your preceptor to determine the need to complete any prerotation background checks and obtain an identification badge, parking permits, start times, dress code, and rotation hours.

- Determine the need to bring copies of your personal immunization records, intern license, verification of HIPAA training, blood-borne pathogen training, basic life-support certification, and other certifications.
- Review directions and amount of time required to drive to the site, including parking.
- Update your professional portfolio.
- Review material on common disease states, practice guidelines, and medications encountered on the rotation. The preceptor may provide a list of materials for you to review before the first day.
- Ensure that your physical appearance and dress will meet the standards of the practice setting.

Generally, this preparation should begin 2 to 3 weeks prior to the start of a rotation. The experiential program office at the college can provide guidance on any prerotation tasks that you should complete.

On the first day of the rotation, you want to present a favorable first impression to the preceptor. This impression will set the stage for a rewarding experience and decrease the chance for a negative relationship between you and your preceptor. Plan to arrive at the site on time, professionally dressed, and well groomed. Any completed prerotation paperwork and records required should be available to hand to your preceptor.

The first day will likely include an orientation to the rotation. During this time, your preceptor will review the activities and assignments that you will need to complete during the rotation; often a calendar indicating the dates these will be due is provided. The orientation is an opportunity for the preceptor to provide his or her expectations for your performance. These expectations often include not only specific assignments to complete but also those related to professional behavior. Some examples related to professionalism may include policies on dress code, tardiness, absenteeism, patient confidentiality, and cell phone usage. This is the ideal time for you to ask any questions to further clarify what is expected for your performance, especially regarding professionalism. In cases where the preceptor has not established clear expectations for professionalism, it may be helpful to discuss your own expectations of yourself, the preceptor, and the rotation.[12] This meaningful discussion between you and your preceptor about what each individual is expecting during the rotation is essential. You will be more likely to meet or exceed expectations for the rotation when you have been involved in defining them. Incidences of unprofessionalism can often be linked back to either the preceptor not adequately expressing his or her expectations for the student or the student not seeking clarification on what is considered acceptable performance. Taking the time at the start of a rotation to discuss these important issues can lead to a positive experience.

QUICK TIP

Create a list of questions to ask the preceptor that address specific professional behaviors expected during the rotation. Use this list as a guide during the orientation with your preceptor.

PROFESSIONALISM DURING ROTATIONS

The day-to-day activities on a typical APPE can be quite demanding and challenging for students. Preparing for patient care rounds, answering drug information questions, patient case presentations, and journal clubs are just a few of the activities that may be required during an APPE. These activities, coupled with long days at the practice site and completing assignments at home, add to the demand placed on students. In addition, you may be involved in other nonrotation activities such as outside employment, preparing for residency or job interviews, and family-related obligations, only adding to your many responsibilities. As a result, a slip in your professional behavior may occur. Generally, this action is not deliberate but a result of your increased demands. The behavior may be embarrassing and you should make a sincere attempt to avoid any future occurrences. An occasional mishap in professionalism can occur with any pharmacist, even those in practice for a considerable length of time. The important point is to acknowledge when your behavior has slipped and quickly rectify the situation in order to avoid a similar occurrence in the future. During these instances, you may want to seek guidance from your preceptor, advisor, or college experiential director.

Professional behavior may also lapse as the end of the APPEs draws near. It is during this time that you may become more focused on graduating, securing a job or residency, and looking forward to starting the next phase of your professional life. As a result, your performance and professionalism may falter during the last 1 to 2 months of the APPEs. This could potentially lead to a failed rotation, which would significantly affect your plans for a successful, timely graduation. Be aware of this and strive to maintain a high level of performance and professionalism during the last few months of the APPEs.

PORTFOLIOS

The Accreditation Council for Pharmacy Education (ACPE) guidelines require that each student maintain a portfolio that documents progressive achievement of competencies throughout the curriculum.[13] A portfolio can best be described as a collection of information representing your academic and professional accomplishments or achievements. Specific contents vary depending on the institution's own requirements or recommendations. Suggested items to include in your portfolio are the following:

- Curriculum vitae
- Career and professional goals
- Licensure or certificates (e.g., intern license, immunization training, medication therapy management)
- List of IPPE and APPE rotations
- Final evaluations from APPE rotations
- Self-assessments of education outcomes
- Reflections on performance or progress
- Samples of completed projects and presentations (e.g., drug information, journal clubs, formal presentations, drug utilization evaluations, patient education materials, research abstracts, posters, publications)
- Recognitions and awards

Your portfolio content should be organized in some type of binder for presentation to others. Although cumbersome for students to carry and maintain, many preceptors find a portfolio quite helpful in getting to know your interests, areas of accomplishment, and skills in need of further development. An alternative to a binder is an electronic portfolio or e-portfolio. Many of the companies that provide educational management software programs for experiential education also offer e-portfolios. These are typically customizable to meet the school's requirements, can be maintained easily by individual students, and are accessible to preceptors on demand. Portfolios are not only viewed by preceptors but may also be presented to potential employers or residency programs. Generally, this would be a condensed version of the primary portfolio containing significant accomplishments and projects (e.g., completed research, publications, and formal presentations).

Regardless of the format, you should be diligent in maintaining your portfolio, thinking of the portfolio as an extension of your own professionalism. A nicely organized, well-maintained, and appealing portfolio provides a positive impression to a preceptor or prospective employer. On the other hand, a disorganized, incomplete portfolio may demonstrate to the viewer a student with a lack of professional presence. You are encouraged to seek feedback from advisors, faculty, and preceptors on the content and appearance of your portfolio.

QUICK TIP

Key tips for maintaining and using a portfolio:

* Assess the content of your portfolio prior to the start of APPEs. Does it contain the most current information and accomplishments?

* Keep your portfolio updated as you progress through the APPEs by adding samples of significant projects and presentations that you have completed.

* Utilize preceptors or advisors to provide feedback on your portfolio.

* Consider creating a condensed version of your portfolio to present to prospective employers or residency programs.

PROFESSIONALISM IN COMMUNICATING AND INTERACTING WITH OTHERS

One of the most important aspects of professionalism pertains to the manner in which the professionals interact with others. Whether it is patients, preceptors, or other healthcare providers, you must display a dedication to communicating in a professional way. Without these skills, important information may be ineffectively conveyed, misinterpreted, or completely overlooked, potentially having a dramatic effect on the health of patients. Throughout the APPE experience, you will be placed in situations that will develop and test your communication skills.

Patients

Communication with patients can be one of the most rewarding and challenging aspects of a career in pharmacy. To excel at this skill, it is imperative that you understand that communication begins before a single word is uttered. Nonverbal cues are often just as important as the content of the conversation. Each interaction should begin by establishing a strong foundation for good communication. Creating a relaxed, open environment can make the conversation flow more easily and increase comprehension. If possible, you should make every attempt to speak to patients on an eye-to-eye level. Talking down to patients may convey a sense of superiority from the practitioner and cause insecurity for the patient. In traditional pharmacy environments, this may entail coming out from behind an elevated counter or glass partition to engage the patient face-to-face. For patients lying in bed, this can be accomplished by pulling a chair up to the edge of the bed for all communications. Ideally, your full attention should be focused on the patient by squarely facing him or her. If you are busy jotting notes on a clipboard or, even worse, sitting with your arms folded across your chest, it may be interpreted as a signal of haste and triviality of the meeting, no matter how well you are able to converse verbally. In most situations, a distance of 3 to 4 feet is deemed optimal for engaging patients and encouraging open and honest discussion, although individual patients may require adjustments based on personal or cultural preferences. Just as the patient will be aware of your nonverbal messages, following these general guidelines will put you in the best possible position to observe and react to the patient's nonverbal cues and adjust each component appropriately.

Once you have created a sound environment for conversation, proper eye contact can be used to maintain a connection and guide the discussion from beginning to end. Like many of the other nonverbal communications skills discussed above, obtaining a delicate balance is crucial and the patient can be an excellent source of clues to the effectiveness of your communication skills. On one extreme, you may use too little eye contact and seem distracted. This is a common problem for students that rely too heavily on notes when performing counseling activities or feel pressured to write down every aspect of a medical interview. On the other end of the spectrum, a harsh or aggressive gaze may be off-putting to the patient as well. When an appropriate level of eye contact is established, nonverbal and verbal encouragement can be used to keep the discussion going. This is a skill that will help you uncover important details that may be left out when less-effective communication skills are employed. The encouragement ranges from a simple nod of the head or reassuring smile to short responses like "uh-huh" or "mm-hmm."

QUICK TIP

Although encouraging cues are an important tool for improving communication, overuse of these interjections can be distracting and disrupt the smooth flow of information.

Once the foundation has been laid for a productive patient encounter with proper nonverbal communication, verbal communication skills are required to effectively collect relevant data and deliver patient education. The opening moments of each encounter set the tone for the rest of the experience. When you enter an exam room, greet a patient at the counter, or answer a telephone call, a warm greeting, proper introduction, and brief explanation of the reason for the conversation can go a long way. When meeting face-to-face with a patient, enter the room with purpose and engage the patient directly. After verifying the patient's identity, you should shake hands with the patient firmly and introduce yourself as a student-pharmacist. Next, an open invitation should be presented to the patient to begin discussing the matters at hand. This is often accomplished with the effective use of open-ended questions that the patient cannot simply answer with short "yes" or "no" responses, effectively encouraging the patient to describe his or her conditions, issues, or questions in greater detail. Although open-ended questions are of vital importance to proper communication, closed-ended questions continue to have a role. When used as a follow-up to an open-ended question, closed-ended questions have a clarifying effect.

CASE QUESTION

M.B. is conducting a patient interview and starts the encounter by asking, "Are you here for your diabetes?" Before reviewing the patient's blood glucose logs, she asks, "Have your sugars been under control?" How could she have rephrased these questions in an open-ended manner?

One of the most challenging areas for students to gain proficiency is in the conveyance of empathy. Empathy is a powerful tool that communicates a deeper understanding of what a patient is feeling and can be used to defuse many difficult situations. The difficulty for most students arises from an inability to divide their attention between the task at hand (conducting a medical interview, counseling a patient, etc.) and actively listening to the concerns of a patient. When students become too invested in completing an assignment or seeing all of the patients on a service, the understated clues that illuminate the patient's point of view are easily missed and the opportunity to form a true bond passes unnoticed. In order to master the ability to convey empathy, you should listen closely to patients' words to identify any description of their current emotions and what circumstances are influencing them. When these feeling words are identified, you should take the opportunity to reflect the patient's emotions back to him or her using a paraphrased version of the patient's own words. Although it may sound simple enough when described this way, the vast majority of patients will not simply express their emotions in a clear, concise statement during a conversation. The subtle hints to a patient's feelings are often fleeting and vague, but when they are identified and reflected back, there is perhaps no better way to obtain the patient's trust.

CASE QUESTION

M.B. is reviewing her patient's medications. After discussing each of the medications, her patient says, "Things are going well but I feel so overwhelmed when I see all of these medication vials." M.B. replies, "Okay," and continues the appointment. How could M.B. properly reflect her patient's emotions?

There are a number of other common pitfalls that students often encounter. Throughout your academic career, you are bombarded with extremely technical explanations of the pathophysiology of disease, mechanism of action of drugs, clinical presentations, and human anatomy. In the classroom, a deep understanding of these topics is vital to excel on exams and achieve a passing grade. When making the transition to the experiential component of the curriculum, however, the complicated minutia often lead to communication difficulties and poor comprehension for patients. First, because of the vast knowledge base you possess, you may feel as though you have already identified the resolution to a patient's problem before collecting all of the relevant information. When students jump to conclusions, they may ask leading questions. As opposed to open- and closed-ended questions, leading questions are asked in ways that are suggestive of the type of answer that should be provided. They can bias an otherwise objective patient interview and lead to improper conclusions, misunderstandings, and, potentially adverse effects on a patient's health. To avoid leading questions, you should approach each interview as objectively as possible. You should avoid making premature judgments and utilize open-ended questions as often as possible to obtain the patient's true perspective.

CASE QUESTION

M.B.'s patient mentions that she has noticed a pain in her legs that has become more problematic in recent weeks. M.B. replies, "The pain feels like numbness and tingling, right?" How could she rephrase her follow-up question to gain a better understanding of the patient's symptoms?

Another potential error that is often made as a result of the type of education most healthcare providers receive is the use of medical jargon when trying to communicate with the lay public. In an academic setting, it is expected that you should explain every detail of very complex processes. Explaining these processes in a similar way to the general public, however, can quickly result in a confused and disengaged patient. It may be difficult at times to gauge the level of a patient's understanding. As described above, a patient's nonverbal cues can be a valuable tool to help identify comprehension problems. Many patients, for fear of sounding unintelligent, do not respond to confusing language by asking for clarification or giving non-verbal clues to their puzzlement. Instead, they may nod enthusiastically as if to demonstrate understanding and say nothing at all. As a result, important information may be lost without proper translation.

One way to avoid health literacy or jargon issues is to wrap up each encounter with some form of "teach-back" evaluation. This strategy involves asking the patient to rephrase the content of the encounter. As the patient attempts to put the main discussion points into his or her own words, you can correct any misunderstandings and verify that the patient has a good grasp on the knowledge presented. Once the teach-back is complete, it is time to signal the end of the encounter. This can be done in a number of ways but should always include one final check for patient questions, a summary of the encounter, and, if applicable, future steps that will need to be taken.

Preceptors

Throughout the experiential component of the curriculum, preceptors will act as teachers, guides, and evaluators. Professional communication with preceptors is not only key to obtaining a passing grade on a rotation but may also have a significant impact on career development by broadening your network, identifying recommendation letter writers, and even being granted job interviews at rotation sites. The earliest opportunity to exceed expectations actually happens before the first day of the rotation. The guidelines for these early communications may vary from institution to institution. It may be wise to consult your institution's APPE handbook for guidance on what type of communication is preferred for preceptors and what time frame is expected for these communications. In general, most students are expected to contact their preceptors 2 to 3 weeks prior to the start of a rotation. Both premature and late contact may be viewed as a professionalism issue. Although e-mail is usually acceptable, some unique sites may prefer other modes of communication. Before your arrival, initial contact should be made to gain an understanding of the expectations for the first day, identify important materials to review, clarify logistical issues, and provide a general introduction to the preceptor. Whenever possible, you should include links to online portfolios and descriptions of past rotations. As with all professional communications, it is vital that you proofread these communications, avoid informalities and slang, and present yourself in the most professional manner possible.

QUICK TIP

Remember that it is also possible to contact your preceptors too frequently. Avoid excessive e-mails or phone calls and collect all the necessary information in an efficient manner.

Once the rotation is underway, one of the most frequent student-preceptor interactions will be in the form of evaluations. Formative evaluations will take place over the course of the rotation and may be informal, such as verbal comments and corrections when a student presents a case, or formal, such as the rubrics used to evaluate patient encounters, case presentations, and journal clubs. Formative evaluations are designed to be a snapshot of a point in time. This type of immediate, directed feedback is vital for students to improve upon specific skills that are being identified. Summative evaluations occur at the midpoint and end of the rotation and are meant to provide an overall assessment of the student's performance.

Proper assessment of performance during APPEs is important in ensuring that you have acquired the practical, clinical, and professional skills needed to be a practicing pharmacist. The assessment process starts with an understanding by students and preceptors as to what the expectations are for successful student performance. The college of pharmacy aids in this process by providing assessment tools that assist in measuring a student's competency in various skills and activities. Depending on the program, these tools can be quite detailed, covering multiple areas of performance. Components of a typical assessment form may include the following:

- Professionalism
- Communication skills
- Drug and disease state knowledge
- Application of clinical skills
- Medication dispensing skills
- Administrative and leadership skills

Under the professionalism component, one likely will find individual behaviors that often can be linked back to the tenets of professionalism. See **Figure 1-2** for an example used by one college of pharmacy.

Figure 1-2. Examples of Professional Behaviors Contained in an APPE Evaluation

* Participates in the process of self-assessment and displays an interest in life-long learning and continuous professional development

* Maintains a professional manner in both appearance and behavior at all times

* Demonstrates courtesy and respect toward others and exhibits self control in all interactions

* Maintains confidentiality

* Displays cultural sensitivity and tolerance

* Arrives on time and prepared for all rotation activities

* Demonstrates appropriate time management skills and the ability to prioritize

* Demonstrates initiative and responsibility for providing patient care and completing assignments

Adapted with permission from Northeast Ohio Medical University College of Pharmacy.

It is vital that proper feedback is sought and obtained from the preceptor while you are on a rotation. Although it does not need to be a formal, written assessment, formative feedback will give you an idea about the overall progress you are making and reduce the chance for an unhappy surprise during summative evaluations. Most institutions train preceptors to perform the necessary evaluations, but there may be instances where you will need to approach the preceptor to obtain feedback. When doing so, avoid any negative or accusatory language. You should simply approach the preceptor and state the desire for feedback in a given area, being as specific as possible. Once the preceptor's expectations are outlined, you will have a better understanding of the requirements for successful completion of the rotation.

Feedback provided by preceptors is a vital tool for improving your practice of pharmacy. Whenever feedback is provided, care should be taken to view the criticism in this way and avoid feelings of personal attack or anger. In situations where serious disagreement exists, the proper channels should be used to take corrective action. This may include discussing the evaluation with the experiential director, a member of the college's administration, or other professors. At all costs, you should avoid aggressive, brash behavior while practicing at a rotation site. You are a representative of the college or school of pharmacy to outside institutions and providers. These unprofessional behaviors cast a negative light on not only you but also your classmates, the college, and the profession as a whole. As described above, situations like these can be avoided when proper formative feedback is received over the course of the rotation.

In some instances, preceptors may also ask students to perform self-evaluations. When evaluating your own performance, it is important to be as objective as possible. Reviewing the expectations outlined in the rotation syllabus or APPE handbook can greatly improve the usefulness and objectivity of self-evaluations. Without knowing what is expected, any self-evaluation would be incomplete at best. In instances where your self-evaluation and your preceptor's evaluations differ, a discussion can be useful in coming to a consensus on a proper resolution to the discrepancy.

At the end of the rotation, you will often have the opportunity to evaluate preceptors and/or rotation sites. Some students may be tempted to give brutally honest evaluations, especially in circumstances where they feel slighted by a poor grade or comment. It is a necessity that these feelings be put aside in favor of a professional, objective, criteria-based assessment of the rotation and its preceptor. The preceptors and the experiential education staff use your feedback as a way to improve learning opportunities for future students. This responsibility should be taken very seriously. Avoid broad generalizations and stick to specific weaknesses that can feasibly be addressed for future students.

Other Healthcare Providers

A number of rotations will place you on a healthcare team that may be made up of a number of different healthcare professionals. The nonpharmacy providers may have limited understanding of the role of a student pharmacist on rotations. When joining such a team for the first time, you should provide a brief introduction of yourself. It is of utmost importance that you are identified as a student and not as a practicing pharmacist. This will help to avoid any inappropriate expectations and create a better learning environment.

As the rotation progresses, you will be able to contribute to the team by making therapeutic recommendations. Before doing so, you should ensure the proper approach is taken. Some preceptors may require each recommendation to be discussed prior to addressing it with the team. Others may feel comfortable allowing you to make recommendations independently. In either case, it is your responsibility to properly vet all recommendations for safety and efficacy issues before bringing them to the team. When relaying the recommendation, you should be thorough yet concise, including all relevant drug, dose, route, and frequency information, along with any pertinent evidence-based or patient-specific rationale. In some situations, even a sound recommendation may be turned down by the team in favor of an alternative intervention. In these situations, it is imperative that you graciously accept the outcome of the recommendation. Unprofessional behaviors such as whining, frustrated outbursts, or exasperated sighs do little to improve the chances of another recommendation being accepted in the future.

Lastly, working with healthcare teams provides many opportunities to discuss specific cases and deliberate on the best possible treatment. These case presentations often occur in hallways, stairwells, and other public areas of the hospital. When discussing specific cases with other providers, extreme caution must be exercised to avoid disclosing any protected health information. Whenever possible, avoid any patient identifiers such as name, date of birth, and geographical identifiers in favor of patient initials. The APPE handbook may offer additional guidelines when discussing patient cases with other members of the healthcare team.

E-Professionalism

One last aspect of professional communication deals with your online persona. With the advent of social networking sites, many students have amassed impressive amounts of postings, photographs, and comments across numerous sites. Varying degrees of privacy protection mean that much of this material can be viewed by patients, preceptors, other healthcare providers, and potential employers. Many students are unaware that a simple search engine query can result in a disturbing amount of information being displayed that may or may not be setting the best example. It is highly recommended that any student who participates in online social networking becomes very familiar with the privacy policies of each site frequented. If privacy settings are available, it may be wise to limit the types of information that are shared with the rest of the community. For sites that do not have such settings, posts, comments, and photographs posted by you and your peers must be closely monitored and edited to preserve your professional reputation. Although student usage of social networking sites is on the rise, so, too, is the use of these sites to evaluate prospective employees. For this reason, e-professionalism must be considered an equivalent component to professional dress, behavior, or communication and must be given equal attention.

References

1. APhA-ASP/AACP-COD Task Force on Professionalism. White paper on pharmacy student professionalism. *J Am Pharm Assoc*. 2000;40:96-102.

2. Chalmers RK. Contemporary issues: Professionalism in pharmacy. *Tomorrow's Pharmacist*. 1997;March:10-12.

3. Hammer DP. Professionalism attitudes and behaviors: The "A's and B's" of professionalism. *Am J Pharm Educ*. 2000;64:455-464.

4. American College of Clinical Pharmacy. Tenets of professionalism for pharmacy students. *Pharmacotherapy*. 2009;29:757-759.

5. Chisholm MA, Cobb H, Duke L, et al. Development of an instrument to measure professionalism. *Am J Pharm Educ*. 2006;70:1-6.

6. Hamer DP, Berger BA, Beardsley RS, et al. Student professionalism. *Am J Pharm Educ*. 2003;67:1-29.

7. American Society of Health-System Pharmacists. ASHP statement on professionalism. *Am J Health-Syst Pharm*. 2008;65:172-174.

8. American Board of Internal Medicine Committees on Evaluation of Clinical Competence and Communication Programs. *Project Professionalism*. Philadelphia, PA: American Board of Internal Medicine; 2001:5-6.

9. Schweers K. Pharmacists score big in Gallup poll—again. *The Dose*. http://ncpanet.wordpress.com/2009/12/10/. Accessed February 4, 2012.

10. American College of Clinical Pharmacy, Roth MT, Zlatic TD. Development of student professionalism. *Pharmacotherapy*. 2009;29:749-756.

11. Hepler CD, Strand LM. Opportunities and responsibilities in pharmaceutical care. *Am J Hosp Pharm*. 1990;47:533-543.

12. Hamer D. Improving student professionalism during experiential learning. *Am J Pharm Educ*. 2006;70:1-6.

13. Accreditation Council for Pharmacy Education. Accreditation standards and guidelines for the professional program in pharmacy leading to the doctor of pharmacy degree. http://www.acpe-accredit.org/pdf/ACPE_Revised_PharmD_Standards_Adopted_Jan152006.pdf. 2007. Accessed February 9, 2012.

SUGGESTED READING

American College of Clinical Pharmacy, Roth MT, Zlatic TD. Development of student professionalism. *Pharmacotherapy.* 2009;29:749-756.

American College of Clinical Pharmacy. Tenets of professionalism for pharmacy students. *Pharmacotherapy.* 2009;29:757-759.

American Society of Health-System Pharmacists. ASHP statement on professionalism. *Am J Health-Syst Pharm.* 2008;65:172-174.

APhA-ASP/AACP-COD Task Force on Professionalism. White paper on pharmacy student professionalism. *J Am Pharm Assoc.* 2000;40:96-102.

Hammer DP, Berger BA, Beardsley RS, et al. Student professionalism. *Am J Pharm Educ.* 2003;67:1-29.

Hammer DP. Professionalism attitudes and behaviors: The "A's and B's" of professionalism. *Am J Pharm Educ.* 2000;64:455-464.

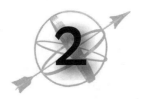

MEDICAL TERMINOLOGY AND ABBREVIATIONS

Katherine M. Cochran, PharmD, and Brandon Mottice, PharmD

CASE

L.K. is an APPE student on her advanced inpatient rotation. After being assigned to follow a patient, L.K. locates the History and Physical and reads that her patient is a 56-year-old male with a "CC of SOB" and a "PMH significant for chronic lung disease." The assessment and plan reveal that the doctor suspects a pleural effusion and has ordered a CXR. While rounding with the team later that morning, the doctor reports that the chest x-ray confirmed the diagnosis of pleural effusion. They performed a thoracentesis that revealed the patient is suffering from a parapneumonic effusion. The doctors discuss that they want to start empiric antibiotics, but they will also perform a bronchoscopy with a C&S so they can narrow down antibiotic therapy, as appropriate. L.K. feels very overwhelmed by all of the medical terminology being used by the physicians. Later that day, she complains to a fellow classmate that they never learned about all of these diseases and tests in pharmacy school.

WHY IT'S ESSENTIAL

A firm knowledge of medical terminology and abbreviations is essential for communication in the world of pharmacy and medicine. The use of medical and professional terminology eliminates ambiguity and provides a common language through which healthcare professionals can communicate. A thorough understanding of the principals used to construct a medical term will allow you to infer the general meaning of terminology, even if the term itself is unfamiliar to you. When communicating in written form, abbreviations can be used to convey ideas in a more efficient way. If used properly, medical abbreviations will help you communicate clearly and concisely.

....

"In order to communicate effectively with fellow healthcare professionals, you need a strong knowledge base in medical terminology."—Student

....

DECIPHERING MEDICAL TERMINOLOGY

A *root word* is the foundation of a medical term. The root establishes the term's basic meaning. In medicine, the root word often refers to a body organ or system. For example, the root of the word *nephrology* is *nephr-*, meaning "kidney." In some cases, more than one root word can be combined to form a compound word. A vowel, called a *combining vowel*, is inserted between the two root words in order to ease pronunciation. The most frequently used combining vowel is *o*; however, other vowels are used as well. For example, when the root word *cardi-*, meaning "heart," is combined with the root word *-vascular*, meaning "blood vessels," an *o* is inserted between the two root words to ease pronunciation. The resulting word is *cardiovascular*, which refers to the blood vessels of the heart. See **Table 1** in **Appendix 2-A** for more examples of root words.

A *suffix* is added to the end of a root word to modify its meaning. A combining vowel is often used to combine the root word with the suffix. For example, when the root word *pulmon-*, meaning "lung," is combined with the suffix *-logy*, meaning "study of," a combining vowel is needed at the end of the root word to ease pronunciation. In this case, the combining vowel is *o* and the resulting word is *pulmonology*, which means "the study of the lungs." **Table 2** in Appendix 2-A lists examples of common suffixes.

A *prefix* is added to the beginning of a root word or a suffix to modify its meaning. In general, prefixes can be combined with the remainder of the word without requiring any change to the root word or suffix. For example, the prefix *hypo-*, meaning "low" or "below normal," can be added to the suffix *-volemic*, meaning "volume of blood," to form *hypovolemic*, which refers to blood volume that is below normal. Along the same lines, the prefix *eu-*, which means "normal," can be combined with the same suffix to form the word *euvolemic*, which refers to normal blood volume. **Table 3** in Appendix 2-A has additional examples of prefixes.

CASE QUESTION

L.K. was overwhelmed by all of the medical terminology the doctors were using. Break down the following medical terms she encountered into their prefixes, roots, and/or suffixes to decipher their meanings: parapneumonic effusion, thoracentesis, bronchoscopy.

PROFESSIONAL TERMINOLOGY

It is essential for pharmacists to develop a working knowledge of common language that can be used to clearly and efficiently communicate with other healthcare professionals. Although medical terminology allows us to communicate disease and diagnosis-related ideas, there are many terms used to navigate the complexities of the healthcare system that do not fall under the category of medical terminology. These words can be referred to as professional terminology. Professional terminology is often related to, but certainly not limited to, reimbursement for services. Terminology related to the dispensing of medications and reimbursement for services is critical to the everyday operations of a pharmacy. Furthermore, it is useful to understand the roles of various governmental agencies in the oversight of healthcare regulations. A strong knowledge of the terms found in **Appendix 2-B** will allow for successful integration into the modern world of pharmacy practice.

ABBREVIATIONS IN THE PHARMACY AND MEDICAL CHART

The modern medical chart contains numerous abbreviations, and it is easy to become overwhelmed at first glance. The use of medical abbreviations offers many advantages within the world of pharmacy and medicine. Abbreviations provide a common universal language for healthcare professionals to communicate effectively. Learning the most common medical abbreviations and their definitions is important, as standardization of these abbreviations prevents errors of ambiguity. If there is not a single interpretation for each abbreviation, there is opportunity for an error to occur. By using the same abbreviations in every hospital and pharmacy across the country, this risk is minimized. Abbreviations also save time. For example, writing "PERRLA" is easier and faster than writing "Pupils equal, round, and reactive to light and accommodation," allowing time to be saved by the writer as well as the reader. Laboratory data may also be written in shorthand, as shown in **Figures 2-1** and **2-2**. See **Appendix 2-C** for more examples of common abbreviations encountered in the pharmacy and throughout the medical chart.

CASE QUESTION

L.K. is struggling with interpreting the abbreviations she encountered on her first day. Can you translate the following medical abbreviations she has encountered: CC, PMH, SOB, CXR, and C&S?

Figure 2-1. Chemistry Panel

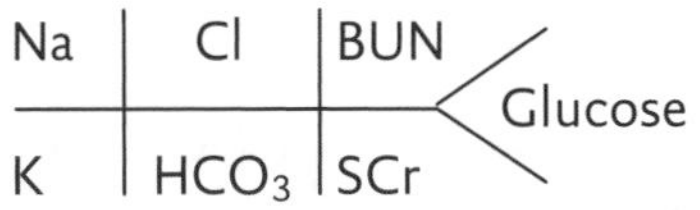

Figure 2-2. Complete Blood Count

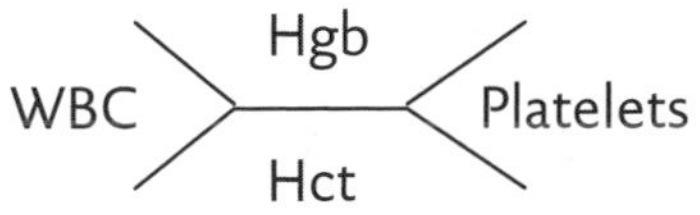

ABBREVIATIONS TO AVOID

Abbreviations have limitations, however. Improper use of medical abbreviations can lead to significant medical errors. Certain abbreviations can be easily mistaken for others, such as "MS" being interpreted as either morphine or magnesium sulfate. Additionally, the use of "trailing zeroes" has been known to result in ten-fold dosing errors. A prescription written for "5.0 mg" could accidentally be interpreted as "50 mg." These are both examples of abbreviations on the Official "Do Not Use" List issued by The Joint Commission (see **Table 2-1**[1]). It is important to become familiar with this list because these abbreviations can still be found in use today.

TABLE 2-1. THE JOINT COMMISSION'S OFFICIAL "DO NOT USE" LIST	
DO NOT USE	USE INSTEAD
MS	Morphine sulfate
MSO$_4$, MgSO$_4$	Magnesium sulfate
Q.D., QD, q.d., qd	Daily
Q.O.D., QOD, q.o.d., qod	Every other day
U, u	Unit
IU	International unit
Trailing zero (X.O mg)	X mg
Lack of leading zero (.X mg)	O.X mg

REFERENCE

1.   The Joint Commission. Official "Do Not Use" List. http://www.jointcommission.org/PatientSafety/
      DoNotUseList/. Accessed February 13, 2012.

SUGGESTED READING

Centers for Medicaid & Medicare Services. Glossary. http://www.cms.gov/apps/glossary/. Accessed February
      12, 2012.

Cohen BJ. *Medical Terminology: An Illustrated Guide*. Baltimore, MD: Lippincott Williams & Wilkins, 2011.

McAuley D. GlobalRPh. Medical Abbreviations. http://www.globalrph.com/medterm.htm. Accessed February
      13, 2012.

MTMS Definition and Program Criteria by the ACMP, AACP, ACA, ACCP, ASCP, APhA, ASHP, NABP,
      National Council of State Pharmacy Association Executives. http://pstac.org/aboutus/mtms.pdf. July 2004.
      Accessed July 22, 2012.

Nutescu EA, Klotz RS. Basic terminology in obtaining reimbursement for pharmacists' cognitive services. *Am J
      Health-Syst Pharm*. 2007;64:186-192.

Stedman's Medical Dictionary for the Health Professions and Nursing. 5th ed. Baltimore, MD: Lippincott Williams &
      Wilkins; 2005.

The Joint Commission. Official "Do Not Use" List. http://www.jointcommission.org/PatientSafety/
      DoNotUseList/. Accessed February 13, 2012.

Thompson JE. *A Practical Guide to Contemporary Pharmacy Practice*. 2nd ed. Baltimore, MD: Lippincott Williams
      & Wilkins; 2004.

U.S. Department of Health and Human Services. Public law 104-191: Health Insurance Portability and Account-
      ability Act of 1996. http://aspe.hhs.gov/admnsimp/pl104191.htm. Accessed July 22, 2012.

APPENDIX 2-A   MEDICAL TERMINOLOGY

TABLE 1. ROOT WORDS	
ROOT WORD/COMBINING VOWEL	MEANING
Aden/o	Gland
Amyl/o	Starch
Angi/o	Vessel
Append/o, appendic/o	Appendix
Arthr/o	Joint
Audi/o	Hearing
Bi/o	Life
Blephar/o	Eyelid
Bronch/o, bronchi/o	Bronchial tube
Cardi/o	Heart
Cephal/o	Head
Cerebr/o	Brain
Chir/o	Hand
Col/o	Colon or large intestine
Cutane/o	Skin
Cyt/o	Cell
Dermat/o, derm/a	Skin
Electr/o	Electricity
Faci/o	Face
Gastr/o	Stomach
Glyc/o	Sugar
Gynec/o	Female
Hemat/o, hem/o	Blood
Hepat/o	Liver
Ile/o, ili/o	Ileum
Immun/o	Immune
Lact/o	Milk
Lapar/o	Abdominal wall; abdomen
Laryng/o	Larynx
Lip/o	Fat
Lith/o	Stone
Lymph/o	Lymph
Mamm/o, mast/o	Breast
Men/o	Menses; menstruation
Mening/o, meningi/o	Meninges
Muc/o	Mucus
Muscul/o, my/o	Muscle
Nephr/o	Kidney

Neur/o	Nerve
Onc/o	Tumor
Opthalm/o	Eye
Or/o	Mouth
Orch/o, orchi/o, orchid/o	Testis
Orth/o	Straight
Oste/o	Bone
Ot/o	Ear
Path/o	Disease
Ped	Child, foot
Phys	Nature
Pleur/o	Pleura
Pod/o, ped	Foot
Presby/o	Old age
Prote/o, protein/o	Protein
Psych/o	Mind
Pulm/o, pulmon/o, pneum/o, pneumon/o	Lungs
Radi/o	X-ray
Rheumat/o	Rheumatism
Rhin/o	Nose
Sinus/o	Sinus
Sphygm/o	Pulse
Thorac/o	Chest
Thromb/o	Clot
Tonsil/o	Tonsil
Trache/o	Trachea
Ur/o	Urination
Vas/o	Vessel

TABLE 2. SUFFIXES

Medical Specialists and Specialties

SUFFIX	DEFINITION	EXAMPLE
-er	One who	Nurse practitioner (one who practices nursing)
-ian	Specialist in a field of study	Physician (a specialist in the practice of medicine)
-iatrics	Medical specialty	Pediatrics (medical specialty dealing with children and their diseases)
-iatry	Medical specialty	Psychiatry (medical specialty devoted to the study and treatment of mental disorders)
-ics	Medical specialty	Orthopedics (specialty in the musculoskeletal system)
-ist	Specialties in a field of study	Pharmacist (drug specialist)
-logist	One who studies	Pulmonologist (one who studies the lungs)
-logy	Study of	Cardiology (study of the heart)

Diagnosis

SUFFIX	DEFINITION	EXAMPLE
-gram	Record or picture	Electrocardiogram (recording of the electrical activity of the heart over a period of time)
-graphy	Process of recording	Radiography (a recording of x-rays passed through the human body)
-meter	Instrument for measuring	Sphygmomanometer (instrument for measuring pulse pressure)
-metry	Process of measuring	Audiometry (process of measuring hearing)
-scope	Instrument for viewing	Laparoscope (instrument used to visualize the inside of the abdominal cavity)
-scopy	Process of visually examining	Bronchoscopy (visual examination of the bronchioles)

Surgical Procedures

SUFFIX	DEFINITION	EXAMPLE
-centesis	Puncture to withdraw fluid	Thoracentesis (procedure in which a needle or tube is inserted into the pleural space to remove fluid)
-desis	Surgical fixation	Pleurodesis (to fix the pleural membrane to the chest wall)
-ectomy	Surgical removal, excision	Appendectomy (removal of the appendix)
-ostomy	Surgically create an opening	Tracheostomy (creation of an opening into the trachea)
-otomy	Cutting into, incision	Laparotomy (cutting into the abdominal cavity)
-pheresis	Remove	Plasmapheresis (removal of solutes from the blood plasma)
-pexy	Surgical fixation	Orchiopexy (surgical fixation of the testicle to the scrotal wall)
-plasty	Surgical repair	Angioplasty (repair of the lumen of blocked blood vessel)
-stomy	New opening	Ileostomy (a new opening from the abdominal wall to the ileum)
-tripsy	Crushing	Lithotripsy (the mechanical crushing of kidney stones)

Disease and Pathology

SUFFIX	DEFINITION	EXAMPLE
-algia	Pain	Arthralgia (joint pain)
-asthenia	Weakness	Myasthenia (abnormal muscle weakness)

-cele	Hernia, protrusion	Meningocele (hernial protrusion of the meninges)
-cusis	Hearing	Presbycusis (impairment of hearing that occurs with age)
-derma	Skin	Scleroderma (hardening of the skin)
-dynia	Pain	Pododynia (foot pain)
-cytosis	Condition of too many cells	Leukocytosis (too many white blood cells)
-ectasis	Dilated, stretched out	Bronchiectasis (widening of the large airways)
-edema	Swelling	Lymphedema (swelling of the lymphatic vessels)
-emesis	Vomiting	Hematemesis (vomiting blood)
-emia	Condition of the blood	Anemia (low red blood cells)
-ism	State of, condition	Hypothyroidism (condition of underactive thyroid)
-itis	Inflammation	Sinusitis (inflammation of the sinuses)
-kinesis	Motion	Hypokinesis (diminished or abnormally slow movement)
-lysis	Destruction	Hemolysis (destruction of red blood cells)
-lytic	Destruction	Thrombolytic (breakdown of blood clots)
-malacia	Abnormal softening	Osteomalacia (softening of the bones)
-megaly	Enlargement, large	Cardiomegaly (enlargement of the heart)
-oid	Resembling	Osteoid (resembling the bone)
-oma	Tumor, mass	Adenoma (tumor of glandular tissue)
-osis	Abnormal condition	Thrombosis (formation of a blood clot in the blood vessels)
-oxia	Oxygen	Hypoxia (deficient oxygen)
-pathy	Disease	Neuropathy (disease of the nerves)
-penia	Deficiency	Cytopenia (deficiency in the number of cells)
-pepsia	To digest	Dyspepsia (disturbed digestion)
-phagia	To eat, to swallow	Dysphagia (difficult or painful swallowing)
-phobia	Fear	Agoraphobia (fear of open spaces or crowds)
-phasia	To speak, speech	Aphasia (loss of the ability to speak)
-plasia	Formation, produce	Hyperplasia (excessive growth of normal cells)
-plegia	Paralysis	Paraplegia (paralysis of the lower extremities)
-pnea	Breathing	Apnea (temporary cessation of breathing)
-rrhage	Bursting forth, outflow	Hemorrhage (outflow of blood)
-rrhagia	Bursting forth, outflow	Menorrhagia (abnormally profuse outflow of menses)
-rrhea	Discharge, flow	Diarrhea (excessive flow of loose stools)
-spasm	Involuntary muscle contraction	Laryngospasm (involuntary contraction of the larynx)
-stasis	Stopping	Cholestasis (obstruction or stoppage of the bile flow)
-toxic	Poison	Nephrotoxic (toxic to the kidneys)
-uria	Condition of the urine	Pyuria (the presence of pus in the urine)

Plural Endings			
SINGULAR ENDING	PLURAL ENDING	SINGULAR EXAMPLE	PLURAL EXAMPLE
a	ae	Vertebra	Vertebrae
en	ina	Foramen	Foramina
ex, ix, yx	ices	Appendix	Appendices
is	es	Analysis	Analyses

ma	mata	Angioma	Angiomata
nx (anx, inx, ynx)	nges	Phalanx	Phalanges
on	a	Ganglion	Ganglia
um	a	Datum	Data
us	i	Embolus	Emboli

TABLE 3. PREFIXES

Numbers or Quantity

PREFIX	DEFINITION	EXAMPLE
Bi-	Two	Biventricular (both ventricles)
Centi-	One hundred, one hundredth	Centimeter (one hundredth of a meter)
Di-	Two	Disomy (two copies of one or more chromosomes)
Diplo-	Double	Diplopia (seeing double of the same object)
Hemi-	Half, partial	Hemiparesis (weakness on one half of the body)
Milli-	One thousand, one thousandth	Millimeter (one thousandth of a meter)
Mono-	One	Monocyte (a phagocytic white blood cell with one well-defined nucleus)
Nulli-	None	Nulliparous (a woman who has had no children)
Pan-	All	Pansystolic (occurring throughout systole)
Poly-	Many	Polyuria (production of too much urine)
Quad-, quadri-	Four	Quadriplegic (a person who is paralyzed in all four limbs)
Tetra-	Four	Tetralogy (group of four)
Tri-	Three	Tricuspid (three points or cusps)

Time, Position, or Direction

PREFIX	DEFINITION	EXAMPLE
Ab-	Away from	Abduct (to carry away)
Ad-	Toward	Adduct (to move toward the middle)
Ante-	Before	Antepartum (before birth)
Ecto-, ex-, exo-, extra-	Out, without, away from	Ectopic (located away from the normal position)
En-, end-, endo-	Within, inner	Endocrine (glands that secrete hormones internally)
Epi-	Above, upon	Epigastric (above the stomach)
Hyper-	Excessive, more than normal	Hyperplasia (an abnormal increase in the production of cells)
Hypo-	Beneath or below normal	Hypotension (blood pressure that is below normal)
Infra-, Sub-	Below, under	Subclavian (beneath the clavicle)
Para-	Near, beside, or abnormal	Paravertebral (adjacent to the spinal column)
Per-	Through, by	Percutaneous (pass through the skin)
Peri-	Around, near	Pericardium (the membrane surrounding the heart)
Post-	After, behind	Postprandial (after meals)
Pre-	Before	Premature (occurring before the appropriate time)
Retro-	Behind, backward	Retroperitoneal (behind the peritoneum)
Super-, supra-	Above, beyond	Supraventricular (above the ventricle)
Sym-, syn-	Joined, together	Synthesis (to combine)
Trans-	Across	Transdermal (across the skin)

Colors

PREFIX	DEFINITION	EXAMPLE
Chlor/o	Green	Chlorophyll (a green pigment found in almost all plants)
Cyan/o	Blue	Cyanosis (bluish discoloration of the skin)
Erythr/o	Red	Erythrocyte (red blood cell)

Leuk/o	White, colorless	Leukemia (cancer of white blood cells)
Melan/o	Black, dark	Melanoma (darkly pigmented tumor of the skin)
Xanth/o	Yellow	Xanthoma (yellow nodule in the skin)

Size and Comparison		
PREFIX	DEFINITION	EXAMPLE
Brady-	Slow	Bradycardia (slow heartbeat)
Dys-	Bad, difficult	Dyspnea (difficulty breathing)
Equi-	Equal, same	Equimolar (the same number of moles)
Eu-	True, good, easy, normal	Euvolemic (normal blood volume)
Hetero-	Other, different, unequal	Heterogeneous (consisting of different parts)
Homo-, homeo-	Same, unchanging	Homeostasis (condition of stability or balance)
Iso-	Equal, same	Isotonic (the same tonicity)
Macro-	Large, abnormally large	Macrocytic (abnormally large cell)
Mal-	Bad	Malabsorption (bad or poor absorption)
Mega-, megalo-	Large, abnormally large	Megacolon (enlarged colon)
Micro-	Small	Microvascular (small vessels)
Neo-	New	Neonate (a newborn infant)
Normo-	Normal	Normotensive (normal blood pressure)
Ortho-	Straight, correct, upright	Orthostatic (caused by standing upright)
Poikilo-	Varied, irregular	Poikilocyte (abnormally shaped red blood cell)
Pseudo-	Fake	Pseudotumor (false tumor)
Re-	Against, back	Reflux (flowing back)
Tachy-	Fast	Tachypnea (abnormally rapid breathing)

APPENDIX 2-B   PROFESSIONAL TERMINOLOGY

Accreditation—A process in which an external organization (an accrediting body) formally evaluates an organization's ability to meet predetermined standards of performance.

Actual Acquisition Cost (AAC)—The actual cost a pharmacy pays in order to obtain a drug after all discounts have been applied.

Adherence—The extent to which a patient implements a treatment plan that was mutually agreed upon by both the patient and the healthcare provider. Adherence implies that the patient plays an active role in the development and execution of a treatment plan. *Compare to "compliance."*

Adjudication—The process of reviewing and resolving an insurance claim.

Adverse Drug Event (ADE)—Any injury that results from the use of a drug, including drug overdoses and adverse drug reactions. *Compare to "adverse drug reaction" and "medication error."*

Adverse Drug Reaction (ADR)—Any harmful, unintended, or undesired effect of a drug after it has been administered at doses typically used for treatment, prophylaxis, or diagnosis. *Compare to "adverse drug event" and "medication error."*

Ambulatory Care—The provision of medical care on an outpatient basis.

Assisted Living—A living arrangement in which patients live on their own in a residential facility but are able to obtain assistance with activities of daily living.

Average Wholesale Price (AWP)—The published price at which wholesalers sell prescription drugs. This price is often used as the basis for pricing prescription drugs.

Beneficiary—A person who receives the benefits of health insurance coverage.

Brand Name—A medication sold under a trademark-protected name.

Capitation—A method of reimbursement in which the healthcare provider is paid a predetermined fee on a monthly or quarterly basis for covered patients; also known as a "per-patient-per-month" rate of reimbursement.

Centers for Disease Control and Prevention (CDC)—The governmental agency responsible for tracking public health trends and controlling the introduction and spread of infectious diseases.

Centers for Medicare & Medicaid Services (CMS)—The federal agency that runs the Medicare program and works with states to run the Medicaid program.

Claim—A form submitted by a healthcare provider or patient to a payer requesting reimbursement of services rendered.

Closed Formulary—A type of formulary in which only drugs listed on the formulary are reimbursed by the plan.

Coinsurance—A method of cost-sharing in which the beneficiary of an insurance plan pays a fixed percentage of the cost of healthcare services. *Compare to "copayment."*

Compliance—The extent to which a patient implements a treatment plan that was prescribed by a healthcare provider. Compliance implies that the patient plays a passive role in following the healthcare provider's treatment plan. *Compare to "adherence."*

Coordination of Benefits—The process of coordinating a patient's benefits when he or she is covered by more than one healthcare plan.

Copayment—A method of cost-sharing in which the beneficiary of an insurance plan pays a fixed dollar amount for a particular service or item. *Compare to "coinsurance."*

Current Procedural Terminology (CPT)—A system developed by the American Medical Association to code and report the services rendered by healthcare providers.

Deductible—A method of cost-sharing in which the beneficiary of an insurance plan pays a fixed amount of yearly healthcare expenses before the payer will reimburse for covered healthcare expenses.

Denial—Refusal to reimburse healthcare services.

Department of Health and Human Services (HHS)—A department of the U.S. government that oversees 11 divisions, including the Centers for Disease Control and Prevention (CDC), the Centers for Medicare & Medicaid Services (CMS), and the Food and Drug Administration (FDA), among others.

Diagnosis-Related Group (DRG)—A system for classifying patients according to the severity of their diagnosis. The system is then used to obtain prospective payment for treatment of patients within that category.

Discharge Planning—A service provided to patients in order to ease the transition from one level of care to another.

Dispensing Fee—A charge added to the price of a drug in order to cover the cost involved in dispensing the prescription.

Drug Enforcement Administration (DEA)—The division of the U.S. Department of Justice that is responsible for enforcing the Controlled Substances Act.

Drug Utilization Evaluation (DUE)—A prospective review of the prescribing, dispensing, and use of a medication. *Compare to "drug utilization review" and "medication use evaluation."*

Drug Utilization Review (DUR)—A retrospective review of the prescribing, dispensing, and use of a medication. *Compare to "drug utilization evaluation" and "medication use evaluation."*

Durable Medical Equipment (DME)—Reusable medical equipment that is ordered by a doctor for use in the home. Examples include walkers, wheelchairs, and hospital beds.

Durable Power of Attorney—A legal document that makes provisions for a patient to designate another person to make healthcare-related decisions on his or her behalf in the event that he or she becomes incapacitated.

Facility Fee—A charge for the use of hospital resources when services are provided in the outpatient department of a hospital. "Facility Fee Billing" is used by pharmacists to bill for services provided in hospital-based clinics.

Fee for Service—The traditional method of reimbursement in which insurance companies pay fees for the services provided to beneficiaries.

Fee Schedule—The maximum fee that a health plan will pay for a healthcare service.

Food and Drug Administration (FDA)—The division of the Department of Health and Human Services that is responsible for ensuring the safety of foods, drugs, vaccines, biological products, and medical devices intended for human and animal use.

Formulary—An approved list of prescription medications that a plan will cover.

Generic Drug—A drug product that is comparable to a brand-name drug in dosage form, strength, route of administration, quality and performance characteristics, and intended use. The generic drug must contain identical amounts of the same active ingredient(s) as the brand-name product and must be proven "therapeutically equivalent" to the brand-name product.

Health Education Data Information System (HEDIS)—A widely used collection of performance measures and their definitions developed and maintained by the National Committee for Quality Assurance (NCQA).

Health Insurance Portability and Accountability Act of 1996 (HIPAA)—A regulation enacted by the U.S. Congress to guarantee patients' rights and protections against the misuse or disclosure of their health information and records.

Health Maintenance Organization (HMO)—A managed care organization where a group of doctors, hospitals, and other healthcare practitioners provide care to beneficiaries for a set payment from the managed care plan every month.

Home Health Agency—A home health aide organization that provides home healthcare services such as personal skilled nursing care, physical therapy, occupational therapy, and speech therapy.

Hospice—A type of care and philosophy that focuses on palliation and supportive care for terminally ill patients.

Incident-to-Billing—A method of obtaining reimbursement for non-physician services, including services provided by a pharmacist, that are provided as an important but incidental part of the physician's service. Often used in non-hospital–based clinics.

International Classification of Diseases (ICD)—The international medical standard diagnostic classification maintained by the World Health Organization (WHO) that provides codes to classify diseases and other health problems.

Joint Commission on Accreditation of Healthcare Organizations—A not-for-profit organization that accredits healthcare organizations in the United States.

Long-Term Care—A variety of services for patients with a chronic illness or disability that help with health or personal needs and activities of daily living over a period of time; this may be provided in the home, in the community, in assisted living facilities, or in a nursing home.

Managed Care—An arrangement in which a health insurance plan contracts between physicians and patients, negotiating fees for service and overseeing the types of treatment given.

Maximum Allowable Cost (MAC)—The highest price allowed for a specific drug under a specific plan.

Medicaid—A joint federal and state program that helps people with low income and limited resources; programs vary from state to state.

Medicare—A federally funded health insurance program for people 65 years of age or older, those under 65 with permanent disabilities, or those who meet special criteria such as end-stage renal disease.

Medication Error—Any mishap that occurs during the prescribing, transcribing, dispensing, or administration of a medication. Medication errors may include, but are not limited to, adverse drug events and adverse drug reactions. *Compare to "adverse drug event" and "adverse drug reaction."*

Medication Therapy Management Codes—CPT codes that are used to bill for medication therapy management services (MTMS). Codes include the following:

99605: Code for an initial MTMS encounter, 15 minutes in length, provided by a pharmacist

99606: Code for subsequent encounters

99607: Code for each additional 15 minutes

Medication Therapy Management Services (MTMS)—Services provided to optimize therapeutic outcomes for patients. These services are independent of the provision of a medication product.

Medication Use Evaluation (MUE)—A method of reviewing the prescribing, dispensing, and use of a medication with the goal of optimizing patient outcomes. *Compare to "drug utilization evaluation" and "drug utilization review."*

National Drug Code (NDC)—A numerical code used to identify drugs that are FDA approved.

Nursing Home—A residence that provides a room, meals, recreation, and help with activities of daily living for patients with physical or mental disabilities.

Occupational Therapy—Services given to help promote health by allowing one to return to doing usual activities, which include bathing, preparing meals, and housekeeping, after an illness.

Open Formulary—A formulary that allows for the use of medications not specifically listed on the formulary, although often at a higher copayment or coinsurance.

Out-of-Pocket Costs—Healthcare costs that are not covered by insurance and must be paid by the patient.

Pharmacy Benefits Manager (PBM)—A third-party administrator who offers services to a customer (such as an insurance carrier or employer) to control drug expenditures.

Pharmacy and Therapeutics Committee (P&T Committee)—A group of physicians, pharmacists, and clinical experts who help develop formularies and preferred drug lists that are clinically suitable and cost-effective for institutions.

Physical Therapy—Treatment of injury and disease by mechanical means such as heat, light, exercise, and massage to help maximize quality of life.

Preferred Provider Organization (PPO)—A managed care organization of doctors, hospitals, and providers who have contracted with an insurer to provide healthcare to those who belong to the network at a reduced rate. Doctors, hospitals, and providers outside of the network can be used for an additional cost.

Preventative Services—Healthcare services designed to prevent illness and keep patients healthy. Examples include immunizations, screening mammograms, pelvic exams, and colonoscopies.

Prior Authorization—A requirement that a physician obtain approval from a healthcare plan prior to a drug being dispensed by a pharmacy to guarantee the appropriateness and cost-effectiveness of the medication for the patient. If not approved, the medication may not be covered by the healthcare plan.

Protected Health Information (PHI)—Any individually identifiable health information, including information regarding a person's past, present, or future physical or mental health, the provision of healthcare to an individual, or the payment for provision of that healthcare. All forms of media, including written, electronic, and oral, are considered protected.

Skilled Nursing Facility (SNF)—A facility that provides skilled nursing care and related services to patients who require continuous care and assistance with activities of daily living but do not require hospitalization.

World Health Organization (WHO)—A specialized organization within the United Nations that is concerned with public health and also maintains the International Classification of Diseases (ICD) medical code set.

Appendix 2-C.   Pharmacy and Medical Chart Abbreviations

Base Solutions	
ABBREVIATION	DEFINITION
aq.	Water
aq. Bull	Boiling water
aq. Dist	Distilled water
D5NS	Dextrose 5% in normal saline
D5½NS or D5-0.45	Dextrose 5% in ½ normal saline (0.45% NaCl)
D5W	Dextrose 5% in water
DW	Distilled water
LR	Lactated Ringer's
½ NS	Half strength of normal saline (0.45% sodium chloride)
NS	Normal saline (0.9% NaCl)
R.L. or R/L	Ringer's lactate

Quantities	
ABBREVIATION	DEFINITION
aa. or ā ā	Of each
Ad	Up to
ad lib.	Freely, at pleasure
amp.	Ampule
Cc	Cubic centimeter
DS	Double strength
f_	One fluid ounce
fl₃ or fldr	One fluid drachm (5 mL)
g or Gm	Gram
Gal	Gallon
Gr	Grain
i	One
ii	Two
iii	Three
IU or iu	International units
L	Liter
M	Minim
m^2 or M^2	Square meter
Mcg	Microgram
mEq	Milliequivalent
mg	Milligram
ml or mL	Milliliter
mOsm or mOsmol	Milliosmole
O.	Pint
oz.	Ounce
PPM	Parts per million

pt.	Pint
q.s.	Sufficient quantity
Qt	Quart
ss.	Half
tbsp.	Tablespoon
tsp.	Teaspoon
U or u	Unit(s)
vol.	Volume

Administration and Preparation	
ABBREVIATION	DEFINITION
A	Before
a.c.	Before meals
a.m.	Morning
ASAP	As soon as possible
ATC	Around the clock
b.i.d.	Twice a day
b.i.w.	Twice a week
c.	With
D	Day
DAW	Dispense as written
disc. or D.C.	Discontinue
disp.	Dispense
div.	Divide
d.t.d.	Give of such doses
e.m.p.	As directed
f. or ft.	Make
h or hr	Hour
h.s.	At bedtime
M	Mix
m. ft.	Mix to make
min	Minute(s)
MR	May repeat
MRX_	May repeat _ times
NG	Nasogastric
noct.	Night
NPO	Nothing by mouth
p.c.	After meals
p.m.	Evening
p.r.n.	As needed
Post	After
post-op	After surgery
pre-op	Before surgery
q¯ or q	Every

q.d.	Every day
q.h.	Every hour
q_h	Every _ hour(s)
q.i.d.	Four times a day
S	Without
S.A.	According to the Art
s.i.d.	Once a day
s.o.s.	If there is a need
stat.	Immediately
t.i.d.	Three times a day
t.i.w.	Three times a week
u.d. or ut dict	As directed
w/	With
w.a. or WA	While awake
Wk.	Week
w/o	Without
X	Times

Preparations or Remedies

ABBREVIATION	DEFINITION
Aq	Water
aur or oto	Ear drops
Cap(s)	Capsule(s)
Chart	Powder
Comp	Compounded
Crm	Cream
EC	Enteric coated
elix.	Elixir
Garg	Gargle
gtt(s)	Drop(s)
inj.	An injection
liq.	Solution
Neb.	Nebulizer
NR	No refills
oint.	Ointment
pil.	Pill
pulv.	Powder
sol.	Solution
suppos.	Suppository
susp.	Suspension
syr.	Syrup
Tab(s)	Tablet(s)
tr.	Tincture

troch.	Lozenge
Ung	Ointment

Methods of Application	
ABBREVIATION	**DEFINITION**
AA	Affected area
a.d.	Right ear
a.s.	Left ear
a.u.	Each ear
AUD	Apply as directed
Dext	Right
e.m.p.	In the manner prescribed
i.n.	Intranasally
IEN	In each nostril
ID	Intradermal
IM	Intramuscular
inj.	Injection
IV	Intravenous
IVP	Intravenous push
IVPB	Intravenous piggy back
o.d. or OD	Right eye
o.l. or OL	Left eye
o.u. or O_2	Each eye or both eyes
o.s. or OS	Left eye
po	By mouth
PR	Per rectum
PV	Per vagina
SC, SQ, subc., or subq.	Subcutaneous
SL	Sublingual
top.	Topically
u.d.	As directed

History of Present Illness (HPI)	
ABBREVIATION	**DEFINITION**
ABW	Actual body weight
AOB	Alcohol on breath
ARF	Acute renal failure
c/o	Complains of
CC	Chief complaint
CP or c/p	Chest pain
DOB	Date of birth
DOE	Dyspnea on exertion
Dx	Diagnosis
ER or ED	Emergency room, department

HA or H/A	Headache
Hx or h/o	History or history of
IBW	Ideal body weight
ICU	Intensive care unit
N/V/D	Nausea/vomiting/diarrhea
Nocturia x_	Urinates _ time(s) during the night
OD	Overdose
PND	Paroxysmal nocturnal dyspnea
PTA	Prior to admission or arrival
SOB	Shortness of breath
s/p	Status post
Sx	Symptoms
TBW	Total body weight
Tx	Treatment
VS	Vital signs
y.o.	Year old

Past Medical History (PMH) and Surgical History

ABBREVIATION	DEFINITION
AAA	Abdominal aortic aneurysm
AF	Atrial fibrillation
AKA	Above-knee amputation
ALL	Acute lymphocytic leukemia
AML	Acute myelogenous leukemia
AODM	Adult-onset diabetes mellitus
ARDS	Acute respiratory distress syndrome
BBB	Bundle branch block
BKA	Below-knee amputation
CA	Cancer or cardiac arrest
CAD	Coronary artery disease
CHF	Congestive heart failure
CLL	Chronic lymphocytic leukemia
CML	Chronic myelogenous leukemia
COPD	Chronic obstructive pulmonary disease
CVA	Cerebrovascular accident (stroke)
DJD	Degenerative joint disease
DM	Diabetes mellitus
DVT	Deep vein thrombosis
HBP	High blood pressure
HD	Hemodialysis
HRT	Hormone replacement therapy
HT or HTN	Hypertension
MI	Myocardial infarction

MS	Multiple sclerosis
MVA	Motor vehicle accident
OT	Occupational therapy
PT	Physical therapy
SZ	Seizure
TIA	Transient ischemic attack (mini stroke)
TKR	Total knee replacement
URI	Upper respiratory infection
UTI	Urinary tract infection

Family and Social History	
ABBREVIATION	DEFINITION
↓	Deceased
A&W	Alive and well
D of A	Drugs of abuse
ETOH	Alcohol (ethanol)
IVDA	Intravenous drug abuse
Ppd	Packs per day
Py	Pack-years
Tob	Tobacco

Medications	
ABBREVIATION	DEFINITION
APAP	Acetaminophen
ASA	Aspirin
BCP	Birth control pills
CCT	Crude coal tar
CPZ	Chlorpromazine
DPT	Diphtheria, pertussis, tetanus
DSS	Docusate
EDTA	Edentate
EES	Erythromycin ethylsuccinate
EPI	Epinephrine
EPO	Erythropoietin
FA	Folic acid
FU or 5-FU	Fluorouracil
HC	Hydrocortisone
HCTZ	Hydrochlorothiazide
INH	Isoniazid
LCD	Coal tar solution
MDI	Meter dose inhaler
MMR	Measles, mumps, rubella
MO	Mineral oil
MOM	Milk of magnesia

MVI	Multivitamin
NTG	Nitroglycerin
OC	Oral contraceptive
Pb	Phenobarbital
PCN	Penicillin
PPD	Purified protein derivative (tuberculin)
PPI	Proton pump inhibitor
SMX/TMP	Sulfamethoxazole/trimethoprim
SSKI	Saturated solution of potassium iodide
TAC	Tetracaine, adrenalin, and cocaine
TCA	Tricyclic antidepressant
TCN	Tetracycline
TMP/SMX	Trimethoprim/sulfamethoxazole
TPN	Total parenteral nutrition
ZnO	Zinc oxide

Laboratory and Diagnosis

ABBREVIATION	DEFINITION
ABG	Arterial blood gas
AFB	Acid fast bacilli
ANA	Antinuclear antibody
ANS	Autonomic nervous system
BMP	Basic metabolic panel
BP	Blood pressure
BS	Blood sugar
BSA	Body surface area
BUN	Blood urea nitrogen
BW	Body weight
C	Centigrade
C&S	Culture and sensitivity
CBC w/ diff	Complete blood count with differential
Cl	Chloride
CT	Computed tomography
CXR	Chest x-ray
ECG or EKG	Electrocardiogram
EEG	Electroencephalography
EF	Ejection fraction
F	Fahrenheit
FBS	Fasting blood sugar
FOB	Fecal occult blood test
GFR	Glomerular filtration rate
GTT	Glucose tolerance test
H/H or "H and H"	Hemoglobin and hematocrit

HCO$_3$	Bicarbonate
Hct	Hematocrit
Hgb or Hb	Hemoglobin
HR	Heart rate
I&O	Input and output
K	Potassium
MRI	Magnetic resonance imaging
Na	Sodium
P	Pulse
Plt	Platelet
RBC	Red blood cell
RR	Respiratory rate
SCr	Serum creatinine
T&C	Type and crossmatch
U/A or UA	Urinalysis
U/S or US	Ultrasound
UUN	Urine urea nitrogen
UV	Ultraviolet
WBC	White blood cell

Review of Systems (ROS)	
ABBREVIATION	DEFINITION
–	Negative
?	Questionable
+	Positive
A & O x3	Alert and oriented to person, place, and time
Abd	Abdomen
AELBM	After each loose bowel movement
ANS	Autonomic nervous system
b/l	Bilateral
BM	Bowel movement
BRBPR	Bright red blood per rectum
BS	Bowel sounds or breath sounds
c.	With
CCE	Clubbing, cyanosis, and edema
CN	Cranial nerves
CNS	Central nervous system
CTA & P	Clear to auscultation and percussion
CV	Cardiovascular
CVAT	Costovertebral angle tenderness
DTR	Deep tendon reflexes
EENT	Eyes, ears, nose, and throat
EOMI	Extraocular movement intact

et.	And
Ext	Extremities
GI	Gastrointestinal
GU	Genitourinary
HEENT	Head, eyes, ears, nose, and throat
IOP	Intraocular pressure
JVD	Jugulovenous distension
JVP	Jugulovenous pulse
LAD	Lymphadenopathy
LUE	Left upper extremity
m/r/g	Murmurs, rubs, gallops
MN	Motor neurons
MS	Mental status
Musc	Musculoskeletal
NAD	No apparent distress
NCAT	Normocephalic and atraumatic
Nd	Nondistended
Nl	Normal
NSR	Normal sinus rhythm
Nt	Nontender
OB-GYN	Obstetrics-Gynecology
PCP	Primary care provider
PERRLA	Pupils equal, round, and reactive to light and accommodation
PNS	Peripheral nervous system
PPI	Patient package insert
PR	Per rectum
PV	Per vagina
r/o	Rule out
Rect	Rectal
ROM	Range of motion
RRR	Regular rate and rhythm
RUE	Right upper extremity
S_1, S_2, S_3, S_4	Heart sounds
SN	Sensory neurons
TM	Tympanic membrane
URI	Upper respiratory infection
USP	United States Pharmacopeia
UTI	Urinary tract infection
Wd	Well developed
Wn	Well nourished
Wnl	Within normal limits

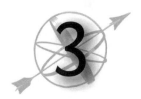

BIOSTATISTICS

Lawrence A. Frazee, PharmD, BCPS, and Mate M. Soric, PharmD, BCPS

CASE

A new antihypertensive agent, appesartan, has been tested in a large randomized, double-blind, placebo-controlled trial consisting of patients at high risk for myocardial infarction. The primary endpoint was cardiovascular death. F.M. has been asked to review the literature supporting the use of appesartan and is having difficulty understanding the statistics involved in the trial.

WHY IT'S ESSENTIAL

The practice of evidence-based medicine depends on the interpretation and application of the results of clinical trials. Without empirical evidence from well-designed clinical trials, decisions about whether a therapy is safe and effective can be made based only on anecdotal experience. *Biostatistics* is the mathematical science that describes observations made during experimentation, helps us to decide whether observed differences are likely to be real, and allows us to describe the magnitude of benefit and harm so that rational therapy decisions can be made. It is important for you to have a basic understanding of biostatistics when evaluating medical literature throughout the APPE rotations and beyond.

SUMMARIZING DATA

Before any statistical test can be performed, the aggregate data from any trial must be summarized. Being able to describe the data allows you to choose the appropriate statistical test and report results in an easy-to-understand way.

Types of Data

In general, *outcome data* are described as categorical, ordinal, or continuous. Categorical variables with only two possible categories are referred to as *binomial* data. Sex is an example of a binomial variable, and mortality is an example of a binomial outcome. A categorical variable with more than two possible outcomes (such as race or ethnicity) is a *nominal* variable. In either case, a categorical variable has no inherent order.

QUICK TIP

Being able to identify the type of data in a trial is vital to ensuring the proper statistical tests are used for analysis.

Ordinal variables have an inherent order, but the specific number has no mathematical meaning. A common example is a 10-point pain scale in which a score of 10 is higher than a score of 9. With this type of data, however, the differences between two numbers on the scale are not necessarily equal, meaning the difference between a 1 and 2 may not be the same as the difference between a 9 and 10.

Continuous data are data that come in the form of any numerical value (as opposed to discrete categories). This category is further subdivided into *interval* and *ratio* data. Temperature on the Celsius scale is an example of an interval variable because a difference of 1°C has the same meaning along the entire scale but the definition of zero is arbitrary. Because of this, a ratio cannot be calculated to express the relationship between outcomes measured on a continuous interval scale. Because 0°C does not mean "no temperature," one cannot say that 50°C is twice as much temperature as 25°C. Conversely, a continuous variable that is measured on a scale with a nonarbitrary value of zero is a ratio variable. The Kelvin scale for measuring temperature is an example of a continuous ratio scale because it contains an absolute zero value. Mass is also an example of a ratio variable because a value of 0 grams does, indeed, mean no mass. Outcomes on this scale can be expressed as a ratio because 50 grams is twice as much mass as 25 grams.

CASE QUESTION

Categorize each of the following variables from the appesartan trial as a binomial, nominal, ordinal, interval, or ratio variable: concomitant use of a beta-blocker, blood pressure reduction, quality-of-life score based on a Likert scale, cardiac survival, recruitment site.

Sometimes data collected on an ordinal or continuous scale can be expressed in a categorical way. For example, a placebo-controlled trial of a new diabetes medicine could present the average change in hemoglobin A1c from baseline with the new medicine compared with placebo. If the average change in hemoglobin A1c with the new medicine was −2.3 points, we know that some patients achieved a greater reduction while some achieved a smaller one. But what if the investigators are not interested in the average change in hemoglobin A1c as much as how many subjects reach the goal hemoglobin A1c of 7%? The study could be designed to report the proportion of patients who reach their goal with the new medicine compared to placebo, thus presenting continuous data on a categorical scale. In fact, most large comparative clinical trials measure outcomes on a categorical scale.

CASE QUESTION

One of the secondary endpoints in the appesartan trial is reduction in systolic blood pressure. How could this continuous outcome be converted into a categorical outcome?

Descriptive Statistics

Before a statistical test can be performed, descriptive statistics must be used to summarize the central tendency of the data. For categorical data, the most straightforward descriptive statistic is the proportion of subjects that fall into each category. When the scale has only two categories (yes or no), there is usually only one proportion reported. For example, a study that has mortality as an outcome will report the proportion of patients in each group that died because this is a binomial outcome (patients either died or survived).

For ordinal and continuous data, an expression of central tendency is needed to describe the outcome. The *mean* (average) has the advantage of being well suited for mathematical manipulation but is also easily influenced by outliers if the data are not normally distributed. The *median*, on the other hand, is the value for which half of the data points are below and half are above. The median has the advantage of not being as influenced by outliers but is not as easy to manipulate mathematically. Lastly, the *mode* is the value that occurs most often in a data set.

The mean is the most common and useful expression of central tendency for continuous data. There are, however, circumstances when the mean may not be appropriate, especially if the data are not normally distributed. It is not uncommon for studies to report the length of hospital stay as a median rather than a mean due to outliers that could skew the results. For ordinal data, such as a pain scale, the median is the most appropriate expression of central tendency, although it is not uncommon to see these outcomes expressed as a mean.

Establishing Statistical Significance

Two processes limit our ability to draw conclusions from clinical trials—bias and chance. *Bias* is a systematic error that tends to skew results in one particular and predictable direction, whereas *chance* is, by definition, a random process. There are several types of bias to be aware of when evaluating the literature, but one of the more common types is selection bias. Most common in observational studies, *selection bias* occurs when patients end up in a particular group based on something other than the variable being studied. An example might be an observational study designed to assess the incidence of tachycardia in patients with acute asthma treated with one of two different beta agonists. If prescribers are more likely to select one particular beta agonist in patients who present with baseline tachycardia (perhaps because of a belief that it causes fewer beta-mediated side effects), it will be difficult to determine whether any observed difference in heart rate after treatment is due to treatment selection or patient selection. Performing statistical tests on the results of a strongly biased clinical trial will do nothing to eliminate bias. If a trial is biased to produce results in one direction, it is likely that our statistical tests will demonstrate statistical difference in that direction because there is a true difference between the groups. The problem is that the difference observed is likely due to something other than the variable under study. The primary method to minimize bias is through rigorous trial design. Prospective randomized group assignment and blinding are two of the most common methodologies employed in this regard.

QUICK TIP

Although clinicians must always be on the lookout for bias, the potential for bias does not necessarily mean that it is present, nor does it mean that the bias is actually skewing the results to a significant degree.

Despite our best efforts at selecting a study population and assigning individuals to treatment groups in an unbiased way, there is still a possibility that the group will differ from the population as a whole. This is often referred to as *random sampling error* and is due to chance. There are two general approaches used to assess the effect of chance on observed outcomes. The first approach is called *hypothesis testing* and produces the well-known "*P* value." The second approach is called *estimation* and is represented by the point estimate and confidence interval.

CASE QUESTION

F.M. has noted that, despite the randomized trial design, the two groups used in the appesartan trial were significantly different with regard to smoking status. What type of error has been identified?

Hypothesis Testing

The proper statistical test allows the clinician to determine with a certain level of confidence whether the observed difference between groups is real or due to random chance. Before we get into the specifics of hypothesis testing, it is important to understand some of the assumptions that underlie statistical testing in biomedical research. Perhaps the best way to understand this is with an example from jurisprudence.

The phrases "innocent until proven guilty" and that guilt must be proven "beyond a reasonable doubt" are most likely familiar to anyone who has seen an episode of *Law and Order*. Where do such phrases come from, and how do they relate to statistical testing? In the American legal system, when a person is accused of a crime, the accused is assumed to be innocent and the prosecutor must prove that he or she is guilty. If the prosecutor is not able to do this, then the defendant cannot be found guilty. The assumption of innocence is intentional because it is borne out of a culture that values freedom. No system will come to the true conclusion 100% of the time, so it must be asked if it is better to convict an innocent person or to acquit a guilty person. Because we place a high value on freedom, the American legal system is designed so that the burden of proof is on the prosecutor. If the amount and magnitude of the evidence is enough to prove the defendant guilty beyond a reasonable doubt, then the jury will return a verdict of "guilty." If there is reasonable doubt regarding the guilt of the defendant, the jury will return a verdict of "not guilty." Notice that in this system, either the defendant is guilty or the jury is unable to say that the defendant is guilty. The jury cannot say that he or she is innocent.

This example is very instructive for understanding hypothesis testing. Biomedical researchers want to be as sure as possible that a treatment is truly effective. They would rather take the chance of saying that an effective treatment is not effective than say that an ineffective treatment is effective. The assumption is that there is no difference in the outcome under study between the study treatment group and the control group (innocent until proven guilty). The burden of proof is on the investigator to prove that the study treatment is more effective than the comparator. If the statistical test shows that the difference between groups is real beyond a reasonable doubt, the investigator will conclude that the treatments are statistically different. If this cannot be shown beyond a reasonable doubt, the investigator must conclude that they are not different. In a classic superiority trial, where the study treatment is compared to placebo or standard treatment, this is accomplished by attempting to disprove the null hypothesis (H_0). The null hypothesis posits that there is no difference in the outcome being studied between groups. If the outcome is mortality and two treatments (A and B) are being compared, then the null hypothesis would be that mortality in treatment group A is equal to mortality in treatment group B. The study is then designed with the goal of disproving, or rejecting, the null hypothesis. This is analogous to assuming that the defendant is innocent and then going to trial to try to disprove or reject this hypothesis. **Figure 3-1** illustrates the comparison between hypothesis testing and jurisprudence.

Avoiding Error

Type I Error

As shown in Figure 3-1, there are four possible conclusions in hypothesis testing, two of them correct and two of them incorrect. A *type I error* is made when a statistical test concludes that two treatments are different when there really is no difference—analogous to convicting an innocent person. The probability of making a type I error is given by the P value.

Let's consider the example of a study that compared the beta-blocker bisoprolol to placebo to reduce postoperative 30-day mortality in high-risk patients undergoing noncardiac vascular surgery.[1] Investigators reported that the incidence of cardiac death at 30 days was 3.4% in the bisoprolol group and 17% in the placebo group, with a reported P value of 0.02. The absolute treatment difference between

Figure 3-1. The Analogy of Jurisprudence and Hypothesis Testing

TRUTH

	GUILTY	INNOCENT
Guilty	CORRECT	ERROR
Not Guilty	ERROR	CORRECT

Verdict from the Jury

JURISPRUDENCE:

1. The accused is considered innocent until proven guilty.

2. The burden of proof is on the prosecutor to disprove/reject #1.

3. The verdict is either "guilty" or "not guilty" but not "innocent."

TRUTH

	DIFFERENT	EQUAL
Different	CORRECT	Type I (α) ERROR
Not Different	Type II (β) ERROR	CORRECT

Conclusion from Statistical Test

HYPOTHESIS TESTING:

1. The treatments are considered equal until proven different.

2. The burden of proof is on the investigator to disprove/reject #1.

3. The conclusion is either "different" or "not different" but not "equal."

---

groups is 13.6% (17 minus 3.4), but what is the likelihood that this difference is real and not due to selecting higher-risk patients in the placebo group by random chance? The answer is the *P* value.

The null hypothesis in this study was that the 30-day mortality would be the same in the bisoprolol and placebo groups, resulting in an absolute treatment difference of zero. The *P* value represents a 2% probability that the mortality difference observed (13.6%) would have been obtained when the null hypothesis (mortality difference of 0%) was, in fact, true. In other words, there is a 2% chance that a type I error was made. In biomedical research, we are willing to accept up to a 5% probability of making a type I error, although this is a completely arbitrary value.

CASE QUESTION

Patients who used appesartan had a mortality rate of 80 out of 1,000 (8%), compared with 100 out of 1,000 (10%) in the placebo group. The corresponding P value was calculated to be 0.005. What is the chance that a type I error has occurred?

P values can be reported in several different ways. Some investigators will report the actual *P* value, no matter what it is. In these cases, a *P* value that is less than 0.05 is interpreted as a statistically significant difference between groups, whereas a *P* value greater than 0.05 is interpreted as a difference that is not statistically significant. Sometimes a significant *P* value is just reported as less than a certain threshold, such as less than 0.01 or less than 0.001, and a nonsignificant *P* value is reported as NS (not significant) if it is greater than 0.05.

Type II Error

Although there are many things to consider when evaluating a study that showed a statistically significant difference, the concept is fairly straightforward. The issue of type II error, however, is a little more difficult to assess in most studies. A *type II error* is made when two treatments are said to be not different (*P* > 0.05) when they really *are* different (analogous to setting a guilty person free). The most common reason this happens is that the observed difference between groups was smaller than expected.

When designing a study, the investigator must make certain assumptions about the difference he or she wants to be able to detect between groups. This expected difference is based on observations from other studies as well as what would be considered a clinically meaningful difference. It is used to calculate the number of subjects that will need to be enrolled to detect this difference statistically. If an investigator believes that there will be a very large difference between groups, it will not take many subjects to prove it. The problem, of course, is that if the investigator uses this small sample size and the observed difference turns out to be smaller than predicted, there will not be enough subjects to say with confidence that the difference was not due to random chance. Having said that, it is also very expensive to conduct large studies, so the investigator must select a difference in treatment effect that is small enough to avoid missing an important treatment effect but large enough to keep the sample size at a reasonable number. The probability of making a type II error (also called beta [β]) is usually set at 0.2. The power of a study is expressed as $1 - \beta$, or 0.8, and is directly proportional to the sample size. Notice that the probability of making a type II error (0.2) is much higher than the acceptable probability of making a type I error (0.05). This is intentional because the burden of proof is on the investigator to demonstrate that there is a difference between groups.

When looking at a clinical trial, how does one determine whether or not a type II error was made? The first thing to understand is that a type II error cannot occur when a statistically significant difference is observed. There is no possibility of erroneously concluding that a treatment effect is not different if your statistical test concluded that it *is* different. So, if the *P* value is less than 0.05, the study was, by definition, powered to detect the difference that was observed and no type II error was made. However, when the *P* value is greater than 0.05, one must consider that the observed difference might be real but smaller than expected, leading to a potential type II error. To illustrate this concept, consider a study in diabetic women with asymptomatic bacteriuria. Patients were randomized to receive antibiotics or placebo to see if treatment could prevent symptomatic urinary tract infections and complications. The investigators concluded that there was no statistically significant difference between the antibiotic and placebo groups in any of the outcomes measured. Is it possible that a type II error was made? To answer this question, one must read through the Methods section of the study to determine how large of a difference the study was powered to detect. The following is excerpted from the Methods section of a study:

> We estimated that the frequency of pyelonephritis among diabetic women with asymptomatic bacteriuria would be twice as high, or 8 percent per year, with a cumulative rate of 25 percent over a period of three years. If this rate was decreased to 5 percent by treatment, consistent with the decrease from 20 to 30 percent to 2 to 3 percent reported with treatment among pregnant women, then 58 women would be needed in each group for the study to have 80 percent power to identify an absolute difference between groups of 20 percent with an a level of 0.05.[2(p1577)]

The study was powered to detect an absolute difference in the rate of pyelonephritis of 20% (25% with placebo to 5% with antibiotics), and the sample size was calculated to detect this difference. If the difference between antibiotics and placebo is real but smaller than 20%, this study would not be powered to detect it. In fact, the incidence of pyelonephritis over 3 years was found to be 0.28 and 0.13 for the placebo and antibiotic groups, respectively, a statistically insignificant difference ($P = 0.13$). If these numbers are compared with the percentages used to calculate the sample size, then the observed treatment difference was 15% (28% minus 13%), smaller than the expected difference of 20%. Because the sample size was based on this predicted difference, it is entirely possible that the observed difference in the incidence of pyelonephritis is real but smaller than expected (a type II error). If the observed difference was found to be statistically significant, it would likely represent a clinically meaningful result, but the only way to address this clinical question would be to conduct a larger trial that is powered to detect a smaller difference.

CASE QUESTION

Based on the primary endpoint described previously, could a type II error have occurred in the appesartan trial?

The Confidence Interval

An alternate way to assess the likelihood that the difference observed in a clinical trial is due to random sampling error is to consider the point estimate of the treatment effect along with an estimate of the statistical precision around that estimate. In reality, the true treatment effect may be less than or more than the point estimate in a single clinical trial, so one must ask about the possible range of values that would be seen if the study was repeated many times. The *confidence interval* is the possible range of values. Most commonly, a 95% confidence interval (95% CI) is reported, meaning that if the study were to be repeated 100 times, the point estimate of the treatment effect would fall within the range 95 times (and, hence, would fall outside the 95% CI only 5 times).

QUICK TIP

The confidence interval can be expressed in absolute or relative terms.

An absolute treatment difference of 0 or a relative risk ratio of 1 would indicate that the outcome was exactly the same in both groups. Therefore, if the 95% CI contains "no difference" (0 for treatment difference and 1 for risk ratio), then it must be concluded that a difference between groups could not be demonstrated beyond a reasonable doubt. Conversely, if the 95% CI does not include the value corresponding to "no difference," it can be concluded that there is a statistically significant difference between groups, with a less than 5% probability of making a type I error. In effect, the 95% CI provides the same information as the *P* value, but it also provides information about the range of possible values as well as statistical power. In addition to providing insight into the chances of committing a type I error, the confidence interval can also shed light on the statistical power of the results. When the sample size is small, the 95% CI is wide because there is a great deal of uncertainty about the precision of the point estimate. As sample size increases (and power increases), there is more confidence in the reproducibility of the observed results, so the 95% CI becomes narrower. The width of the 95% CI can become an important tool for assessing the likelihood that a type II error was made.

Consider the theoretical example in **Figure 3-2**, where the point estimate is represented by the solid circle and the 95% CI by the horizontal lines extending in either direction from the point estimate (upper and lower limits of the 95% CI). In both examples, it must be concluded that no difference between groups could be demonstrated because the 95% CI includes zero. However, in study 2, the 95% CI is large and contains many values that would favor the new treatment. It is entirely feasible that a type II error was made and that this study was underpowered to detect a real difference between groups. On the other hand, the 95% CI in study 1 is narrow, with a significant proportion of values on either side of the "no difference" line. It is much less likely that there is a significant power issue with this study and, if a true treatment difference exists, the magnitude would be relatively small.

Figure 3-2. The 95% Confidence Interval and Statistical Power

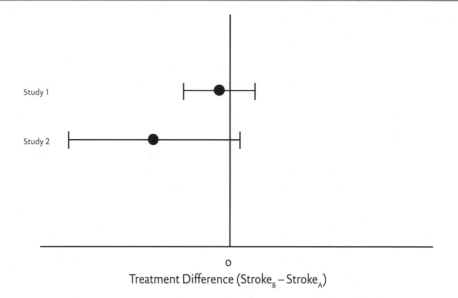

Treatment Difference $(Stroke_B - Stroke_A)$

Two theoretical examples of a study of a new anticoagulant (Drug A) compared with standard therapy (Drug B) for stroke prevention in atrial fibrillation.

EXPRESSING THE MAGNITUDE OF BENEFIT OR HARM

Once statistical significance has been demonstrated appropriately, focus should shift toward characterizing the magnitude of that difference. In some trials, very small differences between study groups may meet the criteria for statistical significance; however, when applied to real-world settings, these minute differences may have little impact on clinical practice. To help students and practitioners differentiate between statistical and clinical significance, a deeper understanding of risk, odds, and other calculations must be obtained.

Take, for example, the hypothetical clinical trial comparing appesartan to placebo for the prevention of cardiovascular death over 12 months. The investigators have identified a cardiovascular mortality rate of 8% (80/1,000 patients) in the treatment group, compared with 10% (100/1,000 patients) in the placebo group, a statistically significant difference. These results can be explained in a number of ways, including a 2% reduction in mortality, a 20% reduction in mortality, or one less death for every 50 patients treated with appesartan for 12 months. Without a solid grasp of the calculations that go on behind these results, you may be easily misled by the results of clinical trials, leading to inappropriate recommendations and potentially poorer patient outcomes.

Absolute Versus Relative Risk

Of all of the calculations discussed in this section, absolute risk is likely the easiest to understand. In clinical trials, *absolute risk* is reflected by dividing the number of patients that met a study outcome by the total number of patients in the group. In our hypothetical trial, 80 of 1,000 patients treated with appesartan experienced the primary outcome of cardiovascular death (an 8% absolute risk of mortality). On its own, absolute risk provides little information about the clinical relevance of an outcome until we compare the two study groups using the *absolute risk reduction* (ARR), which is calculated by subtracting the absolute risks of the two groups. For appesartan, subtracting the 8% risk of death from the 10% risk in patients treated with the placebo results in an ARR of 2%. In most cases, ARR calculations will result in relatively small numbers. As they cannot be artificially inflated, it is typically recommended that clinicians rely on absolute rather than relative results whenever possible.

CASE QUESTION

Absolute risk increase can be calculated using similar mathematics. Appesartan was shown to cause hyperkalemia in 12 out of 1,000 patients, compared to 2 out of 1,000 patients in the placebo group. Calculate the absolute risk increase of hyperkalemia with appesartan.

Despite the fact that it is highly encouraged to use absolute calculations of risk, outcomes are commonly presented in relative terms. The *relative risk*, or *risk ratio*, is calculated by dividing the absolute risk in the treatment group by the absolute risk in the control group. If the absolute risk of the outcome is exactly the same in both groups, the relative risk will be 1. A relative risk greater than 1 indicates that the outcome is more likely to occur in the treatment group, whereas a relative risk less than 1 indicates the opposite. For appesartan, 8% divided by 10% equals a relative risk of 0.80, signifying a lower risk of death with the new antihypertensive compared to placebo. Depending on the type of study and outcome, relative risk may also be reported as a hazard ratio or likelihood ratio.

A related concept is the *relative risk reduction* (RRR), which relates the ARR to the baseline risk in the control group. As discussed earlier, the 8% mortality rate with appesartan is 2% lower than the 10% mortality rate with placebo, resulting in an ARR of 2%. Because the baseline mortality in the control group is 10%, this could be expressed as a relative decrease in mortality of 20% (2% divided by 10%). The RRR will always be numerically larger than the ARR, making the treatment effect appear larger. This same problem can occur when relative terms are used to express the risk increase of an outcome like an adverse effect. For example, a news story may report that appesartan "quadruples the risk of cancer," but a prudent clinician will check absolute risk to identify what may be an increase from only 1 in 100,000 patients to 4 in 100,000 patients, an increase in absolute risk much smaller than would be suggested by the relative risk increase. See **Table 3-1** for additional examples of how absolute risk and relative risk compare to one another.

QUICK TIP

Alternatively, RRR can be calculated by subtracting the relative risk from 1. For appesartan, this calculation would be 1 minus 0.8, resulting in the same 0.2 RRR.

TABLE 3-1. COMPARISONS OF ABSOLUTE RISK, RELATIVE RISK, AND NUMBER NEEDED TO TREAT

RESULTS		RELATIVE RISK REDUCTION	ABSOLUTE RISK REDUCTION	NUMBER NEEDED TO TREAT
TREATMENT	PLACEBO			
1/4	2/4	50%	25%	4
1/40	2/40	50%	2.5%	40
1/400	2/400	50%	0.25%	400
1/4,000	2/4,000	50%	0.025%	4,000

Odds Ratio

Thus far, the discussion has centered on relative and absolute risks. These are two very important calculations; however, they cannot be applied to all types of studies. In fact, of the observational study designs, only cohort studies are able to take advantage of these types of expressions of magnitude. For case-control trials, odds and odds ratios are the primary methods for conveying effect size. In this study design, the investigators choose the number of patients that have and do not have a particular condition or event, artificially setting the prevalence. This sample of patients is not chosen to reflect the actual prevalence of the disease; therefore, it is impossible to calculate a relative risk ratio. If relative risk compares the number of times an event occurs to the number of times it could occur, odds can be said to compare the number of times an event occurs to the number of times it does not occur. Analogous to the odds at a casino, dividing the number of patients experiencing the primary outcome by the number of patients that did not experience it produces the odds of the event. For example, in the trial of appesartan, where 80 out of 1,000 patients experienced death, the odds of death occurring can be calculated by dividing 80 by 920, equaling 0.087. When investigators compare the odds of an outcome between two groups, they are calculating the odds ratio. For the appesartan trial, dividing 0.087 (the odds of death in the appesartan group) by 0.11 (the odds of death in the placebo group) results in an odds ratio of 0.79, a value very similar to the relative risk ratio of 0.80 calculated above.

QUICK TIP

When the incidence of the primary endpoint is low, odds will be very similar to risk calculations. As the incidence grows, especially above 10%, the odds may exaggerate the risks.

Number Needed to Treat or Harm

Popularized by clinicians, the number needed to treat (NNT) and number needed to harm (NNH) calculations provide pharmacists with a simple, easy-to-understand method to evaluate clinical significance. NNT is calculated by dividing 1 by the ARR for a given endpoint. NNH, on the other hand, is calculated by dividing 1 by the increase in risk for a given side effect. The resulting figure is the number of patients that would need to be treated to prevent (or cause) the specific endpoint. Although absolute and relative risks perform a similar function, it is often difficult to apply these calculations to real-world situations and determine if benefits outweigh risks. For appesartan, the NNT for cardiovascular mortality risk can be calculated by dividing 1 by 0.02, resulting in a value of 50. In other words, 50 patients need to be treated with appesartan to prevent one cardiovascular death. This value can be compared to the calculated NNH values to determine if the benefits outweigh the risks of treatment. If the difference in the rate of angioedema between appesartan and placebo is determined to be 0.04%, the NNH would be calculated as 1/0.0004 or 2,500 patients.

QUICK TIP

The number produced by the NNT and NNH calculations should be rounded up to the nearest whole number.

There are a number of important facts to consider about the NNT and NNH calculations. First, not all endpoints can be used to calculate the values. Continuous endpoints, such as blood pressure or hemoglobin A1c, and statistically insignificant results cannot be used in these estimates. Only statistically significant, binomial variables are eligible. Most commonly, these include morbidity and mortality endpoints. Second, the results of the NNT or NNH calculation must be taken only in the context of the trial design. The results cannot be extrapolated to patient populations, treatments, or conditions not included in the trial. In addition to these limitations, students often forget to include the time course of the trial when they report NNT values. For appesartan, our NNT of 50 should also mention that these 50 patients would need to be treated for 12 months, the duration of the trial used to calculate the NNT. Lastly, NNT can help clinicians consider costs of treatment. Multiplying the NNT by the cost of the treatment being evaluated can help you compare the cost-effectiveness of new treatments.

CASE QUESTION

In the adverse events analysis, appesartan was shown to cause hypotension in 210 out of 1,000 patients compared to 50 out of 1,000 patients in the placebo group. Calculate the number needed to harm for this endpoint.

NONINFERIORITY AND EQUIVALENCE TRIALS

Up to this point, the discussion of statistical testing has focused on trying to prove that a treatment is different than a comparator. What if an investigator wants to prove that a new treatment is equivalent or "not worse" than the standard therapy? This is a very common question and is important for a number of reasons. First, if an effective therapy exists for a disease state, it would be unethical to test a new treatment against placebo. This can be illustrated when new anticoagulants are developed for stroke prevention in patients with atrial fibrillation. Warfarin is an established and consistently effective therapy that reduces the risk of stroke in these patients, and any study that included a placebo group would cause some of those patients to experience a stroke. However, warfarin is a difficult drug to use due to interpatient variability in dosage, need for monitoring, and interactions with other medications and foods. If a newer anticoagulant could be developed that was effective, did not require monitoring, did not interact with other medications or foods, and did not require dosage adjustments, this could be a significant advance. Of course, it must be established that this new anticoagulant is at least as effective as the standard therapy.

In a traditional superiority trial, the new agent would be compared to standard therapy with a null hypothesis that there is no difference in the incidence of stroke between groups. Based on the above discussion, this is a problem if the goal is to show that the new therapy is "not worse" than standard therapy. If such a study is conducted and no difference is demonstrated, how can the investigator be certain that a type II error was not made? In fact, a conclusion of "no difference" would be more likely if the study was underpowered with a small sample size. Because we want to be as certain as possible that the new treatment is not worse than the standard treatment, a different approach to trial design is necessary.

Noninferiority (NI) and *equivalence* (EQ) trials are designed to assess whether a new treatment is "not worse than" or equivalent to standard therapy, respectively. For simplicity's sake, we will not consider NI and EQ trials separately. The key to understanding NI trial design is understanding the null hypothesis for this type of study. Whereas a classic superiority trial posits a null hypothesis that the treatments are the same, an NI trial assumes that the new treatment is worse than the standard treatment by some predefined NI margin (Δ). Once the null hypothesis is established, the process of statistical testing is fairly similar to the typical superiority trials as the investigator designs and conducts the study to try to reject the null hypothesis.

QUICK TIP

An equivalence trial can be thought of as a two-tailed NI trial because it seeks to prove that the new treatment is not worse nor better than the comparator, whereas a NI trial seeks only to prove that it is not worse.

Assessing Noninferiority

Whether a new treatment is noninferior to standard treatment is determined by the 95% CI for the treatment difference between groups. Consider a hypothetical study in which a new treatment (drug A) for hyperlipidemia is compared to standard treatment (drug B) with a primary outcome of cardiovascular (CV) events after 5 years of treatment. In a classic superiority trial, the null hypothesis would be that no difference in cardiovascular events exists between treatments, and the study would be designed to reject this hypothesis.

Superiority H_0: CV event (A) – CV event (B) = 0

However, if the goal is to demonstrate that drug A is at least as effective as (or noninferior to) drug B, then the null hypothesis would be that cardiovascular events with drug A are no more frequent than those with drug B plus some predetermined margin (Δ).

Noninferiority H_0: CV event (A) – CV event (B) > Δ

The point estimate of the treatment difference between drug A and drug B will be presented along with the 95% CI around that estimate. For example, suppose the incidence of cardiovascular events with drug A and drug B was found to be 1.3% and 0.9%, respectively. This may be reported as a treatment difference of 0.4% with a 95% CI of –0.6% to 0.8%, but how are these results interpreted?

Because the 95% CI for the treatment difference includes zero, the investigator can conclude that a difference between treatments was not demonstrated. This is not the same as saying the treatments are "equivalent" or that the new treatment is "not inferior." This can be concluded only if it is determined that the upper end of the 95% CI for the treatment difference falls to the left of the predefined Δ. **Figure 3-3** illustrates several different scenarios when interpreting the results of an NI trial. In studying Figure 3-3, it should become apparent that interpretation of the results of an NI trial hinges on where the 95% CI for the treatment difference falls relative to a treatment difference of zero and a treatment difference of Δ.

Figure 3-3. Hypothetical Scenarios of Treatment Differences in a Noninferiority Trial

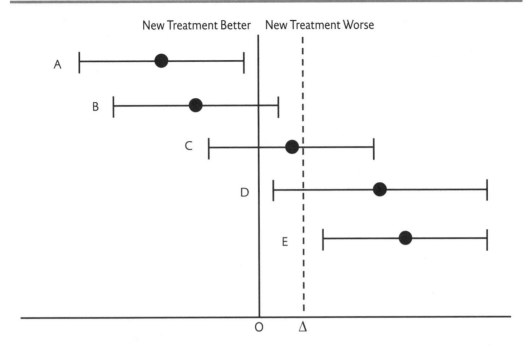

Treatment Difference for Adverse Outcome (e.g., Death)
(New Treatment Minus Standard Treatment)

The point estimate of the treatment difference between the new treatment and standard treatment with 95% CIs.

A. New treatment is superior to standard treatment because the upper end of the 95% CI is to the left of zero.

B. New treatment is noninferior to standard treatment because the upper end of the 95% CI is to the left of the NI margin (Δ).

C. Inconclusive because the 95% CI includes both zero and Δ. The new treatment cannot be called noninferior and is not different (neither inferior nor superior).

D. Confusing because the new treatment cannot claim noninferiority (95% CI includes Δ) and it is inferior (lower end of the 95% CI is to the right of zero).

E. New treatment is inferior to standard treatment.

Source: Adapted from Fletcher MP. Biosimilars clinical development program: Confirmatory clinical trials: A virtual/simulated case study comparing equivalence and non-inferiority approaches. *Biologicals.* 2011;39(5):270–277. Used with permission from Elsevier.

Choosing the Noninferiority Margin

Selection of an appropriate Δ is one of the most important considerations in the design of an NI trial; however, it is often difficult to determine the degree to which a new treatment can be inferior to standard treatment and still be called noninferior. A Δ that is too large can result in a conclusion of NI based on a 95% CI that includes important treatment differences in favor of standard treatment. There are at least two considerations when evaluating whether an appropriate Δ was selected for a NI trial.

First, the Δ should be selected in relative terms. The use of an absolute value for Δ can result in accepting a Δ that is much higher if the incidence of the outcome under study occurs less commonly than expected. For example, suppose that the expected cardiovascular event rate over 5 years was 4% in the study of the new antihyperlipidemic (drug A) compared to standard treatment (drug B). Based on this, an absolute Δ of 1% was selected. Because the 95% CI for treatment difference between groups was less than Δ (−0.6% to 0.8%), it could be concluded that the new treatment is noninferior to standard treatment. There is a problem with this interpretation, however. Notice that the observed event rate of 0.9% in the standard treatment group was much lower than the expected 4% on which the Δ of 1% was based. Because Δ was selected in absolute terms based on an expected event rate more than four times higher than what was observed, the result is a NI margin that is more than twice the event rate observed. In addition, the upper end of the 95% CI of 0.8% means that the new treatment could result in a relative risk of a cardiovascular event that is 89% higher than standard treatment (0.8% divided by 0.9%). If the true cardiovascular event rate is higher than what was observed, then the treatment difference could be much larger than observed in this trial. A Δ that is selected in relative terms is less influenced by event rates that are different than what was expected.

Second, if possible, the Δ should be selected to preserve at least half of the benefit seen with standard treatment compared to placebo. Consider the following statement from a recent trial comparing two antiplatelet regimens for secondary stroke prevention.

> The margin was defined in the following way. Using data from the nonfatal stroke outcomes from the Clopidogrel versus Aspirin in Patients at Risk of Ischemic Events (CAPRIE) trial and from the meta-analysis by the Antithrombotic Trialists' Collaboration, and following the method of Fisher et al., we derived an estimated odds ratio for clopidogrel being better than placebo for the outcome of nonfatal stroke: 1.377 (95% confidence interval [CI], 1.155 to 1.645). Thus, to ensure that the aspirin plus extended-release dipyridamole preserved at least half the effect of clopidogrel, the noninferiority margin was set at 1.075, an effect size equal to half the lower limit of the confidence interval. To reject the inferiority null hypothesis, the upper boundary of the 95% confidence interval for the hazard ratio must lie below the value of 1.075 (an increase of 7.5% in the hazard associated with aspirin plus extended-release dipyridamole).[3(p1240)]

Based on studies of the standard treatment (clopidogrel) with placebo, the investigators determined that the relative odds of stroke with placebo was 37.7% higher than with clopidogrel, with a 95% CI of 15.5% to 64.5%. In order to maintain at least half of this benefit, a Δ that is half of the lower end of the 95% CI was selected, resulting in a relative Δ of a 7.5% increase in the odds of stroke. Therefore, as long as the upper end of the 95% CI for the point estimate of the relative risk of stroke with the new treatment compared with standard treatment was to the left of 1.075 (i.e., all values in the 95% CI are below 1.075), then the new treatment can be called noninferior (as shown in example B in Figure 3-3).

Analyzing Noninferiority Trials

One final issue with NI trials is the use of intention-to-treat (ITT) versus per protocol (PP) analysis. *ITT analysis* outcomes are analyzed in patients based on the group they were randomized to, whether they stayed on treatment or not. *PP analysis* outcomes are analyzed only in patients who remained in the groups to which they were originally randomized. For superiority trials, the ITT analysis is often the favored way to analyze data because it is more like the real world. In essence, ITT analysis biases the results toward no difference and, therefore, makes it more difficult to prove a statistically significant difference between groups. In a NI trial, however, ITT analyses may bias the results in favor of no difference (or NI), making it easier to show that there is no difference between groups. The PP analysis biases results toward the difference between groups, making it more difficult to demonstrate NI in a NI trial. Therefore, for a NI trial, it is appropriate to present both the ITT and the PP analysis and conclude NI if it is true for both types of analysis.

REFERENCES

1. Poldermans D, Boersma E, Bax JJ, et al. The effect of bisoprolol on perioperative mortality and myocardial infarction in high-risk patients undergoing vascular surgery. *N Engl J Med*. 1999;341:1789-1794.

2. Harding GK, Zhanel GG, Nicolle LE, et al. Antimicrobial treatment in diabetic women with asymptomatic bacteriuria. *N Engl J Med*. 2002;347:1576-1583.

3. Sacco RL, Diener HC, Yusuf S, et al. Aspirin and extended-release dipyridamole versus clopidogrel for recurrent stroke. *N Engl J Med*. 2008;359:1238-1251.

SUGGESTED READING

Fletcher RH, Fletcher SW. *Clinical Epidemiology: The Essentials*. 4th ed. Baltimore, MD: Lippincott Williams & Wilkins; 2005.

Hulley SB, Cummings SR, Browner WS, et al. *Designing Clinical Research*. 3rd ed. Philadelphia, PA: Lippincott Williams & Wilkins; 2007.

Motulsky H. *Intuitive Biostatistics*. New York, NY: Oxford University Press; 2010.

Piaggio G, Elbourne DR, Altman DG, et al. Reporting of noninferiority and equivalence randomized trials: An extension of the CONSORT statement. *JAMA*. 2006;295:1152-1160.

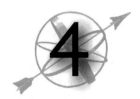

EVALUATION OF MEDICAL LITERATURE AND JOURNAL CLUBS

Lindsay Davison, PharmD, and Jean Cunningham, PharmD, BCPS

CASE

H.G. is a pharmacy student on an internal medicine APPE rotation. At the end of the month, all students on the rotation are required to participate in the pharmacy's journal club. H.G. remembers presenting a handful of journal clubs during pharmacy school, but he has never presented to a roomful of pharmacists before.

WHY IT'S ESSENTIAL

Discussions about journal clubs and medical literature evaluation have been known to cause rapid heart rate, increased blood pressure, and a host of other unfortunate adverse events in otherwise healthy final-year student pharmacists (please note: these data were derived from observational *N* of 1 studies). Alas, have no fear! This chapter is here to save you. You may wonder why medical literature evaluation and journal clubs are considered part of *The Essentials*. Medical literature is what creates the treatment guidelines we rely on as clinicians, and its evaluation is how we can be confident (or not so confident) in a publication's findings. Just as you would not drive a car through an intersection with your eyes shut while the passenger concluded that the coast was clear, you should not accept the author's conclusions of a trial without evaluating the literature. Understandably, you may now be wondering how in the world pharmacists can find the time to evaluate all of the medical literature that impacts their practice. The answer is that they do not. This is where journal clubs come in. A *journal club* is typically comprised of practitioners who meet to critique and discuss recently published medical literature, distributing among a number of practitioners the difficult task of keeping up. While you are on your APPE rotations, you will most likely be asked to become a part of a journal club by reviewing an article and leading the critique—a discussion of the article's strengths, weaknesses, and potential impact on pharmacy practice.

> *"Though literature evaluation can be a difficult skill to master, your rotations offer the perfect environment to put your abilities to the test and build a strong foundation for the rest of your career. Use your preceptors to find and fix any areas in need of improvement and start getting into good habits."—Preceptor*

Note: The views expressed in the chapter do not necessarily represent the views of the agency (Food and Drug Administration) or the United States.

Does This Study Matter to Me?

The process of designing a journal club presentation begins with identifying an appropriate article to present. The age-old question "Does this study matter to me?" is probably the most important one you can ask yourself when surveying the medical literature for an article to present on rotation. If a trial is conducted using a therapy not available to your patients or includes a patient population completely unlike the patients you treat, then reading about it will most likely be a waste of your time. The results of that trial may matter a great deal to other pharmacists but mean nothing to you.

Lesson #1: Do not waste your time. Choosing appropriate journal articles will give you more time to accomplish other tasks and also make your preceptors appreciative that you are providing them with a journal club that they are actually interested in! Interpretations of what matters to a practice site can vary, so do not hesitate to ask your preceptors for guidance when choosing an article. On occasion, a preceptor will direct you toward articles in a certain therapeutic area or within a certain class of drugs. Take this advice and run with it! Use PubMed's medical subject headings (MeSH) terms and limits to your advantage to limit the scope of your search results to match your preceptor's guidance (see Chapter 5 for a review of PubMed searches). Skim over the two to three articles that seem to be the best fit, and if they seem like good options, provide your preceptor with copies. Typically, your preceptor will be more than happy to review your short list of articles and tell you if one stands out as most interesting or impactful on his or her practice.

Finally, if this route is not effective, search the lay press. A general Internet search can help determine if an article you are considering sparked media attention that may have patients making inquiries to your preceptor. For example, if a trial was published in a major medical journal and the nightly news ran a story about how a commonly prescribed drug may reduce cancer risk, the story is definitely going to generate patient interest. Whenever new information is touted to the masses, it represents an opportunity to be one step ahead of the questions that will be coming up in patient encounters.

CASE QUESTION

H.G. is having trouble picking an article to present for his journal club. Where can he turn to get some ideas?

Background and Introduction

Now that you have chosen an article, your evaluation begins before you read a single word of the article. First, the audience at your journal club will expect you to be well versed in the current standards of care for the condition treated in the article and where the investigational agent fits in. Next, you will need to assess the journal that published the article along with its title and authors. Reviewing this information before you dive in to the trial's methods and results will build a strong foundation of knowledge and improve your overall journal club presentation.

Study Context

Before you begin to evaluate your article in detail, you should perform an appropriate literature search to find supplemental materials for the selected article. The introduction section of your presentation, which includes the relevant background information and previous studies, should be about 15% of the total presentation time. This will allow you to put your article into context and describe relevant background data (guidelines, reviews, existing studies on similar agents, etc.). It will also be imperative to find recent publications preceding this article or that have been published since the article was released.

In addition to searching the literature to see what else has been published, make sure you are able to describe the current standard of care in detail. If your article is discussing weight loss therapies, it is expected that you know the lifestyle and drug therapies currently available (including mechanism of action [MOA], efficacy, side effects, monitoring parameters, and cost), the acceptable outcomes, and what the investigational agent may bring to the table. A great place to find this information would be in the guidelines released by relevant organizations. If you are not sure of what guidelines are available, try searching one of the various drug information databases. See Chapter 5 for a discussion on drug information sources.

QUICK TIP

Keep in mind that you will want to cite the original source of all introductory information appropriately. Do not simply cite a drug database or your class notes. Find and cite the primary article.

Finally, you should describe the rationale of the study. Answer the most important question for any presentation, "Why do we care?" Keep your audience in mind. If they are pharmacists, tell them why they should care about this study. The easiest answer is if you are evaluating a study on a new drug. Pharmacists would care because they want to know if the new drug should replace or be added to the current standard of care. You need to put the study into context first and familiarize yourself with the current standards of care, and then you will be able to determine for yourself and your audience why you should care that this study was performed.

The Journal

Although high-quality articles can be published in smaller journals (and vice versa), understanding the peer-review process and relative importance of the journal can give you an idea about the process your article has gone through before reaching you. The best journals will be peer reviewed and targeted toward a specific audience. Each journal has an impact factor that can be used as a surrogate measure for its relevance. In short, the impact factor is one quantitative measure of how often a journal's articles are cited by others, but it does not directly reflect the quality of the articles published. Although some practitioners rely on impact factor to evaluate a journal, others feel this measure of journal exposure can be manipulated and does not reflect quality. Most pharmacy journals have an impact factor of three or less (similar to most practice-specific journals). The "big" journals (e.g., *New England Journal of Medicine*, *Journal of the American Medical Association*, and *The Lancet*) have impact factors above 25. A more thorough evaluation of overall journal quality would look at the diversity of the editorial board, training of the peer reviewers, and number of retracted articles. Unfortunately, this measure does not yet exist, so you are on your own to look up and evaluate this information. Most journals have this information readily available on their websites.

QUICK TIP

Peer review is not a replacement for literature evaluation. Plenty of flawed articles have been published in peer-reviewed journals. You should always perform an evaluation and come to your own conclusions.

The Title

The title of an article is its first impression. It should be unbiased and avoid misleading statements in favor of neutrality. For example, if an article is titled "Reduction in the Risk of Prostate Cancer by 10% with New Diabetes Treatment: The Results of a Randomized, Double-Blind, Placebo-Controlled Clinical Trial," you would automatically think, without even reading another sentence, that this trial would present you with data supporting a drug that reduces the risk of prostate cancer. You are already biased by the title, alone, to think this drug is effective! A more appropriate title would be "An Evaluation of the Efficacy of a New Diabetes Treatment in Reducing the Risk of Prostate Cancer." Now you would need to read on without bias to see whether the treatment was effective. Ideally, the article's title should also avoid using brand names for medications.

The Authors

Next, you will want to look into the authors of the study. Specifically, find out what degrees the authors have, where they practice, and if it makes sense for them to be writing on the topic. If you see a gastroenterologist writing about autism and vaccines, it should make you wonder about the author's expertise. Another helpful step is to search PubMed to identify the author's other publications. This will help you clarify the author's expertise in the topic area. It is recommended that you search at least the first three authors in PubMed. If authored by a study group, find out what else the group has worked on.

STUDY DESIGN AND METHODS

The methods section of any article concisely describes the study's plan. The information provided in this section is the backbone on which the trial is built and usually comprises a large percentage of a journal club presentation.

Common Study Designs

Common study designs include case reports and case series, case-control studies, cohort studies, randomized control trials (RCTs), and meta analyses and systematic reviews. In this chapter, we will focus on the common study designs and provide you with a basic survival guide to noninferiority trials. See **Table 4-1** for a summary of common study designs.

Case Reports and Case Series

These types of studies are typically published to document and communicate clinicians' experiences with particular patients, to share ideas on a subject, or to describe unusual treatments or events, such as a case series or case report of a possible adverse reaction to a drug and how it was treated or resolved. Case reports tell the story of an individual patient's experience, whereas a case series tells the story of multiple patients. These types of publications do not establish causality and are published as food for thought. Case series and case reports need to be analyzed to determine if enough information was given for the reader to re-evaluate the case. Do you know enough about the patient being reported to determine how similar or different your patients may be? These publications can be useful in determining if following the same course of action could be beneficial for your patients. They are often not good choices for a journal club because they are brief, do not provide any methodology or statistical analysis, and do not provide information that can be generalized to a larger patient population.

TABLE 4-1. COMMON STUDY DESIGNS

DESIGN	ATTRIBUTES
OBSERVATIONAL	
CASE REPORT	Description of an unusual or emerging patient situation (e.g., adverse drug event, new potential drug indication, previously unknown drug interaction)
CASE SERIES	Similar to a case report except that similar situations were documented in a small number of patients
CROSS-SECTIONAL	Snapshot of the prevalence of a disease, adverse effect, attitude, etc., at a point in time (e.g., survey research, postmarketing surveillance)
CASE-CONTROL	Patients with a particular outcome are matched with patients who have not experienced that outcome; identifies association between risk factors and outcome
COHORT	Patients with a particular risk factor are matched with patients who do not have that risk factor (may be retrospective or prospective) and followed over time; identifies association between risk factor and outcomes
INTERVENTIONAL	
STABILITY/STERILITY	Various formulations of drugs are assessed for satisfactory continued presence of active drug (stability) and/or freedom from microbial contamination (sterility); typically performed in vitro
PHARMACOKINETIC	Parameters of the drug (e.g., absorption, distribution, metabolism, elimination) are determined; typically performed in healthy volunteers
BIOEQUIVALENCE	Pharmacokinetic parameters of two drugs are compared and assessed for similarity
N OF 1	Effects of a new drug-related intervention are assessed in a single patient; often compared to a historical or cross-over control
NONCONTROLLED CLINICAL TRIAL	A new drug-related intervention is assessed in a situation where a placebo or active control would be unethical or unreasonable
RANDOMIZED CONTROLLED CLINICAL TRIAL	Gold-standard study; determines the cause and effect relationship between a drug-related intervention and an outcome; may use a placebo or active control
META-ANALYSIS	Data from multiple studies are combined, evaluated, and presented; useful in situations where studies assessing similar interventions and outcomes have yielded varied results
PHARMACOECONOMIC	Assesses both clinical outcomes and costs associated with a drug- or practice-related intervention

Case-Control Studies

Case-control studies look at the possible relationship that an exposure or risk factor has with a certain disease or outcome, for example, the association between heart disease and dental cleanings. This study could be designed to evaluate the number of dental cleanings over the past 5 years in patients in two different groups: patients with heart disease and patients without heart disease. The patients with heart disease are the cases, and the patients without heart disease are the controls. The results of this type of trial design would be presented as odds ratios (ORs) because ORs are used to determine the additional risk of developing a particular disease state due to exposure to a certain risk factor. Case-control studies are often performed to make associations because they are efficient and inexpensive, although they cannot be used to establish causality. Selection bias is frequently a confounding factor, and the patients must be matched appropriately to a control for evaluation. This trial design is particularly useful for rare outcomes because you are first identifying the patients who have the rare disease state and then looking retrospectively at the risk factor they may have been exposed to. If you choose to evaluate this type of trial, here are some critique points to consider:

- Are the cases and controls well matched?
- Were the cases and controls evaluated with the same diagnostic tools?
- Were the investigators blinded to whether the patient was a case or a control?
- Did the outcomes occur after the exposure to the risk factor?
- Were the patients similar in their baseline risk of developing the outcome with the exception of the risk factor being evaluated?
- Were patients any more or any less exposed to the risk factor than the general population?

Cohort Studies

Cohort studies are observational studies. This study design allows you to associate various risk factors with the development of an outcome, like a disease. An example of a famous observational study is the Framingham Heart Study.[1] The cohort in the Framingham Heart Study was the population of Framingham, Massachusetts, who did not have cardiovascular disease and had not experienced a heart attack or stroke at the time of the study. This cohort was observed over time to identify risk factors for cardiovascular disease. Although cohort designs are the most effective means of observation and allow the investigators to examine the data prospectively, they are expensive to conduct and generally take a long time to complete. For cohort studies, some critique points to consider include the following:

- Were the patients similar in their baseline risk of developing the outcome?
- Are the inclusion and exclusion criteria clearly stated and reasonable?
- Is the research question clear?
- Was the evaluation of the outcome consistent across all patients?
- Was the study follow-up period long enough to reveal positive and negative effects?

Randomized Controlled Trials

RCTs establish causality (i.e., a cause and effect relationship) and are the most common type of clinical trial presented in journal clubs. An example of an RCT is the comparison of a new cholesterol-lowering medication to placebo or the comparison of a new treatment for gout to the gold-standard therapy. In some cases, it would not be possible to conduct an RCT because of ethical concerns. For example, an RCT would not be designed to evaluate a known teratogenic drug in a population that could become pregnant. RCTs are the most commonly encountered trial design for most student pharmacists and the one that students evaluate most frequently. We will focus on the evaluation of the RCT design throughout this chapter.

Meta-Analyses and Systematic Reviews

Meta-analyses are a great tool for determining the significance of trials that may be too small on their own. Meta-analyses pool the data from these small trials because, together, they may have a large enough sample size or high enough number of events to determine an association. Meta-analyses are also useful for assessing conflicting study results. You must consider the influence of publication bias when evaluating a meta-analysis. Remember, only those study results that were *published* will be included by the researchers conducting the meta-analysis. Therefore, if only positive trials were reported in the medical literature, you already know that the meta-analysis may be biased. Typically, a meta-analysis will present an average of all previously published findings that are pooled in that analysis. The new results of a meta-analysis are often presented as a forest plot, which is a visual representation of the means and confidence intervals of the previously reported studies. In a forest plot, the null value is in the center, and confidence intervals that cross the null value are not significant. Those that lie entirely to the left of the null value are usually negative findings (do not support the treatment studied), and those that lie entirely to the right of the null value are usually positive findings (support the treatment studied).

QUICK TIP

Systematic reviews differ from meta-analyses in that a new statistical analysis is not included. Sometimes, no new conclusions are drawn, no average is given, and a summary of the various articles is presented alone.

The Intended Study Population

One of the first tasks in literature evaluation is to establish what the study's population looks like and whether it mirrors your own. To do so, have a look at the inclusion and exclusion criteria, along with the study setting and time frame.

Inclusion and Exclusion Criteria

The inclusion and exclusion criteria are critical to your understanding of a clinical trial. The criteria that patients had to meet to be included in the trial must be clearly presented. Additionally, all of these criteria must make sense to you and be rationalized by the authors if the rationale is not obvious. If a study excludes patients who use a certain concomitant medication, it must be clear to you why this was done. Is there a drug interaction with that medication? Does that medication affect the disease state being evaluated? If you cannot determine why a certain criterion was used, you must question it and evaluate it further. Inclusion and exclusion criteria should be used to gather a patient population that represents persons with the disease state being evaluated. Most often, the problem with inclusion and exclusion criteria is that they are too stringent and they eliminate what you would think of as the "typical" patient with that disease. A quick way to judge the stringency of the trial's inclusion and exclusion criteria is to look at the percentage of patients included in the study from the population who were screened at the beginning. If only 20% of the patients screened were included in the trial, that means that 80% of the patient population with that disease state was not allowed to participate in the study. When you see a study population that has been whittled down to such a small subset from the original group, you need to take a close look at each of the criteria and determine whether you believe it was appropriate.

Study Setting and Time Frame

The study setting is also an important piece to evaluate. When a trial is conducted in a hospital, you tend to have a sicker patient population, but you also have access to thorough medical and laboratory records. However, if the treatment being evaluated is intended for outpatient use, this would not be an appropriate way to study its effects. An outpatient study has its own set of issues with tracking adherence, getting the study subjects in for follow-up visits, keeping track of adverse events, and more. Many student pharmacists will question whether a pill count is an acceptable method of tracking compliance.

Although patients could be lying about the number of doses they have actually taken, we still accept this method of tracking adherence as adequate because it is the most reliable and inexpensive way to evaluate outpatient adherence. Telephone follow-up visits can be a useful tool for study investigators when they do not need to collect laboratory values, but often studies evaluate surrogate endpoints or biomarkers (e.g., triglyceride levels) that require the patient to come in for blood work.

Studies conducted in a single center, as compared to in multiple centers, also provide you with less generalizable results. When a study is conducted in a single center, you must learn more about what that patient population looks like; is it a population with its own set of unique baseline values and risk factors? When a study is conducted across multiple centers in varying patient populations and in varying locations, you can feel more confident that the study population is diverse and could be more easily generalized to different patient groups. Keep in mind, however, that if a single-center study reflects very closely your patient population, it may be more useful information for you than a multicenter study that includes the types of patients that would never walk through your clinic's door.

CASE QUESTION

H.G.'s journal article was conducted at multiple sites across a number of countries. How might this strengthen the applicability of the trial?

The time frame of the study is extremely important. For example, a study was conducted to evaluate the safety of a weight-loss medication in a patient population with known cardiovascular risk factors. When you read the study, you think that this put the patients at unnecessary risk and is a major study design flaw because you know from the package insert that the medication is contraindicated in patients with known cardiovascular risk factors. Upon further investigation, you note that the study was completed 2 years ago. You check online for the drug's labeling history and find that the product's labeling was not updated to include this contraindication until 1 year ago. Therefore, it was not putting the patients at unnecessary risk at the time of the study because that was not a contraindication at the time. It is also important to note whether significant changes have been made to the standard of care for your study population in the time since the study has been completed. For example, a study of a medication for myocardial infarction patients conducted before the introduction of clopidogrel may not be as applicable in a postclopidogrel world.

Randomization

Randomization is an important part of the RCT. Most student pharmacists, when describing the methods of an RCT, start with the following statement about the methods: "It was a randomized, double-blind, placebo-controlled, clinical trial." We tend to take for granted the study design's strengths included with randomization, blinding, and having a control group. Randomization is important because it attempts, and usually is successful at, distributing evenly between the two groups being analyzed the confounding factors that patients have at baseline. When evaluating the article, you should look at how evenly distributed the baseline characteristics are after randomization. Is there a factor that is more prominent in one group or the other? How could this affect the results of the trial?

CASE QUESTION

H.G. has identified that smoking status differed between the two study groups in his trial. How could this skew the results of the trial?

Blinding

Blinding of a study is important because it prevents the researchers from introducing bias into the results. *Double-blind* means that both the study investigators and the patients were not aware of which treatment they were receiving (active versus control). This ensures that the treatment plan for the patients is not influenced by the knowledge of which treatment they are receiving. Sometimes, double-blinding a study is not ethical. For example, with warfarin treatment, it is critical to patient safety to monitor international normalized ratio (INR) levels, used to determine the clotting tendency of blood, and make adjustments to therapy. Although there is a way to do this and keep a study double-blinded (by using sham INR values in placebo patients), it is sometimes acceptable not to blind clinicians to the fact that certain patients are taking warfarin because of the safety concerns.

Control Groups

A control group is necessary for a comparison to be made and a conclusion to be drawn. Without a control group in an RCT, you would have only an observational study design that could not establish causality. You should evaluate whether a placebo or an active control is appropriate. Take a look at other clinical trials published for similar drugs; do those trials all compare their treatment to placebo? Another great resource is the Food and Drug Administration's (FDA) guidance documents for certain disease states. These documents outline what the FDA expects to see in a clinical trial evaluating a particular disease state when the trial is submitted as part of a New Drug Application. If the FDA recommends using an active control, the investigators should use an active control or provide a strong argument for why they chose to use placebo instead. It is important to note that guidance documents are not published for every type of trial, but they are very useful when they are available. Most often, active controls are used when a placebo group would be considered unethical, such as trials evaluating new anticoagulants for patients with atrial fibrillation. If a placebo control were used in this population, they would be at a significantly increased risk of stroke over the treatment group.

QUICK TIP

Placebo control remains the gold standard for clinical trials because using an active control makes it difficult to tell whether differences between groups were because one drug had a protective effect or the other drug caused additional adverse effects.

Statistics

Next, you want to evaluate how the treatment was analyzed. Although no one expects you to become an expert in statistical analysis, it is important that you are able to determine whether the appropriate statistical tests were used in the analysis. Choosing the right test depends on the type of data that are being collected. Tests such as the Student t test are most appropriate for continuous data, whereas the chi-square test is typically used for categorical data. For more discussion on types of data and statistical tests, see Chapter 3.

There are two main types of analyses that appear in the medical literature: intent to treat (ITT) and per protocol (PP). Fortunately, the names of these analyses are perfectly matched to their definitions. *ITT analysis* evaluates all of the study subjects who were intended to be treated, whereas *PP analysis* evaluates only those study subjects who adhered to the predefined protocol perfectly. Sometimes, ITT analyses are referred to as modified ITT (mITT), simply meaning that a modification has been made to the definition of the ITT population. Most frequently, this modification is to exclude any study subject who did not receive at least one dose of the study medication. This is common practice and should not alarm you. Any time a modification is made to the ITT population, you should evaluate that modification and ask yourself if it matches what you would expect to see in your patient population in clinical practice. For example, you would expect to have your patient take at least one dose of the medication prescribed before you could expect to see any results. However, expecting that your patient consistently takes his or her medication for 1 month straight, makes daily entries in an adverse-event diary, and comes in for follow-up visits on days 1, 2, 3, 6, 9, 10, 20, and 30 may not be realistic for your patient population. When modifications to the ITT analysis are made that are more stringent than you would expect from your average patient, the analysis should be referred to as PP, not mITT.

When ITT analyses are used in a superiority trial, it is thought to be a more "real-world" setting than a PP analysis. ITT is more conservative in demonstrating an effect because it includes all of the study subjects. Take, for instance, a trial conducted to evaluate a type 2 diabetes mellitus medication. Five patients out of 50 took only one dose of study medication and then reported blood glucose levels greater than 300 mg/dL. The other 45 patients took the study medication 80% of the time and experienced consistent blood glucose readings less than 150 mg/dL. When the statistical analysis is performed of this ITT population, it is less likely to show a statistically significant outcome in favor of the study medication because it included the patients who took only one dose of the study drug and continued to have uncontrolled diabetes. This is referred to as the worst-case scenario analysis because the five people who only took one dose of the medication and then had high blood glucose readings are included in the analysis. As a reader, you want to see this because it is reflective of the actual patient population. Some patients are going to receive a prescription and then not ever fill that prescription. This is indicative of real-life medical practice; as an evaluator of this clinical trial, you want to know that this drug is effective despite the inclusion of patients who are not perfect at taking their medications.

Using PP analyses in a superiority trial demonstrates the effect in the "perfect" patient—one who follows instructions, takes his or her medication as prescribed, and reports back to you any and all effects. PP analysis gives you the best-case scenario of how a drug works; it lets you know how well a drug works when taken appropriately and, therefore, is very helpful when evaluating the literature. The danger with PP analysis occurs when it is the only type of analysis available. If we are able to evaluate only the PP analysis, we run the risk of overestimating the treatment effect we will see in our actual patients.

In the setting of noninferiority trials, the most important thing to remember is that the opposite of everything you just read is true! When investigators are trying to demonstrate that one drug is noninferior or the same as another drug, they want to use the analysis that is least likely to demonstrate a large difference between treatment groups. In this case, you want to see only the ITT presented if PP is also presented. An analysis of the group of patients who followed the specified protocol is most likely to demonstrate a difference between two groups and is, therefore, the conservative estimate of noninferiority. When evaluating noninferiority trials, it is important to remember this distinction, as they are less commonly evaluated in journal clubs and student pharmacists often miss this important difference.

QUICK TIP

It is not uncommon to see both an intention-to-treat analysis and per-protocol analysis performed in noninferiority trials.

RESULTS

In the results section of an article, before you get to any primary or secondary endpoints, you should see the baseline characteristics presented. You learned earlier that randomization is intended to disperse the variability evenly between the active and control groups. How well did it do that? Are there outliers in the baseline characteristics, or are the baseline characteristics skewed? It is not important if there are P values presented with baseline characteristics. In fact, it is not recommended that P values be presented with baseline characteristics by the CONSORT (Consolidated Standards of Reporting Trials) group[2] because you must look at the numbers presented and determine if they are clinically significant. Statistical significance cannot be used to guide you. For example, in December 2000, a study was published in the *New England Journal of Medicine* titled "Phenylpropanolamine and the Risk of Hemorrhagic Stroke." This trial concluded in the abstract that "for women, the adjusted odds ratio was 16.58 (95% CI, 1.51 to 182.21; p = 0.02) for the association between the use of appetite suppressants containing phenylpropanolamine and the risk of hemorrhagic stroke..."[3] The conclusion of this trial by the authors was that "the results suggest that phenylpropanolamine in appetite suppressants, and possibly in cough and cold remedies, is an independent risk factor for hemorrhagic stroke in women." That same year, the FDA requested that all drug companies discontinue marketing products containing phenylpropanolamine, citing the risk of hemorrhagic stroke associated with phenylpropanolamine hydrochloride.[4] During your evaluation of the article and your review of the study's baseline characteristics, one baseline characteristic stands out as being its own independent risk factor for stroke: cocaine use on the day of or day preceding the hemorrhagic stroke. Based on this, you might anticipate questions regarding the incidence rate of hemorrhagic stroke with cocaine use in women, similar to the study group. This information may lead you to your own conclusion independent of that of this particular study's authors. Even when your analysis of the overall benefit versus risk leads you to the same ultimate conclusion (in this case, that the benefits of phenylpropanolamine use for weight loss or for nasal decongestion do not outweigh the risks of possible hemorrhagic stroke), it is important to note any flaws or confounding variables in the study you are presenting.

It is also important that the article account for all of the study participants. This is best presented as a flow chart of how many patients were screened, were randomized, dropped out, experienced an adverse event, withdrew consent, etc. Whatever happened to the patient, you need to know.

In the results section, you will present the findings of the primary outcome and, often, the results of some secondary outcomes. It is very important to understand that the study is typically powered to detect only a difference in the primary outcome. The primary outcome should be clearly stated by the investigators and should match what is presented in the methods section. Sometimes, the primary outcome is a composite of a number of endpoints, like major adverse cardiovascular events (MACEs). You should evaluate if there is one that is driving the significance of the results more than the others and discuss this in your critique. For example, if the article's primary outcome is MACEs comprised of myocardial infarction, stroke, and all-cause mortality and 47 patients experience stroke while only 1 patient experiences myocardial infarction and no patients are classified as having all-cause mortality, it would not be appropriate to conclude that all of these endpoints are significant. The overall MACE outcome may have demonstrated statistical significance; however, it is clear that only one of these endpoints was driving the results.

Secondary outcomes should be presented as hypothesis-generating endpoints. It is difficult to draw any firm conclusions from secondary endpoints because trials are not designed to specifically test them, meaning that any interesting secondary finding needs to be analyzed as the primary endpoint in its own trial. Secondary outcomes should be presented only if they are clinically significant to you or worthy of some discussion with your colleagues. Although safety outcomes are important secondary outcomes to address, you will never be able to fully assess safety in a clinical trial. That is why the postmarketing reporting process of adverse events through the FDA's MedWatch program is so critical to our understanding of a drug's benefit-to-risk profile. It is simply impossible to enroll enough patients in a clinical trial to determine all of the rare, infrequent side effects that could be seen with a drug. Additionally, we know that once a product is approved, it is prescribed off label and to patients with additional risk factors that were excluded during the clinical trials. Again, it is important to always present the safety information from a clinical trial, but it must be understood that this information is likely just the tip of the iceberg of what will be seen when the product is on the market and widely prescribed.

CASE QUESTION

H.G.'s trial has a number of secondary endpoints. How can he decide which to present during his journal club?

APPLICABILITY

Now that you are comfortable assessing whether or not a trial applies to your patients, known as *external validity* or *generalizability*, we can talk about how you determine if a study has internal validity. The example provided previously is a good representation of a threat to internal validity. If the confounding variable of cocaine use was driving the increased risk of hemorrhagic stroke, then the study would lack internal validity. This is something that must be discussed and evaluated as part of your literature evaluation of that particular trial. Selection bias is another good example of a common threat to internal validity, and one that is seen frequently with trials for obesity drugs and smoking-cessation therapies. *Selection bias* refers to the bias that occurs when the selected patient group has some sort of tendency. In obesity trials and smoking-cessation trials, this occurs because the patients who enroll in these types of trials are generally those who are already considering weight loss or smoking-cessation programs. The threat to internal validity arises when those patients, regardless of what treatment group they are randomized to, are already more motivated than the average patient that will be prescribed that drug treatment in clinical practice. Selection bias can also result from trial recruitment tactics. If a trial posts flyers to recruit patients only in high-end coffee shops in a wealthy suburb, then it is likely that the patients who will sign up will be wealthy and have access to good-quality health care and other socioeconomic factors that may not be generalizable to your patient population.

Another type of bias that is frequently cited by students is *funding*. You should never cite funding as a bias without providing the answer to "why." A common misconception by student pharmacists is that when a drug company funds a study, there is inherently bias associated with the study's publication. This is not true! Who else would fund a trial of this drug? It makes sense that drug companies pay for the research necessary to prove the safety and efficacy of their treatments. Without a reason *why* you think the study has bias, simply funding a study is a very minor limitation.

For example, in the JUPITER trial, it states that "the trial was financially supported by Astra Zeneca."[5] Listing this as a bias would be inappropriate without listing reasons why you believe this trial could have been biased. This trial concluded that "in…apparently healthy persons without hyperlipidemia but with elevated high-sensitivity C-reactive protein levels, rosuvastatin significantly reduced the incidence of major cardiovascular events." Let's say that in your evaluation you find this conclusion to be sound. However, in doing your research of the authors, you discover that the primary author is also the developer and patent holder of the only test available to measure high-sensitivity C-reactive protein levels. Would this be an instance of bias present in a trial? It certainly could be and should be presented for discussion as such. Some other red flags of study-sponsor bias include situations where the sponsor wrote drafts of the final manuscript, collected and analyzed the data, or made the final decision to publish the article. Sources of sponsor bias of less concern would include providing study medications and providing unrestricted grant funding.

QUICK TIP

Most articles will discuss sources of funding and conflicts of interest in a side bar at the beginning of the article, in the methods section, or in the small print at the end of the article.

A common misconception is the idea of varying levels of significance with results. Sometimes, a difference is identified as "highly significant" or "trending toward significance" and is misleading. The alpha value is established *a priori* and is how the author tells the reader what results will be statistically significant. Let's say that alpha is set at 0.05, meaning that a P value less than 0.05 is significant and a P value greater than or equal to 0.05 is not significant. Saying that P is less than 0.0001 is "highly significant" has no meaning because significance is a "yes" or "no" question. The same is true for authors who conclude that a P value of 0.054 is "trending toward significance." The all-or-nothing nature of statistics means that the endpoint is not significantly different, and stating that it is trending toward significance is misleading.

Another misleading conclusion is the statement that the authors have found statistically significant differences for endpoints other than the endpoint they powered their study to detect. A study is typically only powered to detect one primary endpoint. This is important because in almost all published medical literature, there are conclusions made about secondary endpoints that the study was not powered or designed to detect. The issue with secondary endpoints lies with the repeating of a statistical test and how it dilutes the P value. Essentially, the more statistical tests are performed, the higher the likelihood of a type I error occurring (or concluding that a significant difference exists when there really is no difference). For instance, if a study performs 20 secondary analyses, it almost ensures that one of the tests will demonstrate significance. A 5% chance of a type I error exists with each of the 20 secondary endpoints, adding up to a 100% chance. For this reason, post hoc secondary endpoints, or those endpoints that were not established before the study was initiated, should especially be viewed with skepticism because it is never known how many endpoints were tested before one was found to be statistically significant.

QUICK TIP

A number of statistical maneuvers, called *alpha spending*, can be used to decrease the chance of having a type I error with multiple tests.

It can often be difficult to apply the results of a clinical trial to your specific patient population. Statistical significance does not always clearly show how a new treatment may benefit or harm the patients you are treating. A quick way to translate statistical significance into clinical significance is to calculate the number needed to treat (NNT) and the number needed to harm (NNH). You should present these numbers in the article's critique, whenever possible. It is an easy way for your audience to digest the bigger picture of the results and how they might apply to their patients. You can learn much more about how and when to calculate NNT and NNH in Chapter 3.

Conclusion

The end of nearly every piece of medical literature contains the authors' conclusions. In this section, the authors list the strengths and weaknesses of their trial, along with a final conclusion. You should include each of these sections in your journal club discussion. In addition to the authors' conclusions, your journal club should also include additional strengths, weaknesses, and appropriate conclusions that you uncovered during your literature evaluation process. Review each of the sections described above and identify those aspects that you feel the authors completed effectively and those that did not quite meet expectations. Your conclusion section should also include information about the applicability of the trial and any unanswered questions that remain to be addressed.

Question and Answer Time

The best journal clubs encourage questions. You should encourage the audience to ask questions as well as ask them questions in return. Being prepared is key. If you perform the necessary background research and become well versed in the article, you should be more than capable of answering any questions that come your way. In the event that you are unable to answer a difficult question, assure the audience member that you will perform additional research and provide the answer as soon as possible.

CASE QUESTION

H.G. is asked a difficult question that he did not anticipate. What is the appropriate way to handle this situation?

Journal Club Handouts

As described above, the purpose of a journal club is to allow a group of practitioners to meet, critique, and discuss recently published literature. Often, journal clubs are used as a forum to discuss different views about therapeutic controversies and to keep practitioners current with new evidence and literature. The format of a journal club is usually a verbal presentation, with an emphasis on discussion. Most students will provide the audience with handouts that highlight the study's key parts and discuss how to use the results in practice. The worst kind of handout would be something that simply regurgitates what is already in the study. *Do not do this.* There is nothing more frustrating than to read an article and then attend a journal club where the student almost rereads it to you. *Add insight, content, and application.* **Table 4-2** is a helpful checklist for a successful journal club handout.

References

1. D'Agostino RB, Vasan RS, Pencina MJ, et al. General cardiovascular risk profile for use in primary care: The Framingham Heart Study. *Circulation.* 2008;117:743-753.
2. Schulz KF, Altman DG, Moher D. CONSORT 2010 statement: Updated guidelines for reporting parallel group randomised trials. *J Pharmacol Pharmacother.* 2010;1:100-107.
3. Kernan WN, Viscoli CM, Brass LM, et al. Phenylpropanolamine and the risk of hemorrhagic stroke. *NEJM.* 2000;343:1826-1832.
4. Food and Drug Administration. FDA issues public health warning on phenylpropanolamine. http://www.fda.gov/Drugs/DrugSafety/InformationbyDrugClass/ucm150763.htm. Accessed February 21, 2012.
5. Ridker PM, Danielson E, Fonseca FAH, et al. Rosuvastatin to prevent vascular events in men and women with elevated C-reactive protein. *NEJM.* 2008;359:2195-2207.

TABLE 4-2. JOURNAL CLUB HANDOUT CHECKLIST

BACKGROUND

- ☑ Briefly describes disease state and current guidelines
- ☑ Highlights current therapies available for disease state
- ☑ Discusses rationale for study design and the role of the agent being studied
- ☑ Describes the role of the study sponsor

STUDY OBJECTIVES

- ☑ Summarizes primary objective of study

METHODS

- ☑ Identifies study design
- ☑ Outlines the intervention (medication, dose, duration, etc.)
- ☑ Defines patient population (setting, timing, inclusion and exclusion criteria)
- ☑ States how primary objective is measured and type of variable used (continuous, nominal, ordinal, etc.)
- ☑ Describes relevant secondary objectives
- ☑ Identifies how data are handled (intention to treat, per protocol, or other)
- ☑ Explains if statistical test used is appropriate for the data variable measured
- ☑ Provides prespecified statistical criteria (alpha [level of significance], beta [power], sample size requirements, and delta [if designed to detect a difference])

RESULTS

- ☑ Describes the baseline characteristics of the study population
- ☑ Lists number lost to follow-up, drop out, issues with compliance
- ☑ Clearly states results of primary objective, including P values and confidence intervals
- ☑ Describes relevant or interesting secondary results
- ☑ Highlights significant adverse events associated with therapy

CLINICAL RELEVANCE

- ☑ Calculates NNT and discusses importance of value found, if possible
- ☑ Discusses if findings are clinically significant/relevant and provides rationale

DISCUSSION

- ☑ Highlights study strengths with rationale
- ☑ Discusses study limits with rationale
- ☑ Includes suggestions for future studies

CONCLUSIONS

- ☑ Summarizes overall opinion of trial and makes final recommendation for practice based on results

HANDOUT DETAILS

- ☑ Includes the 6 Cs of drug information: Correct, Conscientious, Complete, Concise, Critical, and Clear
- ☑ Follows presentation format (flows with presentation)
- ☑ Is free of grammatical errors
- ☑ Has professional format and appearance
- ☑ Graphically represents complicated data/uses tables appropriately
- ☑ Expands on information presented
- ☑ References listed appropriately
  - ☑ Includes tertiary references and guidelines for background
  - ☑ Includes any additional references for discussion section (comments, letters to editor, etc.)

SUGGESTED READING

Guidance documents from FDA on trial design available at http://www.fda.gov/RegulatoryInformation/Guidances/ucm122046.htm

Malone PM, Kier KL, Stanovich JE. *Drug Information: A Guide for Pharmacists*. 4th ed. New York, NY: McGraw-Hill Medical; 2012.

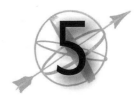

Drug Information Questions

Robert D. Beckett, PharmD, BCPS

CASE

E.B. is a pharmacy student on the first week of her internal medicine APPE rotation. She has been working hard to keep up to date with her patients every morning before rounds and has been pretty successful integrating with the medical team. So far, her role has mostly been performing medication reconciliation and counseling prior to discharge following a hospital protocol. As she electronically documents a warfarin education session performed with her preceptor, she encounters the intern on her medical team who looks very flustered. He sees her, rushes over, and says, "Oh good, a pharmacist. Can amoxicillin cause muscle pain?" E.B. checks her drug information software on her smartphone and quickly responds that it does not and recommends starting acetaminophen 500 mg every 4 to 6 hours as needed for muscle pain.

Why It's Essential

Healthcare professionals and patients look to pharmacists to provide accurate, clear, concise, evidence-based drug information. Pharmacy students on IPPE and APPE rotations will frequently receive requests for drug information. While specialty drug information rotations are often available, skills in drug information are vital to success in all rotations across all practice settings. Developing a comprehensive, systematic approach to answering drug information questions is crucial for success in experiential education, and a strong foundation in drug information can greatly enhance your practice as a licensed professional.

The Seven Step Modified Systematic Approach

Developing a comprehensive, systematic approach to answering drug information questions is the best way to ensure that high-quality, evidence-based information is provided to a patient, healthcare professional, or preceptor. It is paramount that only accurate information is provided, especially when that information will be used to make patient care decisions. Although there are other published systematic approaches to providing drug information, the Seven Step Modified Systematic Approach is a well-recognized, frequently used strategy.[1-4] Although the components of each step are essential to providing high-quality drug information, efforts should be made to achieve a natural flow of professional communication with the requestor and avoid fragmentation of this process, especially as you obtain greater experience.[1]

• •

"Developing my own systematic way to answer drug information questions that come up on rounds has made the process much easier. I used to dread receiving drug information questions until I took the time to think critically about how I was answering them."—Student

• •

Step 1: Identify Demographics

Understanding who will be using the information provided is vital to preparing a meaningful drug information response.[1-4] Although it is often easy to identify the demographics of the requestor if he or she is a preceptor or member of the medical team, you may also receive drug information requests remotely via e-mail or telephone. When receiving a drug information request from an unknown individual, greet that person politely and clarify your role as a pharmacy student. Even though identifying the demographics is listed as the first step in the Modified Approach, it is also appropriate to integrate identification of the demographics throughout the encounter (i.e., Steps 1 through 3). Key information to obtain includes requestor name, education level, affiliation, and role in the context of the question (e.g., patient, caretaker, healthcare provider).

Step 2: Determine Background Information

Once it is clear to whom you are speaking, it is vital to obtain sufficient background information to answer the question.[1-4] This is often a challenging step, as you must identify the most relevant information when very little is given voluntarily. Additionally, the requestor may not understand why specific background information is needed and may pressure you to rush through this process. A good way to approach this challenge is to first ask the requestor whether his or her question pertains to a specific patient. This question enables the requestor to provide an introduction to the situation and allows you to identify relevant background questions based on the type of question being asked. This step is frequently omitted by students and professionals. Clarifying the appropriate background information is essential in determining the true information needed and responding appropriately.[5] Suggested relevant background questions for patient-specific inquiries, based on question type, are provided in **Table 5-1**.[1-4] During this step, it is also important to identify which resources have already been consulted to help clarify the context of the question and possibly prevent duplication of efforts.

• •

"An effective drug information response is completely dependent on gathering appropriate background information from the requestor."—Preceptor

• •

QUICK TIP

For questions received via e-mail, it is often helpful to do a brief literature search before obtaining background information, giving you more context and confidence when discussing the question with the requestor.

One subset of drug information questions that may require a different approach to determining the background information is *assignment-type questions*—in-depth drug information questions assigned as long-term projects to complete throughout the rotation—that are commonly assigned by preceptors of

TABLE 5-1. SUGGESTED BACKGROUND QUESTIONS BASED ON QUESTION TYPE

QUESTION TYPE	SUGGESTED BACKGROUND QUESTIONS
Dosing/Pharmacotherapy	What is the patient's age? Sex? Weight? Height?
	What is the indication for the medication?
	What is the patient's renal function? Hepatic function?
	Is the patient suspected of having an adverse reaction?
	Is the patient well nourished? Taking medications by mouth?
	What other medications is the patient taking? Recently taken?
	Is the patient taking any nonprescription medications? Dietary supplements?
	Does the patient have any chronic disease states? Allergies?
	If female of child-bearing age, is the patient pregnant?
Interactions	Is an interaction already suspected of occurring? Is there a suspected adverse event?
	What other medications is the patient taking? Doses?
	Is the patient taking any nonprescription medications? Dietary supplements?
	When is the patient taking the medication(s)?
	How long has the patient been taking the medication(s)?
	Is intravenous compatibility a concern?
	What is the patient's current medical status?
	What steps have been taken in the management of the patient?
	If female of child-bearing age, is the patient pregnant?
Adverse Reactions	Has a reaction already been experienced? How severe? Has it resolved?
	What were the signs and symptoms of the reaction?
	What other medications is the patient taking? Recently taken?
	Is the patient taking any nonprescription medications? Dietary supplements?
	How long has the patient been taking the medication in question?
	What other medications is the patient taking? What doses?
	Does the patient have any chronic disease states?
	What steps have been taken in the management of the patient?
	Does the patient have any known allergies or intolerances?
	If female of child-bearing age, is the patient pregnant?
Pregnancy/Lactation	How many weeks pregnant is the patient? How old is the breast-fed infant?
	What is the indication for the medication in question?
	What is the patient's age? Sex (if infant)? Weight? Height?
	What is the patient's renal function? Hepatic function?
	What other medications is the patient taking? Doses?
	Is the patient taking any nonprescription medications? Dietary supplements?
	What chronic disease states does the patient have?

clinical and drug information APPE rotations. These questions are less likely to be based on a specific patient, and the background information obtained should reflect that.

CASE QUESTION

E.B. reconsidered her response to the intern's question and determined that the question was being asked about L.R., a patient E.B. has not been following. E.B. identified L.R. as a 57-year-old woman who was started on amoxicillin 3 days ago for a urinary tract infection and has since experienced dull, achy muscle pain. What additional questions should E.B. ask of the intern?

Step 3: Determine the True Question

It has been estimated that up to 85% of questions received at some drug information centers differ in a significant way from the actually researched inquiry and the information ultimately provided to the patient.[6] Frequently, requestors will ask the question in a way that is biased based on individual experience.[1-4,6] For example, if a patient is experiencing an adverse effect, the healthcare provider may associate the adverse effect with the medication started most recently and phrase the question in a restrictive way (e.g., "Can amoxicillin cause muscle pain?"). This association could distract you from considering other medications that may cause an adverse effect several weeks or even years after initiating treatment. It is your responsibility to determine the true question being asked by carefully gathering background information. In the example cited above, the true question might be, "Could any of the patient's medications be contributing to dull, achy muscle pain experienced for the past 3 days?"

QUICK TIP

It may take a couple tries to determine the true question—do not get discouraged, even if you realize that you may be researching the wrong question after several hours of work. It sometimes happens!

Once the true question has been determined, it is important to clarify expectations for a response with the requestor.[1-4] Pharmacotherapy questions requiring in-depth research may take several days to complete, as opposed to adverse effect or dosing questions that could be rapidly addressed using tertiary references. You should determine when a response is needed, considering the context of the situation and input from the requestor. For example, if a question pertains to a patient due to be discharged later in the day, your time frame should consider this information. The requestor's preferred mode of response (e.g., e-mail, telephone) should also be determined.

Step 4: Develop a Search Strategy

Once the requestor's demographics are secured, sufficient background information has been obtained, and the true information needed has been determined, it is helpful to prospectively develop a plan for obtaining the drug information necessary to answer the question.[1-4] In general, a search strategy should flow from tertiary to secondary to, finally, primary information. As alluded to above, many questions can be answered using tertiary references, whereas others will require detailed assessment of the primary literature (see the Resources section below for a complete description of tertiary, secondary, and primary literature). A good search strategy, incorporating the resources described, is vital to providing evidence-based drug information.

Depth of review should depend on the audience, question type, type of information requested, and time frame.[1-4] Additionally, you should consider what resources have already been consulted by the requestor. For example, if tertiary resources have been exhausted, a search of the primary literature may be necessary. Determining whether a question requires review of primary literature is an acquired skill that takes time to develop. Search strategies should consider the resources available from the college/school of pharmacy and from the practice site.[4] Early in your clinical rotation, it is a good idea to inquire about the availability of electronic and print resources and how to access them.

CASE QUESTION

Through her collection of background information, E.B. determined that L.R. has been taking simvastatin 80 mg by mouth daily and lisinopril 10 mg by mouth daily for about 2 years, in addition to her recent prescription for amoxicillin 500 mg by mouth three times daily. Should E.B. consult primary literature, tertiary literature, or both to answer her original question?

Step 5: Evaluate, Analyze, Synthesize

This step describes appropriate action that should be taken once the necessary drug information references have been identified.[1-4]

Evaluate: Every source of information should be assessed prior to use. As a pharmacy student with many responsibilities, it can be tempting to use information from the first source identified; however, careful evaluation will often reveal that a source may not be the most appropriate to use. Every reference should be evaluated for applicability to the question, completeness, and quality of information (see the Resources section for tips on evaluating tertiary resources and Chapter 4 for a detailed discussion of primary literature evaluation).

Analyze: Once a resource has been determined to be useful and appropriate for answering a drug information question, detailed extraction and analysis of the material is essential for compiling accurate information in preparation for a response. It may be helpful to create a chart or table detailing research findings obtained from different references.

Synthesize: Synthesis is the process of reviewing all of the information obtained from various sources and integrating those results in a cohesive way. When compiling information from multiple sources, it can be tempting to list findings in a stepwise format; however, when providing drug information, it is vital to integrate all information obtained into an overarching body of evidence that answers the true question being asked.

QUICK TIP

Consider entering all information from primary literature into a table to allow for rapid evaluation, analysis, and synthesis, particularly if many studies are needed to answer the question.

Step 6: Formulate Response

Various formats for provision of drug information responses are described in the Responses section below. These formats may include memoranda, e-mail, structured discussion, charts and tables, monographs, class reviews, and written papers.[1-4] The format ultimately used for a drug information response will differ greatly depending on the audience, time frame, type of question, and type of information requested; however, there are common qualities (easily remembered with six Cs) that every response should achieve:

Correct: The information provided, most importantly, should accurately reflect the best evidence available. Accuracy of the response will ultimately depend on careful evaluation and analysis of all relevant references obtained. If the accuracy of any information is in question, a good rule is to not dispense that information. Another rule of thumb is to verify drug information with a preceptor prior to distribution.

Conscientious: All relevant evidence obtained during the literature search should be discussed in the response. This is especially important when conflicting results are identified. For example, when researching whether continuous infusion or intermittent bolus is the preferred strategy for delivering pain control to patients receiving palliative care, divergent recommendations can be found. It is your responsibility to provide both sides of the argument and to build a final recommendation based on both sets of information.

Complete: The response should address every facet of the question. If the question was regarding a specific patient, it is the responsibility of the pharmacy professional to identify and suggest resolution for all drug-related problems identified. For example, if the original question concerned a potential drug–drug interaction and an unrelated dosing error was identified, that information should be addressed in the response. Additionally, if a problem was identified with a particular therapy, dose, etc., you should suggest a solution.

Concise: In the effort to provide complete information, pharmacy students often produce drug information responses that become excessively wordy. It is important to use a scientific writing style that provides information as succinctly as possible. Bear in mind that most healthcare professionals are extremely busy, and if the drug information response appears excessively long, they may ignore the recommendations altogether.

Critical: As the information from various resources is discussed, it is appropriate to direct the reader's attention toward major limitations of those resources that were identified during Step 5. For example, if a complicated therapeutic issue has been addressed only via observational studies, it is a significant limitation that will be important for the audience to know. For patient-specific questions, it is critical to compare and contrast the patient with the Food and Drug Administration (FDA)-approved population for a medication or the patient population included in a clinical trial.

Clear: The drug information response should be presented in an understandable way that provides the audience with an unambiguous summary of the research findings and a definitive recommendation for proceeding. Even if there is no obvious single recommendation or if the research findings are conflicting, that information should be stated.

Step 7: Follow-Up

Once the response has been formulated and delivered to the audience, your job is still not done! Facilitating appropriate follow-up is, unfortunately, an area of weakness for many pharmacy students and seasoned professionals. Follow-up should first consist of appropriate documentation, which is vital for reducing liability, assessing the quality of service provided, and facilitating rapid responses to commonly asked questions.[1-4] For a pharmacy student on a drug information rotation, documentation will likely be facilitated in a structured manner. Questions answered in a clinical rounding or operational setting may not be documented in a consistent manner; however, it is a good student exercise to maintain a professional portfolio with a section dedicated to drug information questions answered (with any protected health information removed).

QUICK TIP

Following up with the requestor signals to him or her that you are a professional. It also can help build your self-confidence and personal network!

Additionally, many drug information questions require follow-through to ensure adoption of evidence-based recommendations and answer any further questions that have arisen.[1-4] This is often easily facilitated on clinical rotations that have a rounding component where all team members touch base on a daily basis, but it may be more challenging in a purely distributive setting. Long-term follow-up may be required occasionally if new information has been published since provision of the original response. For this reason, documentation should be reviewed on a regular basis to identify issues that require update.

The Seven Step Modified Systematic Approach is just one example of a methodical way to address drug information questions encountered on all types of rotations.[1-4,6] Although the amount of time dedicated to each step will vary based on the urgency and complexity of the information requested, the general principles should be followed, especially early in your practice experience. As clinical experience is gained, you may develop your own approach to drug information questions; however, it is recommended that it incorporate the basic steps outlined above.

Resources

The use of appropriate resources to address drug information requests is the foundation of the evidence-based practice of pharmacy.[2,4,7] Pharmacy resources may be broadly divided into three categories: tertiary, secondary, and primary literature.

Tertiary Literature

Tertiary literature can be defined as information that is compiled from other references, such as primary literature and other pieces of tertiary literature.[2,4,7] The most common types of tertiary literature a pharmacy student is likely to encounter include prescription drug labeling, drug information databases, reference books, textbooks, medical information databases, and clinical practice guidelines. Information obtained on the Internet is also usually considered to be tertiary literature.

As described above, tertiary literature should always be reviewed early during a literature search.[2,4,7] The advantage of consulting tertiary literature is that it provides context, ideally considering all of the previously conducted research. Additional inherent strengths of tertiary literature include common availability at practice sites and ease of use. Despite these advantages, tertiary literature does have inherent limitations, including a tendency to become outdated quickly as new information is made available and a potential lack of detail regarding more current topics. It is also important to note that the quality of tertiary literature is subject to the completeness of the authors' literature search, potential bias, and level of expertise. It is good practice to check at least two tertiary resources to confirm the accuracy of the information being obtained.

Prior to use, a piece of tertiary literature should be evaluated for its strengths and limitations.[2,4,7] Some questions to consider are the following:

- Are all contributors identified? Are the authors well-published experts in the field?
- Does the publication date limit the resource's usefulness? Has important information regarding the topic been published since this date?
- Is the peer-review and/or editorial process for publication rigorous?
- What is the intended focus of the resource? Is it the most relevant choice for answering your question?
- Is the information referenced throughout? Are these references up to date?

The following sections describe common tertiary references that are useful on IPPE and APPE rotations. It is important to note that this list is not exhaustive.

Prescription Drug Labeling

FDA-approved prescription drug labeling, also known as package inserts or prescribing information, is a valuable resource that may be overlooked by pharmacy students and professionals.[2,4,7] The FDA recently standardized the expected components of the package insert, a change that greatly improved the readability of these materials. Package inserts can be very useful for answering basic patient-initiated questions and simple stability/compatibility questions. They are also an excellent starting point for more complicated inquiries. The most important limitation of information found in package inserts is that it only represents the FDA-approved body of information and does not provide information regarding off-label indications, dosing, etc. Package inserts may be located at the DailyMed website (http://dailymed.nlm.nih.gov), at Drugs@FDA (http://accessdata.fda.gov/scripts/cder/drugsatfda/index.cfm), on the manufacturer website, or physically attached to the product.

QUICK TIP

FDA-approved information is vital for answering many questions; however, you should not stop there if you do not find the information you need. Other tertiary resources will often be more comprehensive.

Drug/Medical Information Databases

A variety of electronic drug information databases provide compendia of information specific to a medication.[2,4,7] Most IPPE and APPE practice sites (and schools/colleges of pharmacy) will have access to at least one database. The greatest strength of these resources, as a whole, is that they contain non–FDA-approved information and are generally very easy to use; however, you should continue to follow the rule of checking at least two sources of information when using them. In studies that have compared these resources with their mobile applications, most have been found to be highly usable; however, Epocrates® products have been associated with a very high level of error and are not recommended as a first choice.[8,9] Additionally, a notable number of errors have been identified in Clinical Pharmacology®.[8,9] Online Facts and Comparisons®, Lexicomp® Online, and Micromedex® have been shown to have a higher accuracy rating, with similar scores for scope and completeness.[8,9] For answering questions regarding dietary supplements, the Natural Medicines Comprehensive Database® and Natural Standard® can be helpful, evidence-based resources. A comparison of the features of the major electronic drug information databases is provided in **Table 5-2**.

Medical information databases are increasingly used in pharmacy practice settings, particularly in health systems. The most popular of these are UpToDate® and DynaMed®. These databases organize medical (and drug) information into specific articles, often addressing not only a broad topic but also specific aspects of that topic (e.g., "diagnosis of hypertension" as opposed to "hypertension"). Articles will often extensively link to each other in a way that makes searching for information about a specific topic relatively easy.[10,11] Medical information databases enable users to rapidly access comprehensive information.[12-14] Despite these advantages, it is important to evaluate these products and their individual articles prior to use. The user should carefully consider the peer-review process and author qualifications. This information may not be readily provided by every product. Additionally, while many products state that they are "continuously" updated, the updating speed (in response to new clinical practice guidelines and primary information) has proven to be quite variable.[15]

Medical information databases are most appropriate for reviewing background information on a topic prior to research or rapidly obtaining information when it is needed immediately. Patient care decisions should be based on a more comprehensive review of the evidence and published clinical practice guidelines in order to ensure that the information used is current.

TABLE 5-2. ELECTRONIC DRUG INFORMATION DATABASE FEATURES

	CLINICAL PHARMACOLOGY	LEXICOMP ONLINE	MICROMEDEX	ONLINE FACTS AND COMPARISONS
Drug Identification Tool	X	X	X	X
Drug Interaction Checker	X	X	X	X
IV Compatibility Checker	X	X	X	X
Link to Drug Shortage Information		X		
Link to Recall Information		X		
Manufacturer Contact Information	X			
Patient Handouts	X	X	X	X
Side-by-Side Comparisons	X		X	X
Mobile Product Available		X	X	X

QUICK TIP

Check with your preceptor to find out his or her views on UpToDate® and DynaMed®. Many preceptors discourage regular use of these resources and may not approve them as listed citations in projects and presentations.

Clinical Practice Guidelines

Clinical practice guidelines are systematic reviews of published evidence conducted by experts in a particular field. Concrete statements are generally given to provide clinicians with evidence-based recommendations that they can apply to individual patients in a systematic, standardized way. Although the system of evidence-based medicine described by the Modified Systematic Approach is *a bottom-up approach* (i.e., the original research question was defined by a patient-specific situation), clinical practice guidelines are usually developed in a *top-down approach*, where the resulting information can be applied to a general patient population.

Like all drug information resources, the information provided in clinical practice guidelines should be evaluated prior to use. You should consider the transparency of the guideline, including conflicts of interest, the process for obtaining consensus, the organization sponsoring the guideline, and the clarity and specificity of recommendations. Additionally, it is important to assess the primary information cited in the guideline to ensure validity. Clinical practice guidelines should also describe the system used to rank the evidence and potential exceptions in terms of patient populations.

QUICK TIP

Carefully consider the sponsoring organization of the clinical practice guidelines. Many are published by local organizations and not intended for regular use at the national level.

It is generally recommended that, particularly on APPE rotations, pharmacy students base therapeutic recommendations on clinical practice guidelines rather than course notes or information from textbooks to provide up-to-date information using resources familiar to other healthcare professionals. A list of helpful clinical practice guidelines is provided in **Table 5-3**. Although clinical practice guidelines should be used by pharmacists and pharmacy students when making interventions and recommendations, it should also be recognized that patient-specific information and circumstances occasionally will preclude compliance with specific recommendations. Evidence-based clinical practice guidelines can be most easily located at the National Guideline Clearinghouse (http://www.guidelines.gov) or by a PubMed search (described in detail in the Secondary Literature section below).

Books

In addition to electronic drug information databases, students will usually have access through their college/school of pharmacy or practice site to a wide variety of books that can be helpful in addressing drug information questions. Books, commonly available in print format, are increasingly becoming available in electronic database format, electronic portable document format (PDF), and interactive e-reader formats. Steps should be taken to ensure that the information provided by books is current.[2,4,7] It takes approximately 1 year from the time content is generated for a book to reach publication; therefore, even recently published books potentially contain outdated information. It is good practice to verify information obtained from books with a second resource, particularly if the information relates to a rapidly evolving field (e.g., human immunodeficiency virus treatment or oncology). Recommended resources to consider are presented by topic in **Appendix 5-A**. Note that the list is not exhaustive and that alternative publications addressing the same topics may exist.

CASE QUESTION

E.B. has decided to reconsult the tertiary literature now that she has obtained sufficient background information. What resources would be best for E.B. to check to determine whether any of L.R.'s medications could be contributing to her muscle pain?

Secondary Literature

Secondary literature includes indexing and abstracting services used to locate primary literature and other journal articles.[2,4,7] The services are usually electronic. Both types of service provide information pursuant to a search of the database(s); the results for an indexing service include the citation of the returned article, whereas abstracting services provide both the citation and an abstract. The strength of secondary literature is that it provides a systematic tool to search the voluminous primary literature available; however, most indexing and abstracting services do not provide direct access to actual full-text articles free of charge. The abstract should never be used as a substitute for obtaining and reading the full-text article.

Searching with Indexing and Abstracting Services

The same general principles may be used to search most electronic indexing and abstracting services.[4,7] Most tools will use a standardized terminology to index each article included in the database. In addition to the general terminology, subheadings may be used. For drugs, subheadings may include "dosing," "administration," "adverse effects," or others. For example, a case report describing dosing of vancomycin for an adult patient with hospital-acquired pneumonia receiving extracorporeal membrane oxygenation may be indexed under the terms "vancomycin/dosing," "hospital-acquired pneumonia," and "extracorporeal membrane oxygenation." Various collections of terms are used, the most important of these being the Medical Subject Headings (MeSH) terms (used by MEDLINE), the United States Adopted Names, and the International Classification of Disease terms. Using the standard indexed terminology is generally preferred for formal literature searches, as it generally produces a more relevant, albeit smaller, list of citations or abstracts. Simply entering a word into the search field will usually return any article containing that word, even if it is not a keyword used to index that article.

QUICK TIP

Resources vary in how rapidly articles are indexed using standard terminology once they have been added to the database.

In addition to using standardized terminology, the use of Boolean operators can greatly improve the relevancy of search results.[4,7] Using the term "AND" returns only articles containing both search terms, "OR" returns articles containing one or both search terms, and "NOT" returns articles containing the first term but not the second. For example, if you were conducting a search for articles related to the example above, you could search for "vancomycin/dosing" AND "hospital-acquired pneumonia" OR "ventilator-associated pneumonia" AND "extracorporeal membrane oxygenation." If standardized terminology is not employed, using "NOT" will eliminate any article that contains the term, even if it is only in passing and not a keyword for the article. It is generally recommended that students attempt several different searches for each desired topic, especially as they develop this skill.

After the use of standard terminology and Boolean operators, the most effective way to improve the relevance of search results is to make use of the limits that may be applied by the searching tool.[4,7] Available limits vary, but most products will allow the users to limit results by publication date, language, and type (e.g., case report, observational study, interventional study, clinical practice guideline). PubMed, a tool used to search MEDLINE, can also limit results by species, text options (e.g., link to free full-text article), sex, and age. The example described above could potentially be limited to articles published in English and describing adults.

CASE QUESTION

E.B. reviewed AHFS Drug Information, Meyler's Side Effects of Drugs: The International Encyclopedia of Adverse Drug Reactions and Interactions, *and* Micromedex. *She found that it is unlikely that amoxicillin or lisinopril would be responsible for L.R.'s muscle pain; however, simvastatin has been associated with muscle pain and rhabdomyolysis months to years following initiation of therapy. She has decided to perform a search of MEDLINE using PubMed to find some more information. What search terms, Boolean operators, and limits could she use to create an effective search?*

TABLE 5-3. COMMONLY USED CLINICAL PRACTICE GUIDELINES

FIELD	GUIDELINE	SPONSORING ORGANIZATION
Cardiology	Antithrombotic and Thrombolytic Therapy: Evidence-Based Clinical Practice Guidelines	American College of Chest Physicians
	Detection, Evaluation, and Treatment of High Blood Cholesterol in Adults (Adult Treatment Panel III)	National Heart, Lung, and Blood Institute
	Guideline for Coronary Artery Bypass Graft Surgery	American Heart Association, American College of Cardiology
	Guideline for Percutaneous Coronary Intervention	American Heart Association, American College of Cardiology
	Guidelines for the Diagnosis and Management of Heart Failure in Adults	American College of Cardiology, American Heart Association
	Guidelines for the Management of Patients with Chronic Stable Angina	American College of Cardiology, American Heart Association
	Guidelines for the Management of Patients with ST-Elevation Myocardial Infarction	American College of Cardiology, American Heart Association
	Guidelines for the Management of Patients with Supraventricular Arrhythmias	American College of Cardiology, American Heart Association, European Society of Cardiology
	Guidelines for the Management of Patients with Unstable Angina/Non–ST-Elevation Myocardial Infarction	American College of Cardiology, American Heart Association
	Guidelines for Management of Patients with Ventricular Arrhythmias and the Prevention of Sudden Cardiac Death	American College of Cardiology, American Heart Association, European Society of Cardiology
	Management of Patients with Atrial Fibrillation	American Heart Association
	The Seventh Report of the Joint National Committee on Prevention, Detection, Evaluation, and Treatment of High Blood Pressure (JNC 7)	National Heart, Lung, and Blood Institute
Endocrinology	American Diabetes Association: Clinical Practice Recommendations	American Diabetes Association
	Medical Guidelines for Clinical Practice for the Evaluation and Treatment of Hyperthyroidism and Hypothyroidism	American Association of Clinical Endocrinologists
Infectious Diseases	Clinical Practice Guidelines for *Clostridium difficile* Infection in Adults	Infectious Diseases Society of America, Society of Healthcare Epidemiology of America
	Clinical Practice Guideline for the Use of Antimicrobial Agents in Neutropenic Patients with Cancer	Infectious Diseases Society of America
	Consensus Guidelines on the Management of Community-Acquired Pneumonia in Adults	Infectious Diseases Society of America, American Thoracic Society
	Guidelines for Antimicrobial Treatment of Uncomplicated Acute Bacterial Cystitis and Acute Pyelonephritis in Women	Infectious Diseases Society of America
	Guidelines for the Management of Adults with Hospital-Acquired, Ventilator-Associated, and Healthcare-Associated Pneumonia	American Thoracic Society, Infectious Diseases Society of America

Infectious Diseases (cont'd)	Guidelines for Prevention and Treatment of Opportunistic Infections in HIV-Infected Adults and Adolescents	Centers for Disease Control and Prevention, National Institutes of Health, Infectious Diseases Society of America
	Guidelines for the Selection of Anti-Infective Agents for Complicated Intra-Abdominal Infections	Infectious Diseases Society of America
	Guidelines for the Use of Antiretroviral Agents in HIV-1–Infected Adults and Adolescents	Department of Health and Human Services
	Infective Endocarditis: Diagnosis, Antimicrobial Therapy, and Management of Complications	American Heart Association
	Management of Patients with Infections Caused by Methicillin Resistant *Staphylococcus Aureus*	Infectious Diseases Society of America
	Practice Guidelines for the Diagnosis and Management of Skin and Soft-Tissue Infections	Infectious Diseases Society of America
	Practice Guidelines for the Management of Bacterial Meningitis	Infectious Diseases Society of America
	Practice Guidelines for the Treatment of Tuberculosis	American Thoracic Society, Centers for Disease Control and Prevention, Infectious Diseases Society of America
Neurology	Evidence-Based Guidelines for Migraine Headache	American Academy of Neurology
	Guidelines for the Early Management of Adults with Ischemic Stroke	American Heart Association, American Stroke Association
	Practice Guideline for the Treatment of Patients with Alzheimer's Disease and Other Dementias	American Psychiatric Association
	Recommendations for the Prevention of Stroke in Patients with Stroke and Transient Ischemic Attack	American Heart Association, American Stroke Association
Oncology	Extensive collections of guidelines for treatment, prevention, and supportive care of oncology patients are maintained by the National Comprehensive Cancer Network and the American Society of Clinical Oncology.	
Psychiatry	Practice Guideline for the Treatment of Patients with Bipolar Disorder	American Psychiatric Association
	Practice Guideline for the Treatment of Patients with Major Depressive Disorder	American Psychiatric Association
	Practice Guideline for the Treatment of Patients with Obsessive–Compulsive Disorder	American Psychiatric Association
	Practice Guideline for the Treatment of Patients with Schizophrenia	American Psychiatric Association
Pulmonology	Global Strategy for Diagnosis, Management, and Prevention of COPD	Global Initiative for Chronic Obstructive Pulmonary Disease
	Guidelines for the Diagnosis and Management of Asthma	National Heart, Lung, and Blood Institute

Available Databases

There are a number of databases that may be used to obtain primary literature pertinent to pharmacy practice. Several of the most important are the following:

- *Cochrane Library:* The content of the Cochrane Library consists exclusively of evidence-based medicine reviews and recommendations, predominantly in the form of meta-analyses. The breadth of topics addressed is large, and the analyses focus on specific clinical scenarios.

- *Cumulative Index to Nursing and Allied Health Literature (CINAHL):* CINAHL provides comprehensive coverage of topics related to nursing and other allied health professions; it can be particularly helpful for pharmacists when their search is specifically related to that discipline. Access to CINAHL is available through many publishers; however, there is significant crossover content with MEDLINE.

- *Embase:* Embase provides broad coverage of topics related to most health professions and related basic sciences (e.g., medicinal chemistry, pharmacology). Embase indexes over 7,500 journals, with greater coverage of international publications than similar products.

- *Iowa Drug Information Service (IDIS):* This indexing service includes full-text articles for over 200 journals, including articles specifically related to drug information. Additionally, IDIS provides access to pertinent FDA and Agency for Healthcare Research and Quality documents.

- *International Pharmaceutical Abstracts (IPA):* IPA was created by the American Society of Health-System Pharmacists and abstracts comprehensive information related to drug information, legislation, technology, and other issues related to pharmacy practice and pharmaceutical sciences. IPA is notable for its inclusion of unpublished conference proceedings and presentation abstracts.

- *MEDLINE:* Maintained by the National Library of Medicine, MEDLINE covers topics relevant to clinical medicine, pharmacy, nursing, dentistry, and other health professions. Additionally, related basic science content is also covered. MEDLINE, one of the most used and comprehensive databases available, abstracts more than 5,000 journals and can be accessed for free using PubMed. (Note: Free full text is not provided for every article.)

If a search of traditional databases has been ineffective, use of Google Scholar should be considered.[7] This search engine provides results related to any scholarly activity published on the Internet. Although Google Scholar can be an effective tool to locate information, including full-text copies of articles, care should be used, as searches often yield a large number and broad range of results.

QUICK TIP

In most cases, use of Google Scholar should be reserved for searches where traditional databases have failed to identify the needed information. Google Scholar searches can easily yield excessive, unrelated information.

Primary Literature

As previously discussed, *primary literature* includes original research and new information not previously processed.[2,4,7] Primary literature relevant to clinical pharmacy practice can be generally divided into observational and interventional studies. *Observational studies* include case reports, case series, cross-sectional/survey studies, case-control studies, and cohort studies. The most important type of *interventional study* for clinical pharmacy practice is the controlled clinical trial; however, other interventional studies, such as pharmacokinetic analyses, bioequivalence studies, stability studies, N-of-1 studies, noncontrolled clinical trials, meta-analyses, and pharmacoeconomic analyses, are often useful as well. For a detailed description of primary literature interpretation and evaluation, see Chapter 4.

Internet

At least 80% of pharmacists report regularly using the Internet to access drug information.[16] The Internet allows users to rapidly access a wide variety of health information and allows that information to be more rapidly updated, disseminated, and applied to practice. Most of the drug information resources described previously in this chapter are available in some type of electronic format that can be accessed on the Internet. This being the case, it is difficult to define the place of the Internet within a formal search strategy. Overall, use of information found on websites, as opposed to peer-reviewed tertiary literature, should be reserved for searches in which traditional sources of drug information have been exhausted. Websites may be particularly helpful in locating information regarding rare diseases and orphan drugs.

Additionally, it is a good idea to become familiar with several appropriate websites for patient referral, should further questions arise. Some examples are the Centers for Disease Control and Prevention (http://www.cdc.gov), Cleveland Clinic Health Information (http://www.my.clevelandclinic.org/health), Healthfinder (http://healthfinder.gov), and Medline Plus (http://www.nlm.nih.gov/medlineplus).

QUICK TIP

Be cautious of any website where the author's identity is unclear and large amounts of information are not cited.

One particular website that bears discussion is Wikipedia, an online encyclopedia that can be accessed and updated by anyone. In recent survey research, 35% of pharmacists reported using Wikipedia to access drug information (only 28% of these respondents were aware that anyone can edit Wikipedia).[17] Although some studies assessing the accuracy of health information obtained on Wikipedia have been favorable, these studies tended to focus on a narrow range of therapeutic areas, considering the breadth of information available on the site.[18] Additionally, preliminary research has suggested that the drug information available in Wikipedia is not only incomplete but also potentially inaccurate.[19,20] Wikipedia should not be used in a professional setting, especially in the clinical care of a patient, considering the multitude of alternative, peer-reviewed, author-identified information available for pharmacists and pharmacy students. Wikipedia also should not be used when preparing presentations or projects encountered during Doctor of Pharmacy coursework.

> *"There is absolutely no role for Wikipedia in a professional practice. I personally will not accept assignments if I become aware that Wikipedia has been used."—Preceptor*

The proliferative amount of medical and drug information on the Internet is undoubtedly useful for answering drug information questions; however, websites should be critically appraised prior to use as there is no standard peer-review process that ensures the validity of information posted on every website.[7] Additionally, there is no requirement that the author, editor, and publisher of content on the Internet differ, increasing the risk for bias. The easiest way to ensure that a website is valid is to identify it as certified by the Health on the Net Foundation (HON), signified by the presence of the HON Code logo.[21] The HON Foundation, a nongovernmental, nonprofit organization, evaluates health-related websites for consistency with eight principles: authority, complementarity, confidentiality, attribution, justifiability, transparency, financial disclosure, and advertising. Additional qualities to consider when assessing a website are its process for adding and updating information, presence of an editorial board, frequency of updating, and professional appearance. HON-certified websites, which may be targeted for healthcare professionals or consumers, are considered to provide high-quality medical information.

QUICK TIP

Be smart when using websites to answer drug information questions. If the website appears to be questionable, it probably is!

RESPONSES

Drug information responses will vary widely depending on the scope and quantity of requested information and the audience; key qualitative components of drug information responses have already been described.

Format

Responses to drug information questions are frequently presented orally, whether in person, during rounds or other patient-care activities, or remotely via telephone.[1] Before providing drug information orally, it is good practice to plan ahead regarding what information will be conveyed during the discussion; most of the time, this will include a systematic summary of the information collected and specific recommendations regarding application of the information. Additionally, depending on the length of time that has elapsed since the original question, an introduction to the question is essential to put the information in context for the audience. Finally, you should consider whether or not to offer a written version of the information. It is suggested to review all information you intend to provide with your preceptor ahead of time, both as practice and to ensure that you are capturing all the necessary information.

Drug information responses can be captured in a number of written formats. Providing information in writing is advantageous in that the reader can refer back to the response; however, it is vital that all written information distributed include the name of the preparer (and preceptor, in the case of a pharmacy student) and the date.[1] Written responses should also provide comprehensive citations. If the response is used at a much later date than it was written, including the original date and citations can help signal to the user whether the information is still appropriate to use or if it is likely out of date.

The following formats, including example questions that could generate the response format, can be useful in answering a variety of drug information questions:

- *E-mail:*[2] If the response is to a very simple question and relatively brief, it can be appropriate to send it via e-mail. More often, e-mail will be used to distribute attached documentation in other formats. The e-mail message itself should be concise and professional. A very brief summary of the information and recommendations contained in the attached document may be provided. *Example question:* What is the renal dose adjustment for dabigatran?
- *Memoranda:*[1,2] A written memo is often the preferred means for responding to drug information. Typically, this document will be up to four pages long. It is suggested to include a brief introduction to the question, as well as any patient data, body of evidence, summary of key points, and recommendations as a standard format. As described above, all information should be appropriately cited. *Example question:* Is tamoxifen a potential treatment option for menstrual migraines for my patient?

- *Monographs:*[22] Drug monographs are typically prepared in response to a request for a formulary evaluation tool; however, on occasion, this format may be useful for organizing information for a very general request for drug information. Most institutions have a standard monograph format that is similar to the FDA-approved prescribing information, with an expanded discussion of clinical evidence. A brief, one-page executive summary is also helpful to provide a broad overview for the reader. *Example question:* Could you provide a detailed overview of the usefulness of fidaxomicin?

- *Class Reviews:*[22] Class reviews can be useful when providing comparative evidence or for organizing detailed drug literature reviews. They may be formatted in a similar manner as a monograph or focus exclusively on clinical trial results and evidence-based guidelines. *Example question:* Could you provide an overview of the evidence for and against using intravenous lidocaine for the treatment of neuropathic pain?

- *Written Papers:* Many preceptors of direct patient care–focused APPEs require students to research a general drug information question and provide information as a written report. These questions are often exclusively focused on a review of the clinical evidence and may be longer than a typical memorandum. It is a good idea to ask the project initiator sufficient background questions about both the question and the expectations for the final project. *Example question:* What evidence is there for the use of probiotics for treatment and prevention of *Clostridium difficile* infection?

Audience

The most important consideration when selecting a response format and writing a drug information response, besides the context of the question, is the target audience.[1,2] In general, drug information responses intended for patients should be brief and easy to read. Often, an oral response supplemented with general, professional patient information is most appropriate. Care should be taken to ensure the response is written at an appropriate reading level, as approximately half of patients read at or below an eighth-grade level.[23] It is difficult to translate reading level to drug information, as responses will inevitably contain multisyllabic terms that are vital to the response. These terms should be included and defined, as necessary. It is suggested to assess the reading level of a patient response qualitatively and to provide written information along with tables, figures, diagrams, and verbal explanation as often as possible.

When providing information for healthcare providers, the individual's role and education level and the depth of the information requested should all be considered.[1,2] The anticipated time frame of the response should also be taken into account. Most drug information questions from nurses and other bachelor-level professionals may be answered orally or via e-mail. Memoranda may be used but should be concise and tailored for the individual. Responses for other pharmacists and other professional-degree or master's-level providers will range from a simple memorandum to a complicated drug-class review. Responses for physicians will also vary widely based on level of experience (e.g., first-year resident versus attending), specialty area, and personal preferences.

QUICK TIP

Sometimes it makes sense to ask the requestor directly what format to use for the response; however, some sites will have a standard process. Become familiar with the expectations of your site.

CASE QUESTION

E.B. has gathered all the information necessary to prepare a drug information response to her question. Based on her findings that simvastatin 80 mg is associated with myopathy and potentially life-threatening rhabdomyolysis, she wishes to recommend alternate therapy and several laboratory measurements for her patient. In what format should she present her findings and recommendations?

Publication

Drug information questions, particularly those received in drug information centers, can often be challenging to answer. Extensive research may reveal therapeutic issues or controversies that would be of wider interest to the pharmacy or health community. In these cases, it may be reasonable to pursue publication of the response. This may be in the form of a case report or article for a drug information–specific column. Several pharmacy publications, including the *American Journal of Health-System Pharmacy*, *Annals of Pharmacotherapy*, and *Pharmacotherapy*, have columns that include drug information–related articles, with topics ranging from patient-specific questions to class reviews.

Articles submitted for publication should be topical, related to new and/or emerging treatments, and of relevance to a wide variety of professionals. Care should be taken to ensure that similar reviews have not been published in the past. It may also be reasonable to contact an editor prior to preparing the response for publication to ensure that nobody else is writing a similar article and determine if the journal is interested in the idea. Publication of a drug information response, in collaboration with a preceptor, is an excellent opportunity for a student on an APPE rotation.

QUICK TIP

Residency program directors love to see prospective candidates with publication experience!

REFERENCES

1. Calis KA, Sheehan AH. Formulating effective responses and recommendations: A structured approach. In: Malone PM, Kier KL, Stanovich JE, eds. *Drug Information: A Guide for Pharmacists*. 4th ed. Chicago, IL: McGraw-Hill Medical; 2011.

2. Gaebelein CJ, Gleason BL. Asking and answering drug information questions. In: Gaebelein CJ, Gleason BL. *Contemporary Drug Information: An Evidence-Based Approach*. Baltimore, MD: Lippincott Williams & Wilkins; 2008.

3. Nathan JP, Gim S. Responding to drug information requests. *Am J Health-Syst Pharm.* 2009;66:706-711.

4. Wright SG, LeCroy RL, Kendrach MG. A review of the three types of biomedical literature and the systematic approach to answer a drug information request. *J Pharm Pract.* 1998;11:148-162.

5. Calis KA, Anderson DW, Auth DA, et al. Quality of pharmacotherapy consultations provided by drug information centers in the United States. *Pharmacother.* 2000;20:830-836.

6. Kirkwood CF, Kier KL. Modified systematic approach to answering questions. In: Malone PM, Kier KL, Stanovich JE, eds. *Drug Information: A Guide for Pharmacists*. 3rd ed. Chicago, IL: McGraw-Hill Medical; 2006.

7. Shields KM, Blythe E. Drug information resources. In: Malone PM, Kier KL, Stanovich JE, eds. *Drug Information: A Guide for Pharmacists*. 4th ed. Chicago, IL: McGraw-Hill Medical; 2011.

8. Polen HH, Zapantis A, Clauson KA, et al. Ability of online drug databases to assist in clinical decision-making with infectious disease therapies. *BMC Infect Dis.* 2008;8:153-162.

9. Clauson KA, Marsh WA, Polen HH, et al. Clinical decision support tools: Analysis of online drug information databases. *BMC Med Inform Dec Making*. 2007;7:7-13.

10. Thiele RH, Poiro NC, Scalzo DC, et al. Speed, accuracy, and confidence in Google, Ovid, PubMed, and UpToDate: Results of a randomized trial. *Postgrad Med J*. 2010;86:459-465.

11. Ensan LS, Faghankhani M, Javanbakht A, et al. To compare PubMed Clinical Queries and UpToDate in teaching information mastery to clinical residents: A crossover randomized controlled trial. *Plos One*. 2011;6:e23487.

12. Goodyear-Smith F, Kerse N, Warren J. Evaluation of e-textbooks: DynaMed, MD Consult, and UpToDate. *Austral Fam Phys*. 2008;37:878-882.

13. Ahmadi S-F, Faghankhani M, Javanbakht A, et al. A comparison of answer retrieval through four evidence-based textbooks (ACP PIER, Essential Evidence Plus, First Consult, and UpToDate): A randomized controlled trial. *Med Teach*. 2011;33:724-730.

14. Fenton SH, Badgett RG. A comparison of primary care information content in UpToDate and the National Guideline Clearinghouse. *J Med Libr Assoc*. 2007;95:255-259.

15. Banzi R, Cinquini M, Liberati A, et al. Speed of updating online evidence based point of care summaries: Prospective cohort analysis. *BMJ*. 2011;343:d5856. doi: 10.1136/bmj.d5856.

16. Hailemskel B, White DP, Lakew DG, et al. Internet as a drug information resource [abstract]. *ASHP Midyear Clinical Meeting*. 2001;36:p-404e.

17. Brokowski L, Sheehan AH. Evaluation of pharmacist use and perception of Wikipedia as a drug information resource. *Ann Pharmacother*. 2009;43:1912-1913.

18. Rajagopalan MS, Khanna VK, Leiter Y, et al. Patient-oriented cancer information on the Internet: A comparison of Wikipedia and a professionally maintained database. *J Oncol Pract*. 2011;7:319-323.

19. Kupferberg N, Protus BM. Accuracy and completeness of drug information in Wikipedia: An assessment. *J Med Libr Assoc*. 2011;99:310-313.

20. Clauson KA, Polen HH, Boulos MNK, et al. Scope, completeness, and accuracy of drug information in Wikipedia. *Ann Pharmacother*. 2008;42:1814-1821.

21. Health on the Net Foundation. HON. http://www.hon.ch/med.html. Accessed February 15, 2012.

22. Malone PM, Fagan NL, Malesker MA, et al. Drug evaluation monographs. In: Malone PM, Kier KL, Stanovich JE, eds. *Drug Information: A Guide for Pharmacists*. 4th ed. Chicago, IL: McGraw-Hill Medical; 2011.

23. Scown SJ. Cancer-patient reading levels in the real world. http://www.onconurse.com/news/reading_levels.html. Accessed February 15, 2012.

SUGGESTED READING

Abate MA, Hildebrand JR. Clinical drug literature. In: Beringer P, DerMarderosian A, Felton L, et al., eds. *Remington: The Science and Practice of Pharmacy*. 21st ed. London, UK: Pharmaceutical Press; 2005.

Gaebelein CJ, Gleason BL. *Contemporary Drug Information: An Evidence-Based Approach*. Baltimore, MD: Lippincott Williams & Wilkins; 2008.

Malone PM, Kier KL, Stanovich JE, eds. *Drug Information: A Guide for Pharmacists*. 4th ed. Chicago, IL: McGraw-Hill Medical; 2011.

APPENDIX 5-A.   SUGGESTED REFERENCE BOOKS

TOPIC	TITLE
Adverse Drug Events	*Drug-Induced Diseases: Prevention, Detection, and Management*
	Meyler's Side Effects of Drugs: The International Encyclopedia of Adverse Drug Reactions and Interactions
	Side Effects of Drugs Annual
Compounding Formulations/Practices	*Allen's Compounded Formulations: The Complete US Pharmacist Collection*
	The Art, Science, and Technology of Pharmaceutical Compounding
	Extemporaneous Formulations
	The Merck Index: An Encyclopedia of Chemicals, Drugs, and Biologicals
	Remington: The Science and Practice of Pharmacy
	Trissel's Stability of Compounded Formulations
	United States Pharmacopeia/National Formulary
Dietary Supplements	*Herbal Medicine: Expanded Commission E Monographs*
	Professional's Handbook of Complementary and Alternative Medicines
	The Review of Natural Products
Dosage Forms	*American Drug Index*
	Red Book Drug Topics
Drug Interactions	*Drug Interaction Analysis and Management*
	Drug Interaction Facts
	Evaluations of Drug Interactions: A Comprehensive Source of Drug Interaction Information
	Stockley's Drug Interactions
Drug Abuse	*Drugs of Abuse*
General Information	*AHFS Drug Information*
	Drug Facts and Comparisons
	Drug Information Handbook
	Drug Prescribing in Renal Failure
	Geriatric Dosage Handbook
	Physicians' Desk Reference
Injectable Products	*Handbook on Injectable Drugs*
	King Guide to Parenteral Admixtures
	Pediatric Injectable Drugs: The Teddy Bear Book
International Products	*Index Nominum: International Drug Directory*
	Martindale: The Complete Drug Reference

Law	*Guide to Federal Pharmacy Law*
	Pharmacy Practice and the Law
Medicine	*DeVita, Hellman, and Rosenberg's Cancer: Principles and Practice of Oncology*
	Goldman's Cecil Medicine
	Harrison's Principles of Internal Medicine
	Diagnostic and Statistical Manual of Mental Disorders
	Merck Manual of Diagnosis and Therapy
	Principles and Practices of Infectious Diseases
	Textbook of Cardiovascular Medicine
Nonprescription Medications	*Handbook of Nonprescription Drugs: An Interactive Approach to Self-Care*
	PDR for Nonprescription Drugs, Dietary Supplements, and Herbs: The Definitive Guide to OTC Medications
Pediatrics	*The Harriet Lane Handbook*
	Neofax
	Pediatric Dosing Guide
Pharmacokinetics	*Applied Pharmacokinetics and Pharmacodynamics: Principles of Therapeutic Drug Monitoring*
	Basic Clinical Pharmacokinetics
	Clinical Pharmacokinetics
Pharmacology	*Basic and Clinical Pharmacology*
	Goodman and Gilman's: The Pharmacological Basis of Therapeutics
Pregnancy and Lactation	*Drugs in Pregnancy and Lactation: A Reference Guide to Fetal and Neonatal Risk*
	Medications and Mothers' Milk: A Manual of Lactational Pharmacology
Therapeutics	*Applied Therapeutics: The Clinical Use of Drugs*
	Pharmacotherapy: A Pathophysiological Approach
	Pharmacotherapy Principles and Practice
Toxicology	*Goldfrank's Toxicologic Emergencies*
	Medical Toxicology
Veterinary Medicine	*Compendium of Veterinary Products*
	Textbook of Veterinary Internal Medicine
	Veterinary Drug Handbook

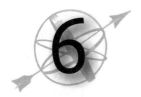

FORMAL AND INFORMAL CASE PRESENTATIONS

Laura A. Perry, PharmD, BCPS

CASE

E.S. is a pharmacy student arriving on her first APPE rotation. Her preceptor has just reviewed her expectations for this rotation. E.S. is nervous because her first assignment is a case presentation, and she has been given very little direction. Her preceptor has only advised her to follow F.S., a patient in room 474, who was admitted last night for elevated blood pressure and to prepare for a formal case presentation to the pharmacy staff the following week. Two days have passed and E.S. has been gathering large amounts of information on the patient, but she is unsure of how to begin organizing the information for her formal case presentation.

WHY IT'S ESSENTIAL

Case presentations are an essential component of student learning because they allow you to strengthen your verbal communication, critical thinking, and clinical reasoning skills. Preceptors use case presentations as a way to evaluate your ability to provide patient care. Once the transition is made from student to practitioner, case presentations become an excellent tool for providing education to pharmacists and other healthcare providers. Furthermore, informal case presentations are part of the daily routine of many healthcare providers. A well-done informal case presentation allows healthcare providers to communicate patient information effectively between one another, learn about unique patient cases, and facilitate collaborative development of care plans. The style and content of case presentations varies according to the purpose of the presentation, the audience, and the amount of time allotted. One approach is described in this chapter.

GENERAL COMPONENTS OF A CASE PRESENTATION

The general components of a case presentation include a discussion of pertinent patient information and current drug therapy and a summary of patient-specific recommendations. The most widely accepted format for organizing a case presentation is the SOAP format, consisting of a presentation of the case information in the following order: subjective, objective, assessment, and plan. Presenting a case utilizing this structured approach ensures the audience is able to follow and comprehend the wealth of information presented, orienting them to who the patient is, the illnesses the patient has, and how they are being managed. The degree of detail provided varies for formal and informal presentations, with more detail being included for formal case presentations than for informal case presentations. Preceptors may have differing opinions of how to best organize patient information into the SOAP format, but a general approach is outlined below.

Subjective Information

Introduction of the patient case involves presenting a variety of information, some of which must be gathered thorough a patient interview at the time of hospital admission or during an outpatient office visit. If the patient is unavailable to communicate, a caregiver may also respond in place of the patient. Subjective information includes the background information necessary to determine possible differential diagnoses, which then direct a thorough patient work up. **Table 6-1** outlines example subjective information that should be obtained and evaluated from the patient's chart.

TABLE 6-1. SUBJECTIVE INFORMATION

SUBJECTIVE INFORMATION	EXAMPLES
Chief Complaint The patient's primary concern upon presentation.	"I feel very dizzy."
History of Present Illness A chronological account of events since the onset of the problem, including significant detail of symptoms and any other pertinent subjective information that may be relevant to the primary problem.	The patient is a 63-year-old man brought in by EMS for altered mental status. According to the family, the patient became dizzy and fell this morning and had an episode of vomiting, after which they called emergency services. EMS reports a systolic blood pressure in the 240s upon their arrival. In the emergency department, the patient was started on a nitroglycerin drip and is being transferred to the medical intensive care unit.
Past Medical and Surgical History A list of previously diagnosed medical conditions and procedures.	CAD with history of STEMI and stent placement CHF (diagnosed 6 months ago) Type 2 DM HTN Appendectomy at age 10
Family History Family history of first-degree relatives.	Both parents had HTN; mother had DM. Father had a heart attack in his early 50s and died in his 70s of a second heart attack. His mother died a few years later of a stroke. One brother, age 60, has HTN, DM, and had CABG 3 years ago.
Social History Information relating to socioeconomic status, alcohol, tobacco, illicit drug use, and lifestyle.	Retired automotive maintainer. Denies tobacco or illicit drug use; drinks one to two beers per day. He has a history of not taking his medications as directed.
Review of Systems A list of questions asked of every patient to uncover clinical symptoms not reported in the initial chief complaint.	Patient denies double or blurry vision, shortness of breath, or abdominal pain. Patient does admit to mild heart palpitations and general weakness.

Abbreviations: CABG = coronary artery bypass graft; CAD = coronary artery disease; CHF = congestive heart failure; DM = diabetes mellitus; EMS = emergency medical services; HTN = hypertension; STEMI = ST-elevation myocardial infarction.

Objective Information

Presented in conjunction with the subjective information, objective evidence is measured by the healthcare team on the patient's arrival to the medical facility. The amount and type of objective information the healthcare team collects will vary depending on the suspected diagnosis. **Table 6-2** outlines example objective information that should be obtained from the patient's chart and evaluated.

CASE QUESTION

To prepare her assigned patient case for presentation, what information will E.S. need to gather and how should she begin organizing this information?

TABLE 6-2. OBJECTIVE INFORMATION

OBJECTIVE INFORMATION	EXAMPLES
Patient Demographics Age Sex Race Height Weight	F.S. is a 63-year-old Caucasian male, 66 inches tall, weighing 105 kg.
Medication List Inpatient medications	*Hospital medications* Nitroglycerin infusion at 200 mcg/min Hydralazine 20 mg q 6 hr prn SBP >160 mmHg Famotidine 20 mg IV q 12 hr Insulin aspart sliding scale q 6 hr Furosemide 20 mg IV q 12 hr 0.9% NS at 50 mL/hr
Home medications	*Home medications* Hydralazine 100 mg tid Procardia XL 60 mg once daily Catapres TTS-1 one patch weekly Simvastatin 20 mg daily Spironolactone 50 mg daily Isosorbide mononitrate 60 mg daily Clopidogrel 75 mg daily Humulin 70/30 50 units bid

Allergies (including reactions)	
Drug or drug class	Penicillin (rash on trunk and extremities)
Inactive ingredients	Latex (hives)
Vital Signs	
Blood pressure	BP 222/170
Heart rate	P 116
Respiratory rate	RR 16
Pulse oximetry	O2 saturation 98%
Temperature	Temperature 37.3°C
Physical Exam	General: Patient appears comfortable but remains confused
Examination by inspection, palpation, percussion, or auscultation	HEENT: Normal conjunctivae, pupils 3 mm and reactive
	Respiratory: Clear to auscultation, no wheezes, rhonchi, or rales
	Cardiovascular: Tachycardic, no murmurs or rubs
	Abdominal: Obese, abdomen soft, nontender, positive bowel sounds
	Neurological: The patient has no localized pain. Positive Babinski sign bilaterally, grip equal on both sides, mild weakness bilaterally
	Extremities: 1+ pitting edema bilaterally
Laboratory Values	
Basic metabolic panel	Na 134, K 4.1, Cl 97, HCO3 15, BUN 33, serum creatinine 1.89, glucose 345
Complete blood count	WBC 13.6, Hb 14.4, Hct 43.8, Plt 326
Others	AST 17, ALT 10
	HbA1c 9.5%
Diagnostic Tests	
X-ray/CT scan/MRI	CT with contrast: No evidence of acute hemorrhage or ischemic stroke.
EKG	EKG: Sinus tachycardia
Others	Echocardiogram: LVEF 40%
Calculations	
Creatinine clearance	CrCl 36 mL/min
Ideal body weight	IBW 63.8 kg
Body mass index	BMI 37.4
Others	MAP 187

Abbreviations: ALT = alanine aminotransferase; AST = aspartate aminotransferase; BMI = body mass index; BP = blood pressure; CrCl = creatinine clearance; CT = computed tomography; EKG = electrocardiogram; Hb = hemoglobin; Hct = hematocrit; HEENT = head, eyes, ears, nose, and throat; IBW = ideal body weight; IV = intravenous; LVEF = left ventricular ejection fraction; MAP = mean arterial pressure; MRI = magnetic resonance imaging; NS = normal saline; P = pulse; Plt = platelets; RR = respiratory rate; SBP = systolic blood pressure; WBC = white blood count.

Assessment

After gathering all essential subjective and objective information, the student must next evaluate the information to determine the patient's problem list, including any drug therapy–related problems. Possible drug therapy–related issues include (but are not limited to) undertreatment or overtreatment of a medical condition, medications without appropriate indications, suspected adverse drug events, or the need for renal dose adjustments. For a full discussion of drug-related problems, see Chapter 13. For each problem identified, an assessment statement can be created that summarizes the important information. This statement usually includes the problem's severity, any precipitating factors, evidence used to rule in the problem, and current treatment status. You must then rank the problems from highest to lowest priority to focus on resolving the problems with the highest priority level first. In most situations, the primary problem will be related to the patient's chief complaint. After the primary problem, other active or uncontrolled medical conditions can be listed in the order of their acuity. If the patient has unmet preventive medicine needs, they can be listed next. Lastly, you may list any controlled or inactive problems. Often, it is not possible for a healthcare team to address all patient problems within a single visit. Prioritizing problems will focus the care plan on the most critical problems, with lower-priority problems being addressed over the next few days, at discharge, or at follow-up visits.

CASE QUESTION

E.S. has determined that F.S. has the following problems: hyperglycemia, hypertensive emergency, coronary artery disease, home medications without identified indications, and well-controlled congestive heart failure. How should she prioritize this patient's problems?

QUICK TIP

Listing unnecessary information may make the assessment long and distract the presenter and listener from the key information. The assessment should focus on pertinent positives and negatives to determine the exact diagnoses from the list of differential diagnoses.

CASE QUESTION

E.S. determines that the primary problem for her patient is hypertensive emergency. She develops the following assessment for this problem: "Moderate to severe hypertensive emergency secondary to medication nonadherence as evidenced by systolic blood pressure in the 240s, dizziness, and altered mental status. Other pertinent findings include 1+ pitting edema, serum creatinine of 1.89, and BUN of 33. CT scan was negative for stroke, and his LVEF is 40%. Past medical history of HTN, CAD, CHF, Type 2 DM, and PAD. Father had a heart attack in his early 50s and died in his 70s of a second heart attack. His mother died a few years later of a stroke. One brother, age 60, has HTN, DM, and had CABG 3 years ago. One cousin, age 55, is in overall good health but may have impaired fasting glucose. Current vitals are blood pressure 122/70 and pulse 116." What information has E.S. included in her problem assessment for hypertensive emergency that may not be pertinent? Has she left out any important details?

Plan

Development of the patient care plan is where students will find themselves spending much of their time and effort. Complete care plans will include goals of therapy, pharmacological recommendations, nonpharmacological recommendations, and patient counseling.

Goals of Therapy

Establishing sound goals of therapy for each problem helps keep the bigger picture of the patient's care in plain view, decreasing the chance for overtreatment or undertreatment. Goals of therapy for each problem should be measurable. Instead of using vague, general statements such as "Control blood pressure," measurable goals of therapy should be chosen, such as "Lower mean arterial pressure by 25% using intravenous antihypertensive medication (patient's current MAP is 187, target MAP is 140) over the first hour. Then, lower blood pressure to 160/100 mmHg over the next 2 to 6 hours. Finally, lower the blood pressure to a target 130/80 over the next 24 to 48 hours." Providing measurable goals will guide the development of drug and nondrug therapy recommendations, as well as monitoring parameters. The focus of most case presentations in the inpatient setting should be on short-term goals; however, long-term goals may be pertinent to some problems, specifically those managed in the primary care setting.

CASE QUESTION

What long-term goals of therapy may be recommended for F.S. to better manage his hypertension at discharge?

Pharmacological Recommendations

As a pharmacy student, the focus of your patient care plan should be on pharmacological recommendations. Pharmacological recommendations should identify and resolve any drug therapy–related issues for each problem, indicating which medications you wish to continue, discontinue, modify, or add. For each medication added or continued, you should provide a complete recommendation, including the drug name, dose, route, frequency, and titration schedule, if applicable. Additionally, a component of the care plan many students struggle with is the development of a rationale for each recommendation. An appropriate rationale should include the benefit or risk of adding, modifying, continuing, or discontinuing a medication, as well as the supportive evidence-based guidelines or primary literature. Most patient problems have more than one correct management approach. Clear and complete rationale for all drug and nondrug therapy recommendations is necessary to inform the audience of the reason for your approach. A well-developed rationale will confirm the accuracy of a recommendation and increase the likelihood that the recommendation will be implemented.

CASE QUESTION

E.S. proposes to discontinue clonidine because it may be harmful to this patient and to start labetalol. Although this is a valid recommendation, E.S. needs to improve the content and rationale of her recommendation. How might she improve the clarity and rationale of this intervention?

Nonpharmacological Recommendations

An effective care plan for many medical conditions involves nonpharmacological therapy alone or in addition to pharmacotherapy. Often, a combination of nonpharmacological and pharmacological therapy provides a more effective approach to patient care than either treatment option alone. Examples of non-pharmacological therapy for chronic medical conditions include (but are not limited to) modifications in diet and lifestyle. For example, recommending the DASH (dietary approaches to stop hypertension) diet and a patient-specific exercise and weight-loss plan is a very important aspect of effective treatment and prevention of elevated blood pressure. Additionally, examples of nonpharmacological recommendations for acutely ill patients include (but are not limited to) proper wound care for a skin and soft-tissue infection or elevating the head of the bed at least 30 degrees to prevent ventilator-associated pneumonia. Targeting modifiable risk factors can avoid additional complications and may even reduce the number and type of medications needed to achieve optimal patient outcomes.

Patient Counseling

Educating patients on all aspects of your recommended care plan can contribute to safe and successful implementation and follow through of each intervention. Counseling a patient may include presenting information on the benefits and risks, proper administration, and proper expectations of each recommendation. With respect to pharmacological therapy, it is important that you educate the patient on how to recognize pertinent drug side effects, as well as any possible complications from known drug–drug, drug–disease, or drug–food interactions. Although there are many possible counseling points to include with each pharmacological or nonpharmacological recommendation, you should limit the amount of education provided at one time to avoid overwhelming the patient.

Monitoring and Follow-Up

Most often, newly added or discontinued medications will be the main cause of adverse drug events. To minimize the chance of causing additional medical problems with your treatment recommendations, complete monitoring plans must be included in the case presentation. Monitoring plans should consist of pertinent clinical signs and symptoms and/or laboratory tests necessary to assess safety and efficacy of the recommended care plan. In addition to listing what needs to be monitored, it is also important to clearly indicate when each of these monitoring parameters should be evaluated at future follow-up. The frequency of monitoring will vary depending on the acuity of the problem and may range from monitoring a parameter continuously (i.e., telemetry), every week (i.e., international normalized ratio [INR]), every 3 months (i.e., hemoglobin A1C), or even every 2 years (i.e., bone mineral density).

FORMAL CASE PRESENTATION

As described above, formal case presentations are often used by practicing pharmacists to provide education to other healthcare providers and by students to demonstrate mastery of the treatment of a given disease state. Compared to the work that is put into developing the patient's care plan, creating and delivering the formal case presentation is a relatively simple task.

Audience

The audience for formal case presentations may consist of just a few pharmacist preceptors or may include attendance by multiple healthcare providers from a variety of disciplines. Check with your preceptor well in advance of the presentation date to make sure you are aware of the audience members. The presentation should be tailored to match the interests and education level of those that will be in attendance. Most commonly, you will be presenting formal case presentations to the pharmacy staff, which will include pharmacists, pharmacy students, and technicians. The case presentation should be designed to tell the audience the story of what you found, what interventions were made, and the final outcome of the patient case. It is also common to be asked questions by the audience at the end of the presentation to clarify information or to expand on the information presented. Be prepared to answer the type of questions that will most likely be asked by the audience.

CASE QUESTION

E.S. has gathered all the necessary subjective and objective information, developed and prioritized a problem list, and developed an evidence-based care plan with appropriate rationale. Her presentation is just one day away. How can she ensure that her presentation will cover this information in the appropriate amount of detail?

Format

When asked to prepare a formal case presentation, you should ask for guidance to guarantee the presentation will meet the expectations of your preceptor. The amount of time allowed for the presentation will assist the student in deciding the most relevant information to include. Time allotted for a formal case presentation varies from 30 to 60 minutes for most APPE sites. In general, formal case presentations should follow the SOAP format outlined above.

In addition to the patient-specific information, a review of the patient's primary disease state should be included in the formal case presentation, most often discussed after the assessment statement. The disease state presentation should outline the pathophysiology, incidence, prevalence, etiology, clinical presentation, proper diagnosis, and possible complications of the primary problem. Following the disease state review, you must provide an overview of current evidence-based treatment guidelines, including pharmacological and nonpharmacological therapy. The outline of drug therapy describes the agents used to treat the disease and may include their mechanism of action, pharmacokinetics, drug interactions, adverse drug reactions, dosing, monitoring, and key patient information. To ensure that your therapeutic review is up to date, a quick literature search for novel treatment options or guideline updates will help you avoid an incomplete presentation. See Chapter 5 for a discussion of literature searches.

Because students are presenting formal case presentations with the goal of telling the audience a story from start to finish, the plan portion of the presentation should include a day-by-day outline of the patient's hospital course. The plan should also critique the treatment course implemented by the medical team. If the treatment plan developed by the medical team differed from the typical treatment regimen outlined during the disease state review, you should rationalize why the team took an alternative approach or identify how the team could improve care for future patients. Furthermore, you should highlight any recommendations that you personally made to the healthcare team.

Following the plan, the final portion of a formal case presentation should be a summary statement. Summary statements allow the presenter to provide an overall impression of the patient case, indicating typical or unique characteristics. Including a summary will provide closure and leave the audience with the final impression and key take-home points you intended to communicate. The conclusion of each case presentation should also include a list of references. You must cite all evidence-based guidelines and primary, secondary, and tertiary literature referenced while completing the patient assessment and plan. Full citation is recommended for most case presentations; however, abbreviated citations may be accepted by some preceptors.

In addition to asking for guidance on content, it is important for the student to confirm with his or her preceptor what technology will be available during the presentation. Many APPE sites prefer students use Microsoft® PowerPoint® to present formal case presentations, with or without a handout for audience members. Other preceptors may request the student present to the audience with only a case handout.

QUICK TIP

Use visual aids during a formal case presentation whenever possible. The use of graphs, tables, and pictures will enhance the presentation of disease background. A great way to outline drug therapy is to develop a drug table to easily compare common treatment options.

INFORMAL CASE PRESENTATION

Audience

Informal case presentations are a part of daily medical rounds. Only a few minutes in length, they allow you to provide a brief summary of the patient case to your preceptor or to the medical team. Additionally, informal case presentations are used by residents, nurses, physicians, and a variety of other healthcare providers at shift change to quickly update each other on what patients are new to the team as well as the progress of patients that the team has been caring for.

Format

The main difference between formal and informal case presentations is the time allotted for the presentation. Although the purpose of formal case presentations is to provide a detailed patient case and disease state review to the audience, informal case presentations are used to streamline communication for day-to-day patient care. The following formats allow for the development of a 3- to-5-minute structured informal case presentation:

SUBJECTIVE, OBJECTIVE, ASSESSMENT, PLAN (SOAP)

SITUATION, BACKGROUND, ASSESSMENT, RECOMMENDATION (SBAR)

FINDINGS, ASSESSMENT, RESOLUTION, MANAGEMENT (FARM)

Unlike a formal case presentation, the information presented to the team is abbreviated to include pertinent information for only the most pressing patient problems. Any of the structured formats above provide a means for development of an easy-to-follow, efficient informal case presentation.

CASE QUESTION

E.S. has successfully presented her formal case presentation to the pharmacy staff with great reviews. For the remaining 2 weeks of her APPE rotation, her preceptor would like her to follow five patients per day and to present each patient informally to him 1 hour before the medical team performs bedside rounds. E.S. is unsure of how she is going to present five cases in 1 hour when it took her 1 hour to present one case. How should her approach to preparing for her informal case presentations differ from her strategy for preparing for her formal case presentation?

Common Pitfalls

Case presentations, both formal and informal, require you to present complex information to an expert audience. It is common for students to be nervous and to be fearful of making mistakes. Recognizing the need to prepare for a case presentation well in advance and setting goals to guide information gathering is the first step to developing a successful presentation. Second, learning from mistakes made on previous case presentations, as well as the mistakes made by other students, is very important. **Table 6-3** contains a list of common pitfalls, or mistakes, that you will want to avoid making.

Table 6-3. Common Pitfalls

COMMON PITFALL	CORRECT ACTION
Not reporting a patient's chief complaint in the patient's own words	Always report a patient's chief complaint in the patient's own words
The patient's chief complaint is hypoglycemia and altered mental status.	The patient's chief complaint is "low blood sugar and feeling out of sorts."
Using poor references	Appropriate references
Outdated textbooks or review articles	Current evidence-based guidelines are preferred over textbooks or review articles
Non–peer-reviewed publications	Clinical trials from peer-reviewed journals
Unreliable websites	Websites monitored by government organizations or well-respected professional organizations
Instructor notes	
Missing data	Perform a complete review of all patient information to avoid missing relevant data.
Not including demographic data	Demographic data, such as patient age, height, weight, and race should be the initial information presented to properly introduce the patient.
Listing all laboratory/diagnostic data	Only list the relevant laboratory/diagnostic data for each problem. Remember, not all abnormal laboratory/diagnostic values may be relevant to every problem. On the same note, some normal laboratory/diagnostic values may be relevant.
Nonmeasurable goals of therapy	Goals of therapy should be the focus of the beginning of every care plan and should be measurable (e.g., goal HbA1C <7%).
Incomplete monitoring/follow-up plan	Every care plan should end with a detailed monitoring plan, including what to monitor and when it should be monitored.

Improper presentation skills	Use fundamental presentation skills.
Reading from slides/notes Poor eye contact	Practice the presentation beforehand, preferably to a pharmacist or pharmacy student. Knowing the presentation well can avoid the need to read from notes and will allow maintenance of eye contact.
Incorrect pronunciation of drug names or medical terms	Always know how to pronounce every drug name and term within the presentation. Look up the proper pronunciation if necessary. Do not guess!
Not knowing your audience	Know the purpose of the presentation as well as the audience. The ideal focus of a presentation to pharmacists may vary from a presentation to physicians or nurses.
Distracting words (i.e., "ummm," "uhhh," "okay," "like," "you know what I mean," etc.) Distracting body movements (i.e., swaying, clicking pen, moving hands constantly, excessive use of laser pointer)	Prior to the presentation, record a video of the presentation or ask for feedback from a willing audience. This will help to eliminate the use of distracting words or body movements. The presenter may or may not pick up on these by practicing alone.
Overuse of slide animation or clip art	If slide animation is used, it should be kept to a minimum. Overuse of slide animation may slow down the presentation or distract the audience.
Wordy slides	Limit content on slides to seven rows of text or less.

SUGGESTED READING

Cipolle RJ, Strand LM, Morley PC. *Pharmaceutical Care Practice: The Patient-Centered Approach to Medication Management Services*. 3rd ed. New York, NY: McGraw-Hill; 2012.

Part II: The Particulars

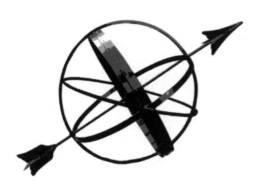

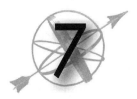

Introductory Pharmacy Practice Experiences

Lori Ernsthausen, PharmD, BCPS

CASE

S.S. is a first-professional-year pharmacy student who has just been assigned to his first IPPE at a nearby community pharmacy. S.S. has worked for several years as a pharmacy technician at a similar community pharmacy in his hometown and is uncertain how this experience will be any different from what he is used to doing at his job. S.S.'s preceptor, a faculty member at the school of pharmacy, spends some time on the first day discussing S.S.'s previous experiences and developing a plan of activities S.S. must complete for school as well as several activities in which S.S. wishes to gain experience. S.S. is feeling a little bit more confident about his IPPE but is still uncertain about whether he will learn anything new.

Why It's Essential

IPPEs are intended to introduce you to the practice of pharmacy, the healthcare system, and the role the pharmacist plays within the healthcare system. You will typically gain experience in community and institutional pharmacy practice and may also have the opportunity to explore other areas of pharmacy practice. The fundamental skills that are cultivated during the introductory experiences are meant to prepare you for the APPEs of the final professional year.

The Accreditation Council for Pharmacy Education (ACPE) sets the standards to which all colleges and schools of pharmacy must conform. All schools are required to have at least 300 hours of IPPEs as part of their doctor of pharmacy degree (PharmD) curriculum. Per ACPE, a majority of the student's time should be divided between community pharmacy and institutional health-system settings (i.e., hospital pharmacy), but time may also be spent in other practice settings (i.e., long-term care, compounding, ambulatory care, etc.). Schools are allowed to use simulation (an activity that replicates pharmacy practice) for up to 60 hours of the 300-hour requirement. Students who attend colleges or schools where simulation training is part of IPPEs may complete experiences with simulation manikins, computer-based simulations, or the use of standardized patients or healthcare providers.

In the most recent accreditation standards and guidelines for the PharmD degree, ACPE put forth a list of domains that are considered abilities students "must have" before entering APPEs (see **Table 7-1**). Students are required to demonstrate these abilities during the completion of their IPPE hours. Although every school of pharmacy must meet the ACPE standards, most programs have unique aspects to their didactic and experiential curriculum that serve to set them apart from others or may be driven by the school's or university's mission, size, location, or proximity to other schools of pharmacy or the teaching philosophy of faculty members. Depending on the school, you may complete IPPEs longitudinally throughout a semester or during a specific block of time. For example, one student may travel every

Thursday afternoon to an IPPE site, whereas another student may complete all required IPPE hours for a given term during a 2-week time period. Not all colleges incorporate simulation activities into IPPEs, although some provide extensive experiences in a simulated environment. Additionally, IPPE students may participate in service learning as part of their IPPEs. This may include involvement in activities with local community partners or agencies during the school year, summer, or other holiday breaks.

Table 7-1. ACPE Core IPPE Domains

CORE DOMAINS

- Patient Safety—Accurately Dispense Medications

- Basic Patient Assessment

- Medication Information

- Identification and Assessment of Drug-Related Problems

- Mathematics Applied to Pharmaceutical Calculations, Compound Medications, Dose Calculations, and Application of Pharmacokinetics Calculations

- Ethical, Professional, and Legal Behavior

- General Communication Abilities

- Counseling Patients

- Drug Information Analysis and Literature Research

- Health and Wellness—Public Health

- Insurance/Prescription Drug Coverage

You will enter your professional program with a variety of pharmacy experience. Some students may have extensive work histories in pharmacies; however, others may have very little or no practical experience. Students may be assigned to IPPE sites that are similar to the site where they work as a paid intern. Although this might seem frustrating, it is important to keep in mind that every practice opportunity in a pharmacy or with a pharmacist preceptor can be a learning experience. It is up to you to make the most out of each site by doing the following:

- Prepare ahead of time.

- Ask questions.

- Get involved.

- Observe and take note of differences in managerial styles, patient care protocols, and dispensing procedures.

Every activity at a site might not be new or unique, but the more experience you gain as a pharmacy intern, paid or unpaid, the more prepared you will be for your APPEs.

A Typical Day

Depending on your professional year and college curriculum, you might find yourself in an IPPE in a community, ambulatory care, or institutional setting, among others. What a typical day might look like will vary from site to site. In general, there are standard activities that you may be involved with at each type of site.

Community

In a community pharmacy, you will most likely be involved with the processing and dispensing of new or refill medications. During this experience, you should become proficient at accurately preparing and dispensing medications and devices and, depending on your year, evaluating the appropriateness of the prescription, taking into consideration patient-specific data and drug information. You may be called on to practice your communication skills by taking prescriptions over the phone, responding to drug information inquiries, or counseling patients on prescription and over-the-counter products. In addition, you may be asked to demonstrate basic calculation and compounding skills.

CASE QUESTION

What opportunities exist in the community pharmacy setting to expand on the previous experiences of a student like S.S.?

Ambulatory Care

In the ambulatory care setting, you will likely practice physical assessment skills, as well as patient interviews and patient counseling. You may also be integrated into the medication reconciliation process or be asked to use your drug information skills to answer questions from patients and healthcare providers. Although not specific to ambulatory care sites, preventative care, wellness programs, assessments, and immunization administration are also potential experiences. Within the ambulatory care setting, you should be challenged to obtain and interpret patient information that relates to the patient's disease management, including the presence of a disease, medical condition, and/or drug-related problems.

Health System

During an institutional IPPE, your responsibilities will likely include unit dose and parenteral medication processing and dispensing and, depending on the site, development of your communication skills through face-to-face or phone interactions with physicians, nurses, and other healthcare providers. Within the institutional setting, you should be introduced to the use of health informatics at the site and the role of technology, especially as it pertains to patient safety. Although you may spend time with the preceptor participating in many tasks in the institutional setting, you might find yourself working closely with a pharmacy technician, resident, or APPE student. Once you have been introduced to the processing and dispensing aspects of institutional pharmacy, some settings may allow you to begin exploring clinical skills in institutional pharmacy, such as daily rounding, pharmacokinetic consults, renal dosing, anticoagulation monitoring, medication reconciliation, and discharge counseling.

QUICK TIP

Before any practice experience begins, the student should inquire about what to expect: typical day, dress code, materials to bring, etc. Each practice site and preceptor will have slightly different expectations, and it is always best to ask the preceptor directly rather than rely on anecdotal reports from other students.

CASE QUESTION

S.S. is excited to begin his first institutional IPPE. He has no experience in the institutional setting and is eager to spend all of his IPPE hours observing the clinical pharmacist on rounds with the medical team. Why is it important that S.S. spend time learning the dispensing aspects of the institution, as well as gain experiences with the clinical pharmacist?

ARRIVING PREPARED

Regardless of whether you are spending several hours at the site on one day or several days at the site consecutively, you should be prepared to jump into assigned tasks and should anticipate questions that may be asked. Preparation on both the student's and preceptor's sides can facilitate a more meaningful experience. **Table 7-2** provides examples of ways in which you can prepare for your IPPEs. As expected, the need for preparation may vary based on your previous experiences (academic and work experience), didactic courses completed in the pharmacy curriculum, and overall communication skills. Preceptors may also have a list of activities and suggested readings that can assist students in their preparation for an experience at a given site.

CASE QUESTION

Based on S.S.'s extensive community pharmacy experience, what preparatory activities would you recommend for him to complete prior to beginning an institutional experience?

Introductory practice experiences provide pharmacy students with the opportunity to apply the knowledge and skills that have been taught in the classroom setting. The experiences gained in your IPPEs will also help build a foundation for the APPEs that follow. Whether you have extensive paid work experience or are entering a pharmacy for the first time, some preparation is required to ensure that you maximize the practice experience.

MEDICATION SAFETY

Although some preceptors or sites may be concerned that integrating IPPE students into their site may pose a risk to patient safety, there are actually several ways in which you may help improve patient safety. For example, at sites where resources are limited, you may facilitate the medication reconciliation process or review of clinical reports that busy pharmacists might not have enough time to complete. When practicing order entry or dispensing, you may be a second or third check that might not normally be present in the process. The opportunity to apply proper techniques and safety protocols in a real-life setting encourages students to employ safe practices at future IPPE and APPE sites. Preceptors should take the time to familiarize you with the site's policies and procedures that relate to safe practices, as well as the technology utilized by a site to improve patient safety, such as automated dispensing robots, automated compounding devices, medication cabinets, and electronic prescribing systems.

CASE QUESTION

What opportunities might S.S. have at an institutional, community, or ambulatory care site to learn about safe medication practices?

TABLE 7-2. TOPICS TO REVIEW PRIOR TO IPPE ROTATIONS

Drug Knowledge	Review top 200 prescription drugs.
	Review top 100 nonprescription drugs.
Drug References	Review what references are available through your university/ college library online and how to use them.
	Consider purchasing smartphone databases or applications (Lexicomp, Micromedex, AHFS Essential, Sigler Drug Cards, MedCalc).
IPPE Requirements	Review your IPPE manual, syllabus, and/or guidelines prior to arriving at your site.
	Always bring a copy of your expectations, objectives, outcomes, competencies, and/or checklist with you for the experience.
Disease State Knowledge	Research your IPPE site.
	Who does the site serve (elderly, indigent, pediatrics, patients on anticoagulants, etc.)?
	What disease states are you most likely to encounter (chronic, acute, both)? You may need to ask your preceptor.
	Are there any identified health disparities in the population that is served?
	Review current practice guidelines for disease states that you are likely to encounter.
Communication	Review counseling techniques taught in classroom/lab (i.e., PAR approach or Three Prime Questions).
	Review written communication techniques taught in the classroom/laboratory (i.e., SOAP notes, FARM notes, documenting clinical interventions, formal drug information responses, journal club, etc.).
Professionalism	Review dress code and professional conduct requirements of school.
	Prior to arriving at the site, inquire about the site's dress code or professional conduct requirements (i.e., white coat, name badge, cell phone policy, etc.).
Dispensing Skills	Review state and federal laws relating to dispensing.
	Review sterile technique and USP <797> requirements.
	Review basic pharmacy calculations.
Medication Safety Skills	Review ISMP Medication Safety Tools and Resources (www. ismp.org).
	Review The Joint Commission National Patient Safety Goals (http://www.jointcommission.org/standards_ information/npsgs.aspx).
Reflection	Review any required portfolio documentation for IPPE.
	Keep a log of activities completed and hours spent at site (these items may need to be formally recorded in experiential management software and/or may be useful when completing an end-of-experience reflection).

Abbreviations: FARM = findings, assessment, resolution, and management; ISMP = Institute for Safe Medication Practices; PAR = prepare, assess, respond; SOAP = subjective, objective, assessment, and plan; USP = United States Pharmacopeial Convention.

SIMULATION

Schools of pharmacy may utilize up to 20% (60 hours) of the IPPE curriculum as structured simulation. Simulation is defined by ACPE as an activity or event that replicates pharmacy practice. Simulation in IPPEs is most commonly used to allow you the opportunity to practice physical assessment and communication skills, as well as to facilitate interprofessional education where pharmacy students are learning alongside other healthcare providers, such as nursing or medical students. Simulation activities may take place on or off campus and usually include a mock scenario (medication reconciliation, patient counseling, medical rounds, etc.) and time for reflection, assessment, or debriefing at the end of the simulation. These activities enable students to learn in an environment where the opportunity to apply skills and knowledge is more like real life than in the classroom or lecture hall, but the risk of harm to the patient is low should a mistake be made.

SERVICE LEARNING

Service learning is another important aspect of IPPEs. Not all schools incorporate service learning into their curriculum; however, those that do may use it to promote health and wellness, facilitate disease prevention, improve the management of diseases and medication therapies, or foster leadership, compassion, and cultural competence. Service learning typically requires the completion of a project or activity outside of the classroom and includes time for self-reflection (which may be written, verbal, or both).

SUGGESTED READING

ISMP Medication Safety Alert!® Newsletters. http://www.ismp.org/newsletters/default.asp

Reiss BS, Hall GD. *Guide to Federal Pharmacy Law*. 7th ed. Delmar, NY: Apothecary Press; 2010.

O'Sullivan TA. *Understanding Pharmacy Calculations*. Washington, DC: APhA Publications; 2002.

Sigler's Prescription Drug Cards. 27th ed. Lawrence, KS: SFI Medical Publishing; 2011. (also available as an iPhone App)

Sigler's Nonprescription Drug Cards. 8th ed. Lawrence, KS: SFI Medical Publishing; 2010.

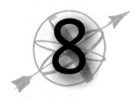

INTERNAL MEDICINE AND OTHER CLINICAL ROTATIONS

Mate M. Soric, PharmD, BCPS

CASE

J.B. is a pharmacy student starting his internal medicine APPE rotation. His preceptor has asked him to begin "working up" the patients on the floor so that he will be prepared for rounds later that morning. J.B. reads through the chart that belongs to the first patient on the list, a 61-year-old man admitted with a congestive heart failure exacerbation. The patient's case is complex, so the medical record is quite large and J.B. spends a great deal of time digging through the various sections looking for important information. Not helping matters, J.B. is repeatedly referring to resources on a desktop computer to help him decipher the various diagnostic tests and evaluate the patient's drug therapy. As a result of the large amount of time spent working up the first case, J.B. is unable to review all of the patients on the list before reporting to his preceptor.

WHY IT'S ESSENTIAL

The internal medicine and specialty APPEs (often called *clinical rotations*) play an important role in the development of critical thinking skills and drug information knowledge for pharmacy students. Regardless of the career goal you have in mind, the ability to evaluate a patient's medical information, identify drug therapy problems, design therapeutic interventions, and communicate recommendations to other healthcare providers are invaluable skills that must be mastered. Few other rotation types allow for the application of these skills on a daily basis.

ARRIVING PREPARED

- Contact the preceptor before the rotation begins for clarification on any required readings, disease states to review, and logistical information (parking, arrival time, etc.).
- Review the rotation syllabus.
- Wear professional dress, including white coat.
- Bring the following items:
    - ☐ Calculator
    - ☐ Pocket reference guides (Drug Information Handbook, Pocket Pharmacopoeia, *Sanford Guide*, etc.) or their electronic counterparts
    - ☐ Clipboard or folder
    - ☐ A patient monitoring sheet

- Review pertinent class notes:
  - ☐ Types of drug-related problems
  - ☐ Presentation skills
  - ☐ Patient interview and counseling skills
  - ☐ Evaluation of drug literature and statistics
- Common disease states to review:
  - ☐ Internal medicine rotations:
    - ◆ Acute coronary syndromes
    - ◆ Atrial fibrillation
    - ◆ Congestive heart failure
    - ◆ Stroke
    - ◆ Hypertension
    - ◆ Thromboembolic diseases
    - ◆ Anemias
    - ◆ Chronic obstructive pulmonary disease
    - ◆ Asthma
    - ◆ Diabetes
    - ◆ Cirrhosis and hepatitis
    - ◆ Pancreatitis
    - ◆ Pain management
    - ◆ Pneumonia
    - ◆ Skin and soft-tissue infections
    - ◆ Urinary tract infections
  - ☐ Cardiology rotations:
    - ◆ Hypertension
    - ◆ Angina pectoris
    - ◆ Myocardial infarctions
    - ◆ Atrial fibrillation and flutter
    - ◆ Paroxysmal supraventricular tachycardia
    - ◆ Ventricular arrhythmias
    - ◆ Torsades de pointes
    - ◆ Atrioventricular and bundle branch blocks
    - ◆ Pericarditis
    - ◆ Systolic and diastolic heart failure
    - ◆ Hyperlipidemia
    - ◆ Valvular diseases
    - ◆ Syncope
    - ◆ Cardiomyopathies

- ☐ Infectious disease rotations:
  - ◆ Complicated skin and soft-tissue infections
  - ◆ Diabetic foot infections
  - ◆ Pyelonephritis
  - ◆ Community-, healthcare-, and ventilator-associated pneumonia
  - ◆ Influenza
  - ◆ Tuberculosis
  - ◆ Infective endocarditis
  - ◆ *Clostridium difficile* colitis
  - ◆ Osteomyelitis and infected prostheses
  - ◆ Human immunodeficiency virus infections
  - ◆ Bacterial and viral meningitis
  - ◆ Invasive fungal infections
  - ◆ Parasitic infections
  - ◆ Sexually transmitted diseases
- ☐ Intensive care unit rotations:
  - ◆ Sedation and pain management
  - ◆ Fluid and electrolyte disturbances
  - ◆ Acute renal failure
  - ◆ Acid–base disorders
  - ◆ Stress ulcer prophylaxis
  - ◆ Delirium
  - ◆ Septic, hypovolemic cardiogenic, and anaphylactic shock
  - ◆ Acute respiratory distress syndrome and ventilator management
  - ◆ Diabetic ketoacidosis
  - ◆ Hypertensive urgencies and emergencies
  - ◆ Acute coronary syndromes
  - ◆ Ventricular arrhythmias
  - ◆ Status epilepticus
  - ◆ Status asthmaticus
- ☐ Psychiatry rotations:
  - ◆ Depression
  - ◆ Anxiety and panic disorders
  - ◆ Bipolar disorder
  - ◆ Schizophrenia
  - ◆ Personality disorders
  - ◆ Alzheimer's and vascular dementia
  - ◆ Delirium

- ◆ Obsessive-compulsive disorder
- ◆ Post-traumatic stress disorder
- ◆ Sleep disorders
- ☐ Oncology rotations:
  - ◆ Breast cancer
  - ◆ Gynecologic malignancies
  - ◆ Prostate cancer
  - ◆ Testicular cancer
  - ◆ Lung cancer
  - ◆ Head and neck cancers
  - ◆ Melanoma
  - ◆ Leukemias
  - ◆ Lymphomas
  - ◆ Colorectal cancer
  - ◆ Multiple myeloma and myelodysplastic syndromes
  - ◆ Tumor lysis syndrome
  - ◆ Pain management
  - ◆ Chemotherapy-induced nausea and vomiting
  - ◆ Management of chemotherapy-adverse drug reactions

CASE QUESTION

What steps could J.B. have taken to improve his first day on an internal medicine rotation?

A TYPICAL DAY

The most common approach to internal medicine and specialty rotations is centered on rounding, or the meeting of a multidisciplinary team to review patients and make recommendations. In general, however, you typically will be required to arrive well before rounds are scheduled to begin. This early arrival allows you to review medical records and fill out monitoring sheets for all of the patients on a given service. Preceptors may also ask you to meet for prerounds, where you will informally present your patients to your preceptor. During this meeting, the preceptor evaluates your ability to interpret patient data and make therapeutic recommendations while giving you a chance to correct any mistakes before rounds truly begin.

At a predetermined time, the entire medical team will meet to begin rounding. The medical team may consist of a number of individuals, including (but not limited to) attending physicians, resident physicians, pharmacists, nurses, social workers, dieticians, and students. The team moves from patient room to patient room, discussing each case, reviewing patient information, and providing care. This is an ideal opportunity for you to be of service to the team. As medication questions arise, you can act as a resource for the team. If drug-related problems are discovered, you can make recommendations to improve patient care. You may also be called on to create presentations on relevant topics to help the team stay up to date on new research and guidelines. Depending on the individual rotation, rounds may take place a few times per week, once daily, or multiple times each day. When afternoons are free, time is spent working on assorted projects, patient counseling, continued monitoring, and attending grand rounds, or formal case presentations to large audiences of healthcare professionals. Typical projects encountered on clinical rotations may include formal case presentations, journal clubs, pharmacokinetic problems, research, manuscript write-ups, drug information assignments, or drug utilization reviews.

QUICK TIP

If there are other students participating in the rotation, use them to pregrade presentations and projects before turning them in to the preceptor. Getting the opinion of nursing or medical students may fill holes that are often missed when addressing only pharmacy issues.

For those rotations that are not located in teaching hospitals, additional techniques may be employed to get students involved in patient care. Instead of traditional rounding between patient rooms, a central location may be used to conduct rounds (also known as *tabletop rounds*). Other hospitals may utilize pharmacy rounds and written communication to convey pharmacy student recommendations.

PATIENT MONITORING AND THE MEDICAL RECORD

The medical record is the primary source of the important information used to evaluate a patient's medication regimen. To make sense of the large amount of information present in this record, monitoring forms are used to place it in an organized, easy-to-follow framework.

The Monitoring Form

Although rotation preceptors may provide you with a monitoring form, students are usually encouraged to find or create a form that they are comfortable with. A high level of comfort with your monitoring form will allow for more efficient transfer of patient data and easier case presenting. If you attempt to use a new monitoring form for each rotation, any time spent with older versions is lost and the process of getting comfortable must begin anew. For a sample monitoring form, see **Figure 8-1**.

QUICK TIP

To shorten the time spent filling out a monitoring sheet, you can come up with your own abbreviation system, but make sure that you decipher your own code before presenting the case to the medical team!

History and Physical

Once a monitoring form has been obtained, you are ready to access the medical record. Whether this document is on paper or in an electronic medical record (EMR) format, patient data are organized into several important categories. Familiarizing yourself with the organizational flow of the chart can also improve the efficiency of patient monitoring, allowing you to work up more patients and be better prepared for rounds.

Figure 8-1. Sample Patient Monitoring Form

Name		Allergies:		Problem List:	
Room	Age				
MRN	Admit				
Ht	Wt	GFR			
CC:		Home Meds:			
HPI:			Notes:		
PMH:					
		ROS:			
FH:		Physical Findings:			
SH:					

Date	Laboratory and Diagnostic Data	Date	Medications and Fluids

---

QUICK TIP

Each site will have a slightly different charting system, ranging from completely paper based to 100% electronic. Get to know the set up of your rotation site and think of ways to overcome any unique obstacles inherent in each system.

Chief Complaint

The History and Physical (H and P) section is usually the starting point for the patient work-up. This document details the presentation and evaluation of the patient at the time of admission. Located at the top, the Chief Complaint (CC) is a record of the patient's presenting symptoms. Ideally, it is a short sentence written in the patient's own words. A common pitfall for students is to use terms like "chronic obstructive pulmonary disease," "cholecystitis," or "hypertensive emergency" when documenting a CC. These terms and other medical jargon should be avoided and replaced with "shortness of breath," "stomach pain," or "blurry vision" whenever possible. If medical professionals lose focus on the patient and, instead, see only a diagnosis, true patient care cannot be provided and important details may be overlooked. For instance, if a patient presents with a CC of abdominal pain and is diagnosed with cholecystitis and treated with an antibiotic that causes abdominal pain, the patient will likely return to seek additional care. If, instead, the patient's CC is well documented and the medical team proactively educates the patient at discharge, a readmission can often be avoided.

CASE QUESTION

J.B. has documented his first patient's CC as "systolic heart failure," just as it was written in the chart. How might J.B. have better described his patient's CC?

History of Present Illness

It is often cited that patient history is 90% of the diagnosis. For this reason, the History of Present Illness (HPI) section of the H and P should not be overlooked. The wealth of patient information within is vital to developing a prioritized problem list, uncovering potential drug therapy problems, and ensuring hidden problems do not go untreated. Although the true burden of diagnosis falls on the physicians of the medical team, pharmacy students can become extremely valuable when they discover potential drug-related causes of a patient's presenting symptoms. In particular, you should closely evaluate a patient's HPI for drug-related adverse events when the team is having difficulty identifying the source of a patient's symptoms.

Past Medical History

To evaluate a patient's current drug regimen, you must have a clear knowledge of all past diagnoses. Without this list, there is no way to identify medical problems that may be contributing to the patient's current illness or to discover those that are undertreated or overtreated. The Past Medical History (PMH) is often the best source for this information. For most diagnoses, it may be sufficient to simply list whether or not they have occurred, but some diagnoses require additional information. For example, it is usually just as important to know the date of a patient's coronary stent placement as it is to know that the patient had a stent placed at all. If possible, you should attempt to identify dates of diagnosis for each entry in this section of the H and P.

QUICK TIP

The HPI and PMH sections of a chart will be full of abbreviations for symptoms, physical findings, and diseases. See Appendices 2-A, 2-B, and 2-C for a review of the most common medical terminology and abbreviations.

Family and Social History

The Family History (FH) and Social History (SH) sections contain information that is valuable for determining a patient's risk for certain conditions. For example, if a patient presents with shortness of breath, a FH positive for unprovoked blood clots and a SH containing significant smoking history would lead the medical team in two very different directions. SH may also include information on a patient's support system, occupation, diet, and daily life. A common term seen in this section of the chart is *pack year* (py). This value is determined by multiplying the number of packs smoked per day by the years the patient has been smoking. For example, a person that smoked two packs per day for 20 years would have a 40-py history.

CASE QUESTION

The SH of J.B.'s patient explains that he is a nonsmoker, only drinks alcohol on rare occasions, works at a desk job in an office supply company, does not exercise regularly, and eats three healthy meals per day with a snack of potato chips after work. What pieces of information in this SH are important with regard to his current presentation?

Home Medications

An obvious section of interest to pharmacy students is the patient's home medication list. A complete, accurate list must be obtained for care to be transitioned from the outpatient to the inpatient setting. Because obtaining this list of medications is often a source of frustration for healthcare professionals, you have another opportunity to become involved in patient care by ensuring the medication list is completed and verified. This can involve patient and family interviewing, contacting primary care providers, or working with local pharmacies. A complete medication list contains all of the prescription information (drug, dose, route, and frequency), but it may also be important to identify when the last dose was taken (for medications taken sporadically) and how long the patient had been taking the medications (to help identify adverse effects of newer agents). Once a list is obtained, you can evaluate it to identify potential drug therapy problems.

QUICK TIP

Not only should you obtain a list of current home medications, but you should also try to identify any recently discontinued agents. Although the patient has stopped taking them, they may still be contributing to drug-related problems.

Physical Exam and Review of Systems

Although the patient's history plays an enormous role in identifying a diagnosis, the Physical Exam (PE) and Review of Systems (ROS) can bring out additional information to help corroborate the findings or discover hidden medical issues. The PE section, organized by body system, will detail any objective findings from an examination of the patient. Clinicians will perform a number of tests that can usually be categorized as inspection, palpitation, percussion, or auscultation. The ROS, on the other hand, is an attempt to catch any last-minute symptoms that the patient may have overlooked in the HPI. Typically starting from the top of the head, the healthcare provider assessing the patient will ask about symptoms of every major body system, attempting to jog the patient's memory for any abnormal symptoms.

QUICK TIP

Look for groups of positive findings in the PE and ROS sections that may corroborate clinical suspicions. For instance, if an infectious process is suspected, look for fever, tachycardia, chills, and night sweats. Abdominal pain accompanied by a lack of bowel sounds and nausea may signify an obstruction. Shortness of breath, chest pain, and an erythematous calf raises suspicions of a deep vein thrombosis that has caused a pulmonary embolus.

Assessment and Plan

The last entry in the H and P is the physician's Assessment and Plan. Although it is important to document the information contained within these sections, it is also important for you to independently evaluate the patient information and design your own assessment and plan. If you blindly accept the assessment and plan of another healthcare provider, there is a significant chance that drug therapy problems may be overlooked and patient care will not be optimized.

CASE QUESTION

When J.B. presents his patient case at prerounds, the preceptor believes that J.B. has missed some important information regarding the physician's findings when inspecting the patient's extremities. In which section of the H and P could J.B. find this information?

Consultations

After an initial assessment, the admitting physician will often ask for advice from specialists and other healthcare providers in the form of consultations (or a consult). These providers will usually see the patient independently and document their findings in a separate note. The organizational structure of a consult is usually similar to the H and P, flowing from CC and HPI to the consulting healthcare provider's Assessment and Plan. The major difference between the two documents is the focus and depth of discussion. Whereas the H and P is a general overview of the patient, a consult tends to focus on a single symptom, diagnosis, or treatment. When the information located in the H and P is too broad and you need specific information, a consult may contain what is required.

Progress Notes

As days pass and additional information is obtained, the medical team will usually document new information in daily progress notes. These notes tend to be considerably shorter than either the H and P or consults, containing only a few pieces of subjective and objective patient information and updates to the original assessment and plan. These notes are valuable to you throughout the course of the patient's hospital stay because they contain the most up-to-date assessments of the patient's condition and the progress toward therapeutic goals.

Laboratory and Diagnostic Tests

Although the H and P, consultations, and progress notes all contain some laboratory and diagnostic test data, they are only summaries of what the healthcare provider deemed relevant. You should not rely on these abbreviated listings. Instead, a section of the medical record will contain all ordered laboratory and diagnostic data. This section must be inspected closely to appropriately monitor the patient's condition, identify drug-related adverse events, and assess the efficacy of current treatments. One mistake often made by students is to simply scan the laboratory data for values outside of the normal range (usually delineated with an asterisk or arrow). Although this strategy significantly reduces the time spent evaluating laboratory results, it can cause you to overlook important findings. For example, in elderly patients, hemoglobin levels may appear to be within normal limits, but a sudden drop of 1 g/dL or more could indicate an acute bleed, even if the value remains in the normal range. If you simply scan the laboratory data for abnormal findings, the bleed may go unnoticed, delaying treatment and putting the patient at risk for serious medical problems. In addition to these issues, some so-called "normal" values are necessary to rule out potential causes of patient symptoms. Additional discussion of specific laboratory tests is presented later in this chapter.

CASE QUESTION

J.B.'s patient has had a D-dimer ordered to evaluate for the presence of a blood clot. The test has come back negative. Why would it be important for J.B. to include this normal laboratory test in his case presentation?

Medication Administration Record

The Medication Administration Record (MAR) contains a detailed listing of when medications are given to a patient. Nurses use this section of the medical record to sign off when a medication is given, identify modifications to the medication schedule, and document missed doses. Two of the most important uses of the MAR for pharmacy students are to verify the authenticity of drug levels and monitor the use of "as-needed" (PRN) medications. If a serum drug concentration reveals an abnormal level, it is important to correlate the date and time of the serum concentration and the last dose of the medication. At times, levels are drawn inappropriately, resulting in inaccurate serum concentrations. To assess the treatment of pain, nausea, or other conditions treated on an as-needed basis, the use of PRN medications can be monitored from the MAR. The use of opioids around the clock is a red flag that may indicate poorly controlled pain.

QUICK TIP

If a patient is not responding to a given medication treatment, it may be wise to check the MAR before declaring it a failure and moving on to another option. Improper administration or a failure to obtain a medication in short supply may be to blame for a less-than-optimal response.

Nursing Notes

Throughout the workday, nursing staff is responsible for documenting a number of important pieces of patient information. Routine vital sign checks, daily weights, pain ratings, and other assessments may be located in a separate section of the patient chart known as the Nursing Notes. Especially in units with a high level of acuity (such as intensive care units), the nurse's documentation may contain the most up-to-date information on the patient's current state of health.

EVALUATION OF LABORATORY DATA AND DIAGNOSTIC TESTS

Laboratory and diagnostic test data are additional tools that clinicians use to evaluate a patient's CC, identify medical problems, and monitor therapy for both safety and efficacy. Although the greatest emphasis should be placed on patient history, these pieces of objective information can offer additional clues when working up a patient. When abnormal test results are obtained, it is important to place them in the clinical context of the patient's case to avoid simply treating a laboratory value in favor of treating the patient as a whole person. It should also be noted that reference ranges for most laboratory tests vary from institution to institution. Please refer to your rotation site's laboratory information when evaluating these data. See **Appendix 8-A** for a quick reference for common laboratory tests.

QUICK TIP

The Suggested Reading section at the end of this chapter lists in-depth resources that cover the interpretation of laboratory data.

Common Diagnostic Tests

Clinicians will use a number of diagnostic tests to aid in the diagnosis of a patient, in addition to the laboratory tests described in Appendix 8-A. The list of available diagnostic tests is long, and this chapter will focus on a brief overview of only the most commonly ordered tests.

Imaging

A view of an organ or body system can be invaluable when attempting to identify a possible cause of patient symptoms. Instead of using invasive techniques, however, technology has allowed clinicians to have a look at the internal organs of their patients without taking them to the operating room. One of the earliest imaging techniques was X-ray imaging, in use since the late 19th century. X-ray radiation can penetrate the body and is absorbed to varying degrees by different tissues. Larger amounts of X-ray photons are absorbed in denser materials, such as bone, and smaller amounts are absorbed in more porous materials, such as soft tissue. Images can be taken of nearly any part of the body, but they are most commonly taken of the chest, abdomen, and extremities, giving clinicians a clear view of what is happening beneath the surface.

Taking the X-ray one step further, *computed tomography* (CT) *scans* use the old technology of the X-ray to take a series of planar images (or slices) of a patient that can be arranged together with the help of a computer to create a three-dimensional image. The resulting series allows clinicians to "scroll" from a patient's head to toes to view both hard and soft tissues. To make the resulting image clearer, patients will often receive a contrast dye that increases the opacity of softer tissues or liquids and enhances the image quality.

More recently, the technology of *magnetic resonance imaging* (MRI) has given clinicians a new avenue to obtain images of soft tissues that typically give poor results under X-ray. The MRI uses powerful magnetic fields to alter the alignment of cellular nuclei. When a radiofrequency is applied, this alignment is displaced and causes the release of energy that can be translated to an image. The major benefits of this technology include a lack of radiation and better imaging of soft tissues, although patients must be able to lie still for extended periods of time within the small, noisy tube of the MRI scanner, conditions that often require patient sedation or use of anxiolytics. In addition to these limitations, patients with implanted materials may not be able to have the imaging performed if they are magnetically active.

QUICK TIP

Certain transdermal patches contain small amounts of metal and must be removed before performing an MRI scan.

Lastly, patients may also avoid the potentially damaging effects of radiation if they can undergo imaging via ultrasound technology. This form of imaging uses high-frequency sound waves to obtain images of tissues and organs. Although the images are much less clear than those seen with MRI, the technology is much more affordable, is readily available, and may be sufficient for a number of applications, such as cardiac imaging and screening for deep vein thrombosis.

CASE QUESTION

What types of noninvasive imaging techniques are available to assess J.B.'s patient's heart function?

Cardiovascular Tests

Perhaps the simplest of cardiovascular tests is the *electrocardiogram* (EKG or ECG). Obtained by placing a series of leads on the chest, arms, and leg, the EKG measures the electrical activity of the heart. The tracing that is produced as a result can be used to evaluate everything from the heart's rhythm, rate, and size to the presence of a myocardial infarction, pericarditis, and adverse drug effects.

QUICK TIP

EKG leads are very sensitive to movement. If a patient does not lie still during the test, the resulting tracing may contain "artifact," or changes to the EKG based on patient movement and not alterations in cardiac conduction. EKG artifact often resembles ventricular fibrillation.

If a patient presents with complaints of chest pain, clinicians may choose to perform a *stress test*. This test requires a patient to exercise on a treadmill or with the aid of pharmacological agents in an attempt to recreate the circumstances that cause symptoms of ischemia. As the heart is "stressed," an EKG and, possibly, an imaging study of the heart are performed to capture what is happening at the level of the coronary arteries. Although a negative stress test cannot rule out the possibility of myocardial ischemia, the test is a noninvasive option in the diagnosis of coronary artery disease.

Slightly more invasive than a stress test, *coronary catheterization* involves threading a small catheter from the femoral or radial artery into the coronary vasculature. Radiopaque dye can then be injected directly into the small blood vessels and images can be taken to identify narrowing of the arteries, signifying the presence of an atherosclerotic plaque. If significant blockages are discovered, a diagnostic procedure can quickly become therapeutic if the cardiologist inserts a stent to open the narrowing arteries.

Respiratory Tests

The most basic of pulmonary tests, *pulse oximetry* is a noninvasive way to assess the degree of oxygenation a patient is achieving. To obtain a reading, a source of infrared light is placed on a thin portion of the patient's body, typically a finger. A probe on the other side of the device can calculate the percentage of oxygenation based on the amount of light reaching the other side of the patient. Although decreased oxygenation can be the result of a number of disease states, pulse oximetry allows for the rapid detection of worsening pulmonary function.

A *ventilation-perfusion* (V/Q) *scan* is a form of imaging study that is unique to the respiratory system. Two sets of images are taken of the patient's lungs and pulmonary vasculature. First, the patient is asked to inhale radiolabeled tracers before an image is taken of the lung field. Next, contrast dye is injected into the pulmonary vasculature and a second image is taken of the blood flow. Under normal circumstances, these two images should match one another, with the vasculature reaching all of the areas with proven ventilation. In the case of a pulmonary embolism, portions of the vasculature may be occluded by the clot, causing a mismatch between the two images and a diagnosis of a pulmonary embolus. Although the V/Q scan is still in use today, it is quickly being overtaken by CT angiography, using the CT technology discussed above to look specifically at the pulmonary vasculature for emboli.

QUICK TIP

V/Q scans are still utilized in patients with poor renal function that cannot tolerate the contrast needed to perform a CT scan of the pulmonary vasculature.

Slightly more invasive than the tests described above, *bronchoscopy* involves inserting a camera into the bronchial tree to look for any abnormalities. In most cases, a flexible bronchoscope is inserted into the nose or mouth of a patient and advanced into the bronchus. In addition to simply obtaining images, tissue or fluid samples also may be obtained for further evaluation or culture. Bronchoscopy is, at times, a therapeutic procedure when the clinician uses the bronchoscope to remove secretions, insert stents, or perform ablative procedures.

Gastrointestinal Tests

A common, noninvasive test used to visualize the gastrointestinal tract is the *barium study*. Because barium sulfate is a radiopaque substance, it is administered to a patient and coats the hollow components of the gastrointestinal tract. When an X-ray image is taken, the dense barium allows for visualization of these typically hard-to-capture organs. When administered via an oral suspension, the barium swallow study can identify patients at risk for aspiration of food particles. If the large intestine needs to be evaluated, a barium enema may be prepared.

Similar to bronchoscopy, slightly more invasive scope procedures can be performed in the gastrointestinal system as well. Called *endoscopy* when visualizing the upper gastrointestinal tract and *colonoscopy* when used to visualize the large intestine, the procedures are largely similar. If necessary, tissue samples can be obtained for further investigation, as is often the case when polyps are discovered in the colon. In addition to visualizing the intestines, endoscopes can also examine the pancreatic and biliary systems in a procedure called an *endoscopic retrograde cholangiopancreatography* (ERCP). With the advent of less-invasive imaging techniques such as MRI, ERCP is rarely performed.

Central Nervous System Tests

Similar to the EKG, electrodes can be placed on the surface of the scalp to measure the electrical activity of the brain. Called *electroencephalography* (EEG), the resulting tracings can be used to identify seizure activity and diagnose its type. If the location of the seizure activity can be pinpointed with an EEG, a patient may become a candidate for a surgical intervention to remove the source.

In certain instances, clinicians require access to a patient's cerebrospinal fluid. Most often, this is to diagnose meningitis or cancer or to administer medications directly into the central nervous system. Called a *lumbar puncture*, this invasive test requires patients to lie on their side in the fetal position. By bringing their legs toward their chest, the spaces between the vertebrae are widened, allowing for the insertion of a needle and withdrawal of a small amount of cerebrospinal fluid for evaluation.

DEVELOPING AND IMPLEMENTING A PHARMACEUTICAL CARE PLAN

Once all of the pertinent patient data has been collected and analyzed, it is time to design a pharmaceutical care plan that addresses patient needs. A complete plan includes goals, rationale, monitoring parameters, patient education, and follow-up, in addition to simply recommending medication regimen alterations.

Goals of Treatment

Before a single medication is ordered, the endpoint of therapy must be identified. By beginning with the end in mind, clinicians can ensure that all members of the healthcare team, including the patient, have realistic expectations, that outcomes can be measured, and that an appropriate time frame is established. All good therapeutic goals contain the same elements: they are specific to a medical problem, contain measureable parameters, are realistic, and contain a time frame for completion. When any of these components are missing, the therapeutic goal is incomplete and may lead to patient misconceptions, inappropriate drug therapy decisions, or even adverse effects. For example, a nonspecific goal of "better memory" in patients with Alzheimer's dementia may lead to a patient's false expectation of the benefits of cholinesterase inhibitors. On the other hand, a lack of measurable parameters may be a cause of medical treatment that lasts beyond the therapeutic intention of the prescriber, as is the case in patients treated with granulocyte colony-stimulating factor beyond the point of white blood cell count recovery. Lastly, it is vital to include the patient when establishing goals of therapy. When the patient participates in the process of goal development, important expectations and preferences can be uncovered that would otherwise go unnoticed.

QUICK TIP

Common goals of therapy include cure, control of symptoms, slowed progression, and prevention of a disease.

CASE QUESTION

J.B. has failed to document a therapeutic goal for his patient with congestive heart failure. Compose a complete goal of treatment for his patient.

Therapeutic Interventions and Rationale

To fulfill the goals of therapy, actions must be taken to optimize the patient's drug therapy. The types of interventions employed to reach these goals are numerous and may include initiating drug therapy, altering dosage, discontinuing drug therapy, ordering laboratory tests, or considering nonpharmacological interventions, among others. When recommending alterations to the drug therapy regimen, a complete order should be communicated to the prescriber, with the drug name, dose, route, frequency, and, whenever possible, duration included in the recommendation. Exact doses should be used in the place of dose ranges.

In addition to making recommendations, including evidence-based rationale for the decisions made can drastically improve the chances of having prescriber-approved recommendations. Citing national guidelines, local protocols, and primary literature serves as both a final check of your recommendations and a means to prove the need for an intervention.

CASE QUESTION

J.B. has recommended the addition of spironolactone 25 to 50 mg to this patient's medication regimen. How can this recommendation be improved?

Patient Education

Patient education, although often an afterthought in the inpatient setting, must be completed if the patient is to understand the treatments being implemented and adhere to them after discharge. A well-informed patient is often a safer, healthier patient, and, for these reasons, you can play an important role in improving patient education regarding medication therapy. In addition to the typical education that includes the names, doses, and indications for all new medications, clinicians will include unique pieces of information about the specific drugs being added. For example, when initiating hypothyroidism treatment, it is important to mention the unique administration requirements of levothyroxine. When discussing adverse drug reactions, the discussion should be limited to only the most common or particularly important reactions. A complete review of all adverse events will likely be time consuming and only serve to frighten patients into nonadherence. Also included in the educational component of the therapeutic plan are any nonpharmacological treatments that a patient may use to control his or her medical problems. Diet, exercise, and other nonpharmacological treatment strategies may be just as, if not more, important than medical management for a number of conditions.

QUICK TIP

If possible, medical jargon should be avoided during patient education to increase the chances of patient understanding and adherence.

Monitoring Parameters and Follow-Up

Both safety and efficacy of medical treatments must be closely monitored to ensure a satisfactory outcome. Similar to the goals of treatment, the parameters outlined in this section of the treatment plan must be specific, be measurable, and include a time frame for evaluation. Patient signs, symptoms, laboratory data, and diagnostic tests may all be included as monitoring parameters. For certain endpoints, such as blood pressure and blood glucose, follow-up evaluation may occur within 24 hours, whereas other parameters, such as thyroid function and cholesterol levels, are slower to react to changes in medication therapy. When following patients throughout their stay, the monitoring parameters should begin to mirror the goals described earlier in the care plan. If the parameters do not appear to be improving or are, in fact, worsening, a re-evaluation of the medication regimen is necessary to correct any issues impeding the patient's progress toward recovery.

CASE QUESTION

J.B.'s spironolactone recommendation has been presented to his preceptor during prerounds, but he has not included monitoring parameters. Design a set of monitoring parameters for this new medication.

ROUNDING

After the pharmaceutical care plan has been compiled, you are prepared to attend a prerounding session with your preceptor. In general, prerounding will require you to present each case being monitored. If the data gathering performed beforehand was complete, you should have all of the necessary information to answer your preceptor's questions and present a complete case. If there is missing information, however, there is still time to perform further investigation before the true rounding experience begins. In cases where there are multiple students on rotation with a single preceptor, the students that are not presenting a case should listen carefully and take notes on their peer's case presentation. They may be called on to contribute to the discussion and develop recommendations for patients that they have not monitored personally.

At a prespecified time, the multidisciplinary team will be asked to assemble for rounds to begin. Because the team is made up of a number of different practitioners, this is an excellent opportunity for pharmacy students to participate in both learning from the members in those professions and providing education regarding drug therapy. Upon arrival, you should introduce yourself to the team with both your name and role on the team. As the team moves from patient to patient, you should listen intently and contribute to the discussion whenever possible. Do not hesitate to ask questions if there is a topic with which you are unfamiliar, but avoid becoming burdensome to the team. There will be situations in which the team may ask you to provide support by educating patients, retrieving medical literature, or presenting a variety of drug topics. You should ensure the turnaround time on these requests is timely and the projects are complete. No doubt, there will be situations in which you may not be sure of the appropriate answer to a clinical question. It is of utmost importance that you are honest with the team; do not guess about matters regarding patient care and assure the team that you will perform the necessary research to find the answer.

CASE QUESTION

J.B. is asked to identify the benefits of adding spironolactone to the patient's medication regimen. He answers that he thinks "it will make the patient's heart failure better." How should J.B. handle a situation in which he does not have a clear answer?

When the team's rounds reach a patient with drug therapy problems, you should utilize the pharmaceutical care plan to articulate all of the important components of the treatment plan. Using the skills described in Chapter 6, a short case presentation may be appropriate to provide relevant background information on the patient case. Provide the team with a complete recommendation, including goals, the intervention itself, rationale, monitoring parameters, and follow-up. Be prepared to defend the recommendation using pertinent patient information that was gathered in the subjective and objective sections of the plan. It should be noted, however, that even when a sound recommendation is made, the prescriber may choose an alternative intervention. After ensuring proper understanding of the recommendations, you should remain professional in these situations and avoid aggressive or confrontational behavior.

DOCUMENTATION

Some rotations may give you the opportunity to document interventions or recommendations in the patient chart. It is important to recognize that anything that is a part of the record is a legal document. For this reason, you must follow all protocols and procedures of the institution. There are a number of different techniques used to document recommendations, including SOAP, SBAR, FARM, and others. SOAP notes, which contain subjective, objective, assessment, and plan sections, are one of the most commonly used documentation schemes and are familiar to most students. SBAR, an abbreviation for situation, background, assessment, and recommendation, along with FARM, an abbreviation for findings, assessment, resolution, and management, are used less often but may still be encountered while on rotations, along with any number of other schemes.

Regardless of which format you choose, there are a number of guidelines that you should follow:

- Flowery language should be avoided in favor of clear, concise statements. The notes should be kept as short as possible while still containing all relevant information. Most healthcare providers are extremely busy, and long notes are often overlooked.

- Although they may shorten note length, unapproved abbreviations should be avoided to decrease the chance of misinterpretation of the note.

- Avoid documenting personal opinion or speculation in favor of evidence-based recommendations.

- Like other recommendations, written suggestions should be worded carefully to avoid making the prescriber feel attacked or inferior.

- Always ensure that the note is placed in the appropriate chart by including the patient's demographic data, the date, the time, and the author's signature.

SUGGESTED READING

Cipolle RJ, Strand LM, Morely PC. *Pharmaceutical Care Practice: The Clinician's Guide*. 2nd ed. New York, NY: McGraw-Hill; 2004.

Groopman J. *How Doctors Think*. Boston, MA: Houghton Mifflin; 2007.

Lee M. *Basic Skills in Interpreting Laboratory Data*. 5th ed. Bethesda, MD: American Society of Health-System Pharmacists; 2013.

Schmidt J, Wierczorkiewicz J. *Interpreting Laboratory Data: A Point of Care Guide*. Bethesda, MD: American Society of Health-System Pharmacists; 2011.

APPENDIX 8-A.   COMMON LABORATORY TESTS

CHEMISTRY PANEL

Blood chemistry is one of the most common tests obtained in the inpatient setting. In general, there are seven major components to a chemistry panel: sodium, potassium, chloride, carbon dioxide (or bicarbonate), blood glucose, blood urea nitrogen (BUN), and serum creatinine. The utility of these tests is far-reaching and applicable to many different disease states and drug therapies.

Sodium

- Adult reference range, 135 to 145 mEq/L
- Major role in fluid balance, maintaining cellular osmolality, and nervous system conduction
- Patients with both increased and decreased sodium levels may present with central nervous system findings, such as confusion, unsteady gait, agitation, lethargy, coma, or even death.
- May be elevated by
  - Increased sodium intake
  - Loss of free water
  - Diabetes insipidus
  - Lithium
  - Colchicine
- May be decreased by
  - Decrease in total body sodium
  - Increases in body water
  - Congestive heart failure
  - Renal impairment
  - Syndrome of inappropriate antidiuretic hormone
  - Diuretics
  - Aldosterone antagonists
  - Carbamazepine
- Hyperglycemia may cause falsely reduced sodium levels. The following equation can be used to correct the sodium level:

  Corrected Sodium = Measured Sodium + [(Serum Glucose - 100/100) x 1.6]

Potassium

- Adult reference range, 3.5 to 5 mEq/L
- Primary role is in nervous system depolarization, especially in skeletal and cardiac muscle
- Patients with increased or decreased levels are at risk for developing cramps, muscle twitching, EKG changes, and cardiac arrhythmias.

- May be elevated by
  - ☐ Renal impairment
  - ☐ Angiotensin converting enzyme (ACE) inhibitors
  - ☐ Angiotensin receptor blockers (ARBs)
  - ☐ Aldosterone antagonists
  - ☐ Potassium supplementation
- May be decreased by
  - ☐ Diminished potassium intake
  - ☐ Diuretics
  - ☐ Laxatives
  - ☐ Corticosteroids
- May be falsely elevated by red blood cell lysis
- Low magnesium levels must also be corrected before hypokalemia will improve.

Chloride

- Adult reference range, 95 to 105 mEq/L
- Mainly transferred around the body in a passive manner
- May be elevated by
  - ☐ Dehydration
  - ☐ Acidosis
- May be decreased by
  - ☐ Fluid overload
  - ☐ Alkalosis
- Due to passive transport, any medication that alters sodium levels may influence chloride ions.

Serum Bicarbonate

- Adult reference range, 24 to 30 mEq/L
- Measures both the base (bicarbonate) and acid (carbon dioxide) components of the blood's primary buffer system
- May be elevated by
  - ☐ Alkalosis
  - ☐ Loop diuretics
  - ☐ Thiazide diuretics
- May be decreased by
  - ☐ Acidosis
  - ☐ Acetazolamide

Blood Glucose

- Typical blood glucose levels will vary depending on a number of factors, including time of day, time of last meal, and content of last meal.

- Fasting blood glucose is usually drawn before a patient has had breakfast in the morning.
  - Adult reference range, <100 mg/dL
- Postprandial glucose level is obtained 2 hours after the beginning of a meal.
  - Adult reference range, <140 mg/dL
- May be elevated by
  - Diabetes
  - Improperly obtained level (such as nonfasting level or a level drawn earlier than 2 hours post-prandially)
  - Active infection
  - Corticosteroids
  - Thiazide diuretics
  - Atypical antipsychotics
  - Niacin
- May be decreased by
  - Nutrition issues
  - Inappropriate doses of diabetes medications such as insulin, sulfonylureas, or meglitinides
- For additional information regarding glucose levels and diabetes, see the Glucose Metabolism section below.

Blood Urea Nitrogen (BUN)

- Adult reference range, 7 to 20 mg/dL
- Produced when proteins are broken down and is primarily removed by the kidneys
- May be elevated by
  - Gastrointestinal bleeding
  - Muscle damage
  - Kidney impairment
- May be decreased by
  - Malnourishment
  - Liver dysfunction
- The relationship between BUN and serum creatinine can be indicative of the type of renal issues a patient may have:
  - If the ratio of the two values is greater than 20:1, the likely source of the problem is prerenal, such as dehydration.
  - For ratios less than 20:1, potential intrinsic or postrenal disease should be considered.

Serum Creatinine

- Adult reference range, 0.5 to 1.4 mg/dL
- Because it passes almost entirely into the urine via glomerular filtration, it can be used as a surrogate marker of kidney function.

- May be falsely elevated in patients with above-average muscle mass
- May be falsely reduced in frail, elderly patients and patients with limb amputations
- A number of equations may be used to convert serum creatinine levels into an estimation of glomerular filtration rate (GFR):
  - Cockcroft–Gault
  - Modification of Diet in Renal Disease (MDRD)
  - Schwartz formula

COMPLETE BLOOD COUNT AND OTHER HEMATOLOGICAL TESTS

The complete blood count, or CBC, is a quick way to evaluate potential signs of infection, bleeding, or other disorders. Concentrations of white blood cells, hemoglobin, hematocrit, and platelets are the typical components of a CBC. When ordered with a differential, additional information may be obtained, including a breakdown of the number of neutrophils, lymphocytes, eosinophils, and basophils.

White Blood Cell Counts

- Adult reference range, 4,500 to 11,000 cells/mm^3
- Elevated in response to infections
- Certain patient populations may have a blunted white blood cell response.
  - The presence of immature white cells (called *bands*) may be a sign of infection in these patients.
- May be falsely elevated in patients taking corticosteroids
- May be decreased by
  - Sepsis
  - Cancer
  - Chemotherapeutic agents
- A differential can give clinicians additional insights into a patient's condition that are not possible to obtain with a simple CBC.
  - Elevated neutrophil counts typically occur in bacterial infections.
  - Eosinophilia is often the result of an allergic response or parasitic infections.
  - Lymphocytes are elevated in viral infections.

Hemoglobin

- Adult reference range, 12.0 to 16.5 g/dL
- Assesses oxygen-carrying capacity of a patient's red blood cells
- Need additional tests to identify the cause of the anemia
  - Mean corpuscular volume (MCV) (adult reference range, 80 to 100 fL/cell) and mean corpuscular hemoglobin (MCH) (adult reference range, 26 to 34 pg/cell) can be used to evaluate red blood cell size and color, respectively.
  - In iron-deficiency anemia, the red blood cells produced are smaller in size and pale, or microcytic and hypochromic.

- ◻ In vitamin B_{12} or folate deficiency, red blood cells appear normal in color but are often large in size, or megaloblastic.
- ◻ If the red blood cells appear normal in size and color, the cause of the anemia may be the destruction of the cells (hemolytic anemia), acute blood loss, or anemia of chronic disease.

Platelet Count

- Adult reference range, 150,000 to 450,000 cells/mm³
- Measures a patient's ability to form a blood clot
- Risk for bleeding is not significantly elevated until levels fall below 50,000 cells/mm³.
- May be reduced by
  - ◻ Heparin-induced thrombocytopenia
  - ◻ Chemotherapy
  - ◻ Linezolid
- Additional lab tests are needed to evaluate the function of the clotting cascade.
  - ◻ International normalized ratio (INR) measures the effect of warfarin.
  - ◻ Activated partial thromboplastin time is used to monitor the effect of heparin.

URINALYSIS

When examining the results of a urinalysis, positive findings may be lost in the numerous components reported.

Macroscopic Analysis

- Leukocyte esterase, an enzyme produced by white blood cells, is indicative of an infection.
- Nitrites, a byproduct of gram-negative bacterial metabolism, are also indicative of an infection.
- Glucose and ketones in the urine may portend of poor glucose control or diabetic ketoacidosis, respectively.
- Proteinuria and hematuria are signs of kidney damage.
- Bilirubin in the urine may predict hepatic dysfunction.

Microscopic Analysis

- Culture and sensitivity remains the gold standard for detecting a urinary tract infection, although this process takes time.
- Actual counts of white blood cells and bacteria can be performed under microscopic analysis.
- Epithelial cells identified in the microscopic analysis suggest a contaminated urine sample was collected.

THYROID FUNCTION TESTS

One potential underlying cause of many different clinical syndromes is thyroid dysfunction. Hypo-thyroidism may masquerade as depression or congestive heart failure, whereas hyperthyroidism may resemble atrial fibrillation or resistant hypertension.

Free Thyroxine

- Adult reference range, 0.8 to 1.5 ng/dL

- Relationship between free thyroxine and thyroid stimulating hormone can be used to identify primary versus secondary thyroid problems.

Thyroid Stimulating Hormone (TSH)

- Adult reference range, 0.25 to 6.7 milliunits/L

- Is primary test used to assess treatment for hypothyroidism

  □ An elevated TSH is a sign that the central nervous system is calling for the production of additional thyroid hormone.

  □ When TSH is low, doses of thyroid hormone are likely too high.

- Monitoring of therapy takes place at 8- to 12-week intervals after initiation and dose titrations.

LIVER FUNCTION TESTS

The laboratory tests known as liver function tests are the aspartate aminotransferase (AST), alanine aminotransferase (ALT), and alkaline phosphatase. These enzymes can be found primarily in hepatocytes and are leaked into the bloodstream when damage occurs to the liver. The cutoff for a positive finding is an elevation three times the upper limit of normal. Although the AST, ALT, and alkaline phosphatase tests are known as the liver function tests, they are actually measures of liver dysfunction, or damage to hepatocytes. Elevated bilirubin and ammonia levels, elevated INR and activated partial thromboplastin time, and decreased albumin are all potential signs of a failing liver.

Aspartate Aminotransferase (AST)

- Adult reference range, <35 units/L

- Elevated in response to liver damage, such as alcoholic liver disease, hepatitis, or medication toxicity

Alanine Aminotransferase (ALT)

- Adult reference range, <35 units/L

- Elevated in many of the same situations as the AST

Alkaline Phosphatase

- Adult reference range, 30 to 120 units/L[3]

- Although it may be elevated in the same situations as the AST and ALT, it is traditionally the hallmark of obstructive liver disease.

CARDIOVASCULAR TESTS

Cardiovascular diseases continue to be a leading cause of hospital admissions. In addition to a number of diagnostic tests and imaging studies, laboratory values can aid clinicians in the diagnosis of cardiovascular diseases such as acute coronary syndromes and congestive heart failure.

Troponin

- Adult reference range depends on subtype and assay used

- Found primarily in the cardiac tissue

- In the setting of myocardial infarction, levels begin to rise in approximately 4 hours and peak in 24 hours.

- A series of three levels are drawn every 4 to 8 hours after admission.

- Renal function can have a significant impact on circulating troponin levels, making clinical decision making difficult.

Brain Natriuretic Peptide (BNP)

- Adult reference range, <100 pg/mL

- Released in response to increased circulating blood volumes or pressure

- Often elevated in patients with congestive heart failure

- Influenced by renal function, age, and patient weight

  ☐ N-terminal proBNP, a precursor to BNP, is less likely to be affected by patient age and weight.

- May also be elevated in cases of pulmonary embolism, cor pulmonale, and severe pulmonary hypertension

GLUCOSE METABOLISM

Blood glucose control is usually closely monitored in patients with and without diabetes in the inpatient setting. Obtaining point-of-care glucose levels allows clinicians to evaluate short-term glucose control that is heavily influenced by a number of factors. Long-term control may be assessed using a hemoglobin A1c level. When blood glucose control is exceedingly poor, patients with diabetes are at risk for developing diabetic ketoacidosis, a healthcare emergency that must be identified and treated before serious, long-lasting consequences take place.

Hemoglobin A1c

- Adult reference range, <6%

- In patients with diabetes, considered controlled when <7%

- Expressed as a percentage, measures the amount of glucose that has been incorporated into hemoglobin molecules

- Roughly proportionate to the average serum glucose levels over 3 months

Serum Ketones (Beta-Hydroxybutyrate)

- Adult reference range, <0.4 mmol/L

- Urine ketones are used as a screening tool for diabetic ketoacidosis, although a positive finding is not definitive.

  ☐ May be increased in the setting of starvation, high-fat diet, or certain medications

- Serum ketones are much more conclusive evidence of diabetic ketoacidosis.

ARTERIAL BLOOD GASES

A staple of intensive care units, arterial blood gases are a necessary (and often painful) test used to identify acid–base disorders. The components of an arterial blood gas are the blood pH, partial pressure of oxygen, partial pressure of carbon dioxide, and serum bicarbonate.

Serum pH

- Adult reference range, 7.35 to 7.45
- Due to compensation, a normal serum pH may not eliminate the possibility of an acid–base disturbance.

Partial Pressure of Carbon Dioxide

- Adult reference range, 36 to 44 mmHg
- Acts as an acid in the body
- Elevated in cases of respiratory acidosis
- Reduced by hyperventilation
- Compensatory mechanisms will rapidly reduce carbon dioxide in patients with metabolic acidosis.

Serum Bicarbonate

- Adult reference range, 21 to 28 mmol/L
- Acts as a base in the body
- Reduced in cases of metabolic acidosis
- Compensatory mechanisms will slowly increase serum bicarbonate in patients with respiratory acidosis.

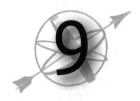

HOSPITAL OR HEALTH-SYSTEM PHARMACY

Dale E. English II, PharmD, FASHP, and John E. Murphy, PharmD, FCCP, FASHP

CASE

F.C. is a pharmacy student beginning a health-system pharmacy APPE rotation in a hospital setting. While going through the student orientation process during the first morning of the rotation, her preceptor is interrupted by one of the other pharmacists asking for assistance. When checking the compounded sterile products that morning, the pharmacist discovered a vancomycin 2-gram intravenous piggyback (IVPB) prepared for a patient. The orders state that the dose is to be infused over a 1-hour period. The pharmacist wants to get confirmation on the appropriateness of the dose and infusion duration for the patient for whom it was prescribed. F.C. is asked to assist the pharmacist in obtaining the information necessary to make this determination.

WHY IT'S ESSENTIAL

As the landscape of healthcare and the profession of pharmacy continue to change, it is important to consider both the challenges and opportunities that the changes create. Pharmacy students and practicing pharmacists must remain competent and confident in their skills as clinical practitioners to participate fully in the many patient care opportunities that are currently available, as well as those that develop over time.

Health-system pharmacy practice in hospitals and other settings is often a required core rotation that provides a foundation on which the education of new pharmacists is grounded and is also a key component on which some other APPE rotations are based. Thus, the skills you should be exposed to and master are vital not only for positive patient outcomes in hospitals but also for overall healthcare quality in a variety of settings. You should make the most of the health-system pharmacy APPE rotation to better understand the entire patient care process, from prevention of disease, to hospital admission, discharge, and follow-up. This process should be viewed as a continuous cycle that, if done correctly, minimizes hospital admissions and readmissions while maximizing patient outcomes.

Full understanding of the concepts relating to sterile technique, pharmaceutical calculations, pharmaceutical compounding, and pharmacokinetic monitoring are critical to enhancing the safety of patients and are fundamental to ensuring the appropriate distribution of the correct medications in the exact dosage and dosage form. Medication-use evaluations are also a component of patient safety that focus on retrospective review of treatment patterns to determine if the patterns are appropriate or if interventions should be made to improve overall treatment.

A Typical Day

A wide variety of activities exist in this type of rotation. You will most certainly be exposed to the dispensing and compounding of medications, along with a number of other clinical and patient safety experiences. The setting for the rotation may be a central pharmacy or, increasingly, decentralized pharmacies throughout the institution. In addition to fulfilling the role of pharmacy technician and pharmacist, there may also be opportunities to experience services provided by other health professionals, such as respiratory therapy, nursing, laboratory, and surgery, among other ancillary departments. Lastly, some rotations give students early exposure to clinical experiences on patient floors. A review of Chapter 8 should help prepare you when this option is presented.

A variety of studies have documented the importance of the types of pharmacists' services that are commonly the focus of hospital and health-system rotations.[1,2] The core services routinely provided in institutional settings are also documented in surveys conducted by the American Society of Health-System Pharmacists (ASHP).[3-5] For example, pharmacokinetic monitoring and renal dosing services are provided in more than 90% of surveyed institutions, with more than 75% of these allowing pharmacists to order initial drug concentrations and adjust doses. Further, staff pharmacists, rather than specialists, generally provide these services. The ASHP national surveys also indicate that pharmacists increasingly participate in therapeutic interchange, standardization of infusion concentrations, and optimization of the technology, such as bar coding, automated dispensing, and computerized prescriber order entry.

> *"The practice of individualized medicine is the forefront of optimal patient care. Designing medication regimens to fit the specific needs of each individual patient goes beyond just the selection of the medication. It includes determining the timing, dosing, and frequency of each drug, of which pharmacokinetics often plays an extensive role. For pharmacy students, learning and understanding pharmacokinetics is critical for future pharmacy practice."—Student*

Arriving Prepared

- As with all rotations, contact the preceptor several days before the rotation begins to ask about required readings, specific coursework to review, and logistical information (e.g., parking, expected hours, where and when to meet on the first day).
- Review the rotation syllabus.
- Arrive professionally dressed, including wearing a white coat.
- Bring a device for performing calculations, including natural log (ln) functions.
- Bring electronic or pocket reference guides.
- Bring some type of electronic or paper notebook for recording information.
- Review pertinent class notes:
  - ☐ Basic and clinical pharmacokinetics
  - ☐ Principles of therapeutic drug monitoring
  - ☐ Therapeutic ranges and common doses for medicines routinely evaluated with drug concentration measurements

- Approaches to dose adjustments for patients with diminished renal function
- Sterile and nonsterile compounding
- Pharmacy calculations
- Medication error prevention and quality assurance
- Personnel management
- Presentation skills
- Patient interviewing and counseling skills
- Technology in healthcare systems
- The impact of the following on medication dosing:
  - Aging
  - Reduced renal or hepatic function
  - Various diseases
  - Obesity
- Drug and food interactions

PHARMACY CALCULATIONS

Your health-system or hospital pharmacy rotation offers the ideal setting to utilize your skills in pharmacokinetics, renal dosing, and other pharmacy-related calculations. By applying what you have learned in the classroom to real-life patients, you can have a significant impact by individualizing medication regimens to minimize adverse events and maximize outcomes.

Applied Pharmacokinetics

Typical activities associated with applying pharmacokinetic principles to the care of individual patients may include the following:

- Daily review of drug concentrations measured in the hospital to determine if they are within the commonly accepted therapeutic ranges
- Reviewing patient charts to determine characteristics that might impact the pharmacokinetics of a drug in question, such as estimated renal and hepatic function, potential drug–drug or drug–food interactions, and patient weight, age, and sex
- Predicting concentrations based on the drug's population pharmacokinetic values and the patient's characteristics
- Evaluating the accuracy of measured concentrations, such as determining whether concentrations were drawn at the time scheduled or if the dose was given at the correct time (particularly important when predictions of concentrations are far from those measured)
- Scheduling ordered drug concentrations
- Determining the need for additional monitoring of drug concentrations, other laboratory tests, and patient outcome measures

CASE QUESTION

What are two important pieces of patient-related information that will help determine if the 2-gram dose is appropriate for the patient?

You should be versed in the use of the pharmacokinetic formulas (see Appendix 9-A) that form the basis of calculations used for the various dosing situations, should possess a basic understanding of therapeutic drug monitoring principles, should know the commonly accepted therapeutic range for drugs that may be monitored at the institution (see Appendix 9-B), and should have a good understanding of the outcomes expected for the drugs that are routinely monitored. It is important to have ready access to information on pharmacokinetic population values for the drugs that are monitored (i.e., clearance, volume of distribution, and half-life), as well as information on how patient characteristics and drug–drug or drug–food interactions may impact the population values. The information is available in textbooks, or the pharmacokinetic values can be found in the product information (package insert) or primary literature.[6,7]

QUICK TIP

Predicting measured drug concentrations based on population values helps students learn how often the predictors are reasonably accurate and gives a sense of their utility or lack of utility when determining a dose and schedule for desired steady-state concentrations of a drug. Unfortunately, errors in the system of drug administration often impact concentrations more than variability of the patient compared to the population. A missed dose or a concentration drawn at the wrong time can create large differences in predicted and actual concentrations, even if the patient fits the population values closely.

QUICK TIP

A variety of individuals will be important to appropriately assess measured drug concentrations and patient outcomes. Get to know individuals in the laboratory that can help troubleshoot unusual concentrations. Phlebotomists are critical to drawing concentrations at the right time. Finally, nurses that administer the medications can let you know if the doses were given off schedule.

When students participate in the pharmacokinetic monitoring of patients, typical activities will vary according to how patients are identified for consultation or for dosing and monitoring recommendations. For example, in a more passive service, where formal consultations do not originate from a prescriber's request, pharmacists may monitor all drug concentrations measured in the institution and follow up on those that are above or below the drug's generally accepted therapeutic range. In this approach, a trip to the patient's floor to review a chart will prepare you to provide suggestions to the pharmacist in charge. These recommendations might include such actions as altering a dose, schedule adjustment, or additional monitoring.

QUICK TIP

Having a specific monitoring form for evaluating patients on whom therapeutic drug monitoring is being performed can add consistency and efficiency in following patients. Depending on the institution, this information may or may not be recorded in the chart or on department-specific forms.

CASE QUESTION

Where can F.C. go to determine her patient's renal function and weight so that she can help her preceptor answer the vancomycin dosing question?

QUICK TIP

Nurses are allowed a margin of time (typically ±30 minutes) for administering scheduled medications without having to report the dose as given early or late. Thus, even though a dose is reported as being given on time, it may actually have been administered at a slightly different time. For many drugs, this does not cause significant problems. When peak and trough concentrations are ordered for drugs with infusion times that could overlap the drawing time, however, changes in start time can influence proper assessment of the patient.

Renal Dosing

Most hospital pharmacy departments in the United States provide a renal dosing program. In such programs, the pharmacy is alerted when estimated or actual creatinine clearance (CrCl) (or glomerular filtration rate) for a patient falls below a certain value. This then triggers an examination of the patient's medication record to determine whether he or she is receiving medications primarily eliminated by the kidneys. A pharmacist may then make a recommendation for the dose to be decreased, dosing interval to be increased, or some combination of the two, to reduce the risk of toxicity caused by higher drug concentrations. In some cases, these recommendations also result in the institution's reduced medication costs. A survey of critical care and nephrology pharmacists indicated that the most frequently adjusted drugs/categories included (among the top five rankings) aminoglycosides, vancomycin, enoxaparin, piperacillin/tazobactam, and carbapenems.[8]

Dosing adjustments may be determined from recommendations in the drug's package insert, texts with renal dosing information, or use of common formulas that take into account the fraction of a drug dose eliminated by the kidney.[9] To participate fully in a renal dosing program, you should be able to predict CrCl from serum creatinine and understand the factors that impact the quality of these predictions.[10]

To adjust a dose or interval based on the drug's fraction excreted unchanged (f_e) and a patient's estimated or actual CrCl, the following formulas may be used. For this case, assume that a drug with an f_e of 0.8 is commonly given as 1 gram every 8 hours in normal renal function (e.g., >100 mL/min). The patient you are reviewing for dosing has a CrCl estimated at 30 mL/min. To determine the dose, the following steps are taken:

$$Q = 1 - \left\{ f_e \left(1 - \frac{CrCl_r}{CrCl_n} \right) \right\},$$

where Q is the adjustment factor, f_e is the fraction of a dose excreted unchanged by the kidney, $CrCl_r$ is the patient's CrCl, and $CrCl_n$ is "normal" CrCl (assumed to be 120 mL/min). Thus,

$$Q = 1 - \left\{ 0.8 \left(1 - \frac{30}{120} \right) \right\} = 0.4.$$

Based on this, the patient should receive 40% of the normal dose per unit of time. Because the normal dose is 3 grams per day (given as 1 gram every 8 hours), the daily dose for this patient should be $3 \times 0.4 \cong 1.2$ grams.

The approach taken could be to cut each dose to 40% of normal or to lengthen the dosing interval. Because this type of dose adjustment is not an exact science, some rounding is feasible. If just the dose is altered, you might recommend 400 mg every 8 hours (or round to 500 mg every 8 hours).

To alter dose and interval, the equation is

$$Dose_r = Q \times \frac{Dose_n}{\tau_n} \times \tau_r$$

where $Dose_r$ is the dose in reduced renal function, $Dose_n$ is the dose in normal renal function, τ_r is the interval to be used in reduced renal function, and τ_n is the interval used in normal renal function. If you decided to increase the interval to 12 hours, the dose would be

$$Dose_r = 0.4 \times \frac{1000 \text{ mg}}{8 \text{ hours}} \times 12 \text{ hours} = 600 \text{ mg (you might recommend 750 mg).}$$

There are a number of important assumptions to using this approach that are beyond the available space for this chapter but should be studied.[8]

Other Calculations

In addition to the calculations used in pharmacokinetic dosing and renal adjustment, you must master many other types of calculations to be effective in ensuring patient safety and optimal outcomes. Activities related to such calculations may include the following:

- Determining the correct amount of drug to put in an admixture or other compounded product based on percent or proportion
- Knowledge of appropriate dose ranges based on patient characteristics such as age and weight
- Appropriately calculating doses, quantities for compounded prescriptions, and infusion rates to deliver prescribed dosing

A firm understanding of these and other calculations is critical as you directly determine the values or as you verify the calculations of others. Tenfold errors are far too common when doing critical calculations, and all those involved in performing them must be aware of the potential pitfalls.

CASE QUESTION

What must be known about the vancomycin IVPB to accurately determine the infusion rate to deliver the entire 2-gram dose over a 1-hour period?

There are two important issues to consider before you would decide how to accurately determine the infusion rate. They focus on whether the 2-gram dose is appropriate for the patient and whether a 2-gram dose and the volume of fluid that the dose is placed in should be infused over a 1-hour period. The first answer is beyond the scope of this discussion and largely depends on the infection, desired vancomycin concentrations, and patient's size and renal function. The second depends on the drug infusion time and the concentration of the final product. Giving a large amount of solution over a short period of time is acceptable for many patients but may be detrimental for patients on a fluid restriction.

Assuming that the dose would be given as written, calculating the infusion rate requires knowledge of the volume of liquid in the IVPB. The 2-gram dose would likely have to be reconstituted from bulk (about 20 mL of final solution) and then put in a 500-mL bag, which is a commonly available size. If the final volume is 520 mL, then the infusion rate would be calculated with the following equation:

$$\text{Rate} = \frac{520 \text{ ml}}{60 \text{ minutes}} = 8.67 \text{ mL/min.}$$

The final rate will depend on the number of drops per milliliter delivered. The calculation would be

Rate = mL/min x gtts/mL = gtts/min.

If the pump or tubing delivered 20 drops/mL and was calibrated according to drops/time,

Rate = 8.67 mL/min x 20 gtts/mL = 173 gtts/min.

MEDICATION PREPARATION

One of the pharmacy department's fundamental responsibilities is the accurate and safe preparation of medication products for patient use. As a student, no health-system or hospital rotation would be complete without a chance to compound products and verify the compounding of others.

Aseptic Technique and Compounded Sterile Products

Aseptic technique and compounded sterile products (CSPs) involve a vast array of knowledge and resource utilization. Depending on the individual institution and the needs of their patients and healthcare providers, pharmacy departments may be required to provide a wide range of products and services associated with CSPs, including the following:

- Intermittent IVPBs (e.g., antibiotics, antiepileptics, antivirals, electrolyte replacements)
- Continuous intravenous (IV) solutions (e.g., maintenance or hydration fluids, hemodynamic stabilizing medications, narcotic infusions)
- Chemotherapeutic agents
- Total parenteral nutrition
- Sterile irrigation fluids
- Eye drops
- Ear drops

Preparation of CSPs is a foundational and critical aspect of daily pharmacy activities. The Centers for Disease Control and Prevention maintain reports on their website of CSPs that have led to the spread of infection and can provide insight into breaches of quality control (www.cdc.gov). Knowledge of the U.S. Pharmacopeia's (USP) Chapter <797> is a key requirement to ensure that CSPs are of the highest quality and lowest risk for the patients who need to receive them. It is important to have a solid knowledge of the specific legal requirements of the state in which your rotation is occurring as they pertain to CSPs and the requirements of USP Chapter <797>.

The USP Chapter <797> standards were established in the early 1970s because of bacterial contamination of parenteral products resulting in thousands of cases of sepsis and hundreds of deaths. These events brought about the need for a higher standard of compounding quality. Although there were several governmental and nongovernmental groups that put forth efforts to raise the standards of compounding quality, it was not until January 1, 2004, that USP Chapter <797> became official. This became the first official and enforceable sterile preparation–compounding standard in the United States.[11-14]

USP Chapter <797> is an extensive guide that provides information on numerous areas of the sterile compounding process. Items detailed in this chapter include but are not limited to:

- Personnel training, garbing, and cleaning
- Hazardous drugs
- Radiopharmaceuticals
- Allergen extracts
- Definitions
- Immediate-use CSPs
- Single-dose and multiple-dose containers
- Personnel competency and evaluation
- Aseptic work practices
- Cleaning/disinfection
- Elements of quality control
- Environmental sampling (microbial air and surface testing)
- Abbreviations and acronyms

The procedural and environmental quality practices necessary for licensed healthcare professionals to assign risk level and beyond-use dating to CSPs, along with the engineering controls (sterile products room, laminar airflow hood, etc.) required, are also described in specific detail.[11-14]

It is important for you to note that USP Chapter <797> is enforceable only by the Food and Drug Administration, unless the board of pharmacy in the state in which you are practicing has adopted this chapter into its regulations. However, any other regulatory or accrediting bodies (e.g., The Joint Commission) may consider USP Chapter <797> the national standard by which they judge healthcare organizations and pharmacies that compound sterile preparations.[11-14]

Nonsterile Compounding

An important, albeit somewhat fading, piece of the pharmacist's workload is the compounding of nonsterile products. Although it is becoming less of a focus in contemporary pharmacy practice, nonsterile compounding is still a key area of daily pharmacy practice that you should be comfortable with and ready to execute when given the chance.

The processes, procedures, and techniques for compounding nonsterile products are quite similar to those associated with sterile compounding. You should have knowledge of basic pharmaceutical compounding and good manufacturing procedures. Similar to sterile compounding, nonsterile compounding regulations can be found in USP Chapter <795> and USP Chapter <1075>, which specifically deals with good compounding practices. These chapters will provide you with a solid foundation to ensure the highest quality and safety of compounded preparations for your patients.[14,15]

USP Chapter <795> will provide you with a clear understanding and distinction between what is considered a *manufactured product* (a product produced by a pharmaceutical company) and *compounded preparation* (a product prepared by a pharmacist). This differentiation is extensively discussed throughout USP Chapter <795>, helping delineate when compounding becomes manufacturing by individual pharmacists or pharmacies. Other areas detailed in USP Chapter <795> include but are not limited to the following:

- Responsibility of the compounder
- Facilities and equipment
- Stability of compounded preparations
- Sources of ingredients
- Acceptable strength, quality, and purity
- Compounded preparations
- Compounding process
- Compounding records and documents
- Quality control
- Verification
- Patient counseling

Repackaging

Although you may be familiar with preparing a medication for dispensing in your typical outpatient encounter, the inpatient dispensing of medication takes on a slightly different arrangement. Medication distribution is done in a unit-dose or unit-of-use fashion in which each dose is packaged separately. Many medications may be available from the manufacturer in this manner, but there are others that pharmacy personnel may need to repackage. As we continue to move healthcare toward a more computerized age, the inclusion of machine-readable barcodes on all medications is another reason that repackaging occurs. The repackaging of manufacturer's bulk medication bottles can be a regularly occurring activity in many hospital or health-system pharmacy departments. You should be prepared to actively participate as the technician preparing repackaged medications or the pharmacist verifying the activity by being well versed in the legal requirements of institutional repackaging, recordkeeping, and policies necessary to maintain the highest level of integrity of the repackaged products.

MEDICATION-USE EVALUATIONS

Medication-use evaluation (MUE) is a performance improvement method that focuses on evaluating and improving medication-use processes with the goal of optimal patient outcomes. Given the continual need to provide our patients with the highest level of care, these activities are a vital component to ensuring we continue to meet these needs and expectations. It is important to realize that MUEs, although they are often taught on these rotations, are not unique to hospitals or health systems and may be utilized by a wide variety of practice settings.[15]

MUEs examine the entire medication-use process (prescribing, preparation, dispensing, administration, and monitoring of medications) and how these functions impact quality of care. These evaluations may look at entire therapeutic classes of medications or single medications at a time. MUEs may be initiated for a multitude of reasons, including the following:

- Medication or medication classes are posing a high health risk because of interactions with other medications, foods, disease states, or diagnostic tests.
- Medication or medication classes are highly utilized or costly.
- Medication or medication classes are associated with a high risk for adverse reactions.
- Medications are being considered for formulary addition, retention, or deletion.

Given the above information, you may identify indicators that may bring medications or medication classes to your attention to consider initiating an MUE, such as adverse events, patient readmission rates for treatment failures, pharmacist interventions, and nonformulary requests.[14,15]

MUEs use a multifaceted approach that also focuses on the system of medication use, working to identify not only actual medication-related problems but also potential problems. Students are often utilized to complete MUEs that identify, resolve, and prevent medication-related problems that would result in less-than-optimal patient outcomes associated with medication use. MUEs can also be a valuable tool for maintaining cost-effective healthcare.[15] You should consider the importance of MUEs that have been published over the years, such as the Beers Criteria, utilized throughout pharmacy practice to avoid the use of potentially inappropriate medications in the elderly.

The MUE process should be an interdisciplinary, collaborative process that includes, at minimum, a physician, pharmacist, nurse, and administrator. When other experts in their respective healthcare disciplines bring a unique perspective to a given process, they should be included as part of the team. Pharmacists, given their training and expertise, should take a leading role in MUEs. Their responsibilities should include development and management of MUE processes that align with the organization's goals and resources. The responsible pharmacist also has an obligation to interpret and present the findings of the MUE, along with suggested improvements to all affected healthcare providers and staff.[14,15]

The MUE process is not immune to the continual need of process improvement and should be reviewed regularly for continued effectiveness and areas of improvement. You should be aware of common pitfalls that may render a MUE process ineffective, including the following:

- Lack of medical staff representation
- Unclear roles and responsibilities for individual members
- Lack of communication as it pertains to the MUE process, its importance to the health system, and its goals
- Ineffective documentation, member involvement, or follow through
- Ineffective data retrieval or information management[15]

As you can see, the MUE process is extensive and requires an interdisciplinary approach to maximize its effectiveness. You, as the future medication expert, are a necessary component to optimizing the use of medications within your health system, but this can only be done by successfully working with your other healthcare colleagues (physicians, nurses, administrators, etc.) to enhance medication-related patient outcomes.

OTHER ACTIVITIES

Be prepared to immerse yourself in all the activities that hospital and health-system pharmacists participate in during the typical workday. The activities described above may only scratch the surface of all the activities you will be exposed to. In addition to the tasks described above, order entry or order verification is the traditional means by which pharmacists verify the appropriateness of the prescriber's medication request against the patient's other medications, disease states, and current overall health status. These are vital processes to ensure the most effective medication-related outcomes for patients. Depending on the hospital's or health-system's specific requirements, some pharmacists may participate in other daily activities, such as code blue (cardiac resuscitation) emergencies, therapeutic substitution of medications, medication reconciliation, patient education for high-risk medications, and discharge medication counseling. These are all areas that you should inquire about and get involved in when the opportunity is available. You must realize that the hospital or health-system setting contains a wide variety of activities that pharmacists take part in each and every day and taking advantage of as many of these opportunities as possible will allow you to gain insight into potential areas of practice. Approaching each day with a positive outlook and high level of curiosity will provide you with the opportunity to maximize your hospital or health-system experience.

REFERENCES

1. Bond CA, Raehl CL. 2006 National Clinical Pharmacy Services Survey: Clinical pharmacy services, collaborative drug management, medication errors, and pharmacy technology. *Pharmacotherapy.* 2008;28:1-13.

2. Bond CA, Raehl CL, Patry R. Evidence-based core clinical pharmacy services in United States hospitals in 2020: Services and staffing. *Pharmacotherapy.* 2004;24:427-440.

3. Pedersen CA, Schneider PJ, Scheckelhoff DJ. ASHP national survey of pharmacy services in hospital settings: Dispensing and administration—2011. *Am J Health-Syst Pharm.* 2012;69:768-785.

4. Pedersen CA, Schneider PJ, Scheckelhoff DJ. ASHP national survey of pharmacy services in hospital settings: Prescribing and transcribing—2010. *Am J Health-Syst Pharm.* 2011;68:669-688.

5. Pedersen CA, Schneider PJ, Scheckelhoff DJ. ASHP national survey of pharmacy services in hospital settings: Monitoring and patient education—2009. *Am J Health-Syst Pharm.* 2010;67:542-558.

6. Winter ME, ed. *Basic Clinical Pharmacokinetics.* 5th ed. Philadelphia, PA: Lippincott Williams & Wilkins; 2010.

7. Murphy JE, ed. *Clinical Pharmacokinetics.* 5th ed. Bethesda, MD: American Society of Health-System Pharmacists; 2011.

8. Dowling TC, Matzke GR, Murphy JE, et al. Evaluation of renal drug dosing: Prescribing information and clinical pharmacist approaches. *Pharmacotherapy.* 2010;30:776-786.

9. Matzke GR, Dowling TC. Renal drug dosing concepts. In: Murphy JE. *Clinical Pharmacokinetics.* 5th ed. Bethesda, MD: American Society of Health-System Pharmacists; 2011:73-87.

10. Winter MA, Guhr KN, Berg GM. Impact of various body weights and serum creatinine concentrations on the bias and accuracy of the Cockcroft-Gault equation. *Pharmacotherapy.* 2012;32:604-612.

11. Buchanan E, Schneider P. *Compounding Sterile Preparations.* 3rd ed. Bethesda, MD: American Society of Health-System Pharmacists; 2009.

12. The ASHP Discussion Guide on USP Chapter <797>. http://www.ashp.org/s_ashp/docs/files/discguide797-2008.pdf. Accessed September 13, 2012.

13. Shrewbury R. *Applied Pharmaceutics in Contemporary Compounding.* 2nd ed. Englewood, NJ: Morton Publishing; 2008.

14. Thompson J. *A Practical Guide to Contemporary Pharmacy Practice.* 3rd ed. Philadelphia, PA: Lippincott Williams & Wilkins; 2009.

15. American Society of Health-System Pharmacists. ASHP guidelines on medication-use evaluation. *Am J Health-Syst Pharm.* 1996;53:1953-1955.

SUGGESTED READING

American Society of Health-System Pharmacists. ASHP guidelines on medication-use evaluation. *Am J Health-Syst Pharm.* 1996;53:1953-1955.

American Society of Health-System Pharmacists. Discussion Guide on USP Chapter <797>. http://www.ashp.org/s_ashp/docs/files/discguide797-2008.pdf.

Ansel HC. *Pharmaceutical Calculations.* 13th ed. Baltimore, MD: Lippincott Williams & Wilkins; 2009.

Hansten PD, Horn JR. *The Top 100 Drug Interactions: A Guide to Patient Management*—2012 edition. Freeland, WA: H&H Publications; 2012.

Lee M. *Basic Skills in Interpreting Laboratory Data*. 5th ed. Bethesda, MD: American Society of Health-System Pharmacists; 2013.

Murphy JE, ed. *Clinical Pharmacokinetics*. 5th ed. Bethesda, MD: American Society of Health-System Pharmacists; 2011.

Schmidt J, Wierczorkiewicz J. *Interpreting Laboratory Data: A Point of Care Guide*. Bethesda, MD: American Society of Health-System Pharmacists; 2011.

United States Pharmacopeia 35 — National Formulary 30. Chapter 795. Pharmaceutical Compounding — Non-sterile Preparations. Rockville, MD: The United States Pharmacopeial Convention; 2011.

United States Pharmacopeia 35 — National Formulary 30. Chapter 797. Pharmaceutical Compounding — Sterile Preparations. Rockville, MD: The United States Pharmacopeial Convention; 2011.

Winter ME, ed. *Basic Clinical Pharmacokinetics*. 5th ed. Philadelphia, PA: Lippincott Williams & Wilkins; 2010.

APPENDIX 9-A.   PHARMACOKINETIC EQUATIONS

The following equations can be manipulated to solve for an unknown part of the equation when the other values are known. S = fraction of dose that is parent compound; F = bioavailability fraction

For additional information, see Murphy JE. Introduction. In: Murphy JE. *Clinical Pharmacokinetics.* 5th ed. Bethesda, MD: American Society of Health-System Pharmacists; 2011:xxix-xxxvii.

Determining K from Two Known Concentration-Time Points in the Elimination Phase

1. $k = \dfrac{\ln(C_i \div C)}{t_\Delta}$

    or (with no C points when $t_{1/2}$ is known or estimated)

    $k = \dfrac{0.693}{t_{1/2}}$

Determining Half-Life from K, the Elimination Rate Constant

2. $t_{1/2} = \dfrac{0.693}{k}$ or $t_{1/2} = \dfrac{0.693}{(CL \div V)}$

Dose to Provide a Desired Concentration (C_Δ or C_0) Immediately After the Dose

3. $D = \dfrac{C_\Delta \bullet V}{S \bullet F}$ or $D = \dfrac{C_0 \bullet V}{S \bullet F}$

Concentration at Any Time *t* After a Single IV Bolus Dose

4. $C = \dfrac{S \bullet D}{V}\left(e^{-kt}\right)$ or $C = C_0 \bullet e^{-kt}$

Concentration at Any Time *t* After Some Initial Concentration (C_i)

5. $C = C_i \bullet e^{-kt}$

Concentration at Steady State on an IV Infusion at Rate *Ro*

6. $C_{ss} = \dfrac{S \bullet Ro}{CL}$ or $C_{ss} = \dfrac{S \bullet Ro}{k \bullet V}$

Average Concentration (Approximately Halfway Between Peak and Trough) at Steady State on a Dose (D) Given Every τ Hours

7. $C_{ssavg} = \dfrac{S \bullet F \bullet D}{CL \bullet \tau}$ or $C_{ssavg} = \dfrac{S \bullet F \bullet D}{k \bullet V \bullet \tau}$

Concentration at Any Time *t* After an IV Bolus Dose Given Every τ Hours

8. $$C = \frac{S \bullet D}{V\left(1-e^{-k\tau}\right)}\left(e^{-kt}\right)$$

Concentration at Any Time T After the End of a Short Infusion Given Over t′ Time Every τ Hours—At Steady State

9. $$C = \frac{S \bullet D}{k \bullet V \bullet t'} \frac{\left(1-e^{-kt'}\right)}{\left(1-e^{-k\tau}\right)}\left(e^{-kT}\right)$$

Average Steady State Concentration for a Drug with Capacity-Limited Excretion

10. $$C_{ssavg} = \frac{(Km)\left(\dfrac{S \bullet F \bullet D}{\tau}\right)}{Vm - \left(\dfrac{S \bullet F \bullet D}{\tau}\right)}$$

Dose and Interval to Produce Desired C_ssavg for a Drug with Capacity-Limited Elimination

11. $$\frac{S \bullet F \bullet D}{\tau} = \frac{(Vm)\left(C_{ssavg}\right)}{Km + C_{ssavg}}$$

Fraction of Steady State Achieved (f_ss) at Time *t* After the Start of Dosing (Usually as Infusion)

12. $$fss = \frac{C}{Css} = 1 - e^{-kt}$$

Css = C/(1 - e^{-kt}) can be used to estimate the steady state concentration from a measured concentration *t* time after the start of dosing.

APPENDIX 9-B.

THERAPEUTIC RANGES OF DRUGS IN TRADITIONAL AND SI UNITS

DRUG	TRADITIONAL RANGE	CONVERSION FACTOR[a]	SI RANGE
Acetaminophen	>5 mg/dL toxic	66.160	>330 μmol/L toxic
N-Acetylprocainamide	4–10 mg/L	3.606	14–36 μmol/L
Amitriptyline	75–175 ng/mL	3.605	180–720 nmol/L
Carbamazepine	4–12 mg/L	4.230	17–51 μmol/L
Chlordiazepoxide	0.5–5.0 mg/L	3.336	2–17 μmol/L
Chlorpromazine	50–300 ng/mL	3.136	150–950 nmol/L
Chlorpropamide	75–250 μg/mL	3.613	270–900 μmol/L
Clozapine	450–? ng/mL	0.003	1.38–? μmol/L
Cyclosporine	100–200 ng/mL[b]	0.832	80–160 nmol/L
Desipramine	100–160 ng/mL	3.754	170–700 nmol/L
Diazepam	100–250 ng/mL	3.512	350–900 nmol/L
Digoxin	0.5–1.2 ng/mL	1.281	0.6–1.5 nmol/L
Disopyramide	2–6 mg/L	2.946	6–18 μmol/L
Doxepin	50–200 ng/mL	3.579	180–720 nmol/L
Ethosuximide	40–100 mg/L	7.084	280–710 μmol/L
Fluphenazine	0.5–2.5 ng/mL	2.110	5.3–21 nmol/L
Glutethimide	>20 mg/L toxic	4.603	>92 μmol/L toxic
Gold	300–800 mg/L	0.051	15 μmol/L
Haloperidol	5–15 ng/mL	2.660	13–40 nmol/L
Imipramine	200–250 ng/mL	3.566	180–710 nmol/L
Isoniazid	>3 mg/L toxic	7.291	>22 μmol/L toxic
Lidocaine	1–5 mg/L	4.267	5–22 μmol/L
Lithium	0.5–1.5 mEq/L	1.000	0.5–1.5 μmol/L
Maprotiline	50–200 ng/mL	3.605	180–720 μmol/L
Meprobamate	>40 mg/L toxic	4.582	>180 μmol/L toxic
Methotrexate	>2.3 mg/L toxic	2.200	>5 μmol/L toxic
Nortriptyline	50–150 ng/mL	3.797	190–570 nmol/L
Pentobarbital	20–40 mg/L	4.419	90–170 μmol/L
Perphenazine	0.8–2.4 ng/mL	2.475	2–6 nmol/L
Phenobarbital	15–40 mg/L	4.306	65–172 μmol/L
Phenytoin	10–20 mg/L	3.964	40–80 μmol/L
Primidone	4–12 mg/L	4.582	18–55 μmol/L
Procainamide	4–8 mg/L	4.249	17–34 μmol/L
Propranolol	50–200 ng/mL	3.856	190–770 nmol/L
Protriptyline	100–300 ng/mL	3.797	380–1140 nmol/L
Quinidine	2–6 mg/L	3.082	5–18 μmol/L
Salicylate (acid)	15–25 mg/dL	0.072	1.1–1.8 mmol/L
Theophylline	10–20 mg/L	5.550	55–110 μmol/L

Thiocyanate	>10 mg/dL toxic	0.172	>1.7 mmol/L toxic
Valproic acid	50–100 mg/L	6.934	350–700 µmol/L
Warfarin	1–3 mg/L	3.243	3.3–9.8 µmol/L

[a] Traditional units are multiplied by conversion factor to get SI units.

[b] Whole blood assay.

Source: Reprinted with permission from Traub SL. *Interpreting Laboratory Data.* 2nd ed. Bethesda, MD: American Society of Health-System Pharmacists; 1996:397.

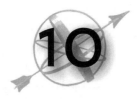

Community Pharmacy

Daniel Krinsky, MS, RPh, and Stacey Schneider, PharmD

CASE

L.B. is a pharmacy student starting his first day in a community pharmacy APPE rotation. His preceptor has told him that he will be spending the morning in the pharmacy doing routine tasks the pharmacist performs to dispense prescriptions. His afternoon will be spent doing a medication therapy management (MTM) visit with a previously scheduled patient, along with other patient-focused activities. As part of his morning routine, L.B. will be required to do a return-to-stock audit on previously filled prescriptions, answer and make physician phone calls, counsel patients on new prescriptions, address drug utilization review (DUR)/clinical issues during the filling process, and perform over-the-counter (OTC) consults. All of these tasks will require L.B. to review patient pharmacy records and obtain information as needed from other practitioners. L.B. has never worked in a community pharmacy and is nervous about his ability to complete these tasks.

Why It's Essential

Welcome to the world of community pharmacy—a continually changing arena in which to practice pharmacy. Finding ways to constantly balance the changing demands of the healthcare system and those of the retail market makes the community pharmacist position one of the most challenging and rewarding positions in the profession. The goal of the community pharmacy experiential rotation is to provide you with an opportunity to practice contemporary pharmacy in a community setting. Because a majority of graduates from pharmacy schools will practice in a community pharmacy setting, it is critical for you to obtain as much experience as possible in a structured learning environment prior to graduation to build skills, knowledge, and confidence.

Although we have numerous "controlled" simulation activities built into the on-campus curriculum, nothing compares to real-world experiences. Students typically learn the basic elements of how to practice and manage patients in the community pharmacy setting through these campus activities, their internship, and their IPPE rotations, but the APPE rotation brings everything together in 1 to 2 months and places the student on the front line. You see how a pharmacy staff manages everything from handling the prescription verification process and managing difficult patients to developing and delivering medication therapy–management services.

> *"What I experienced during my rotation was much more dynamic than what I do during my internship. I now see how I can apply what I've learned in school and what's possible when I become a pharmacist."—Student*

●●●

"Don't settle for the status quo. If you're not being challenged by your preceptor, ask about ways to get more involved."—Preceptor

●●●

Arriving Prepared

The following is a checklist of recommended actions prior to day 1 of your APPE community pharmacy rotation:

- Contact the preceptor ahead of time and ask for information on required readings, disease states to review, and logistical information (parking, location, etc.).

- Obtain a general understanding of the types of personnel working and the basic layout of the pharmacy. These issues are discussed in more detail in the next section.

- Formulate your own personal objectives for the rotation and determine what goals you would like to accomplish; however, ensure they are consistent with the site's objectives.

- Dress professionally; white coat and appropriate identification are mandatory at sites.

- Check with your preceptor to see if pocket reference guides or their electronic counterparts are allowed.

- Review pertinent topics prior to your first day, including drug therapy problems, patient interviewing, counseling skills, drug literature review, and statistical interpretation.

- Be familiar with the most recent treatment guidelines. These include, but are not limited to, the Seventh Report of the Joint National Committee on Prevention, Detection, Evaluation, and Treatment of High Blood Pressure (JNC 7); the Third Report of the Expert Panel on Detection, Evaluation, and Treatment of High Blood Cholesterol in Adults (Adult Treatment Panel III, or ATP III); Standards of Medical Care in Diabetes from the American Diabetes Association (ADA); and Guidelines for Diagnosis and Management of Asthma from the National Heart Lung and Blood Institute (NHLBI).

- Become familiar with MTM services that might be offered. Additional detail is discussed in the MTM Consultation section later in this chapter.

- Understand the importance of the different types of communication that may be necessary.

- Be prepared for OTC consultations.

●●●

"Preceptors appreciate when students approach the rotation with a genuine interest in learning and participating, regardless of preconceived ideas, what they've heard, or where they feel they'll end up practicing after graduation."—Preceptor

●●●

A Typical Day

A typical day during your community pharmacy APPE rotation will involve dispensing, patient-focused activities, and work on projects.

Dispensing activities in the community pharmacy might encompass the following:

- Assisting with processing prescriptions
- Addressing DUR and clinical messages
- Patient counseling
- OTC consults
- Phone calls to physician offices to clarify prescriptions or obtain answers to questions
- Assisting with various audits
- Immunizations (where allowed by law)

Patient-focused activities in the community pharmacy might encompass the following:

- Comprehensive medication reviews (CMRs) with patients as part of an MTM visit—either in the pharmacy or through a home visit
- Wellness screening programs (inside and outside the pharmacy)
- Community outreach events, such as presentations to nursing home residents or community organizations
- Immunization clinics
- Physician office visits to promote pharmacy-specific products and services

Projects may include the following:

- Preparing for and delivering a journal club article
- Preparing for and delivering a case presentation
- Writing a newsletter article for healthcare professionals
- Developing a community-focused presentation
- Preparation for other patient care–focused activities

DISPENSING PROCESS

You will be expected to demonstrate effective pharmacy practice skills in order to assist with the dispensing process. This description is based on the authors' experiences and discussions with other community pharmacists. Almost all community pharmacies employ the following types of individuals:

- Pharmacists: staff and management-level professionals could be in your pharmacy.
- Pharmacy technicians: some may be certified through the national Pharmacy Technician Certification Board (PTCB) and others via state requirements; some will not be certified at all. These individuals are trained to assist the pharmacist in many activities related to prescription processing and customer service.
- Clerks: entry-level staff that are not involved in any activities related to the processing of a prescription. These individuals are usually responsible for running the cash register or similar activities.

Each of these individuals plays an integral role in every activity that takes place within the pharmacy. It is imperative that tasks be matched as closely as possible to the various individuals in the pharmacy and that everyone works together, as the volume of work can be quite challenging to manage, even with optimal teamwork and workflow. Your preceptor should find ways to introduce you to the staff and integrate you into the workflow in the appropriate areas at the appropriate time.

L.B. would like to familiarize himself with prescription processing on his first day. Which of the pharmacy personnel would be the most appropriate to shadow?

Prescription Processing

Most pharmacies are designed to facilitate optimal workflow and maximize work output with minimal movement throughout the physical structure. **Figure 10-1** shows an example of a pharmacy layout, with all the critical sections needed for pharmacy activities, including the prescription drop off, a terminal for order entry, workspace for prescription assembly, a pharmacist's verification terminal, and an area for patients to pick up prescriptions.

Figure 10-1. Schematic Illustrating a Common Community Pharmacy Set Up and Workflow

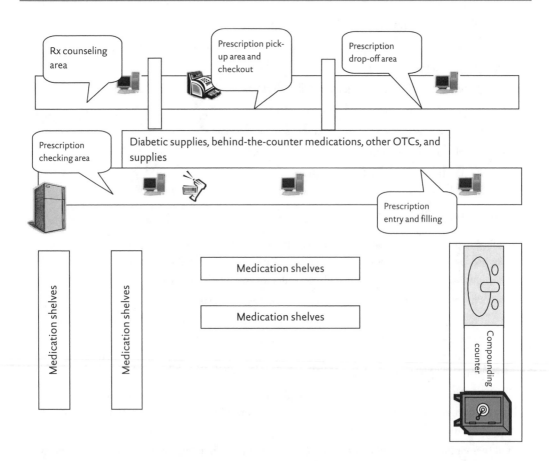

Prescription processing begins at a computer terminal with a software program for prescription entry and processing, label and patient advisory leaflet printing, and maintaining patient profiles and insurance information. The primary prescription entry station, often staffed by a student or technician (although sometimes staffed by a pharmacist), will be located close to the drop-off area. Prescriptions come into the pharmacy in various ways, such as by fax, phone call, voicemail message, e-prescribing, or patient drop-off. For patients who present prescriptions in person, you should also obtain information about allergies, insurance coverage, and contact information. Oftentimes, much of this information will be obtained from a prescriber's office when prescriptions are phoned into the pharmacy. As a student, your ability to participate in taking phoned-in prescriptions and retrieving prescriptions from the voicemail system is state-specific. If you are involved with phoned-in prescriptions, be sure to follow the "repeat back" policy to verify every piece of information when speaking with a prescriber or prescriber's agent. When listening to recorded messages, review the message at least twice to verify all information. Once all of the necessary information has been obtained, the prescription is ready to be entered into the pharmacy computer system by a pharmacist, student, or technician.

Close by, the prescription assembly area is where all the paperwork and prescription information is put together. This is where the medication is counted, the bottle is labeled, and all components are prepared for the pharmacist to check. A great deal of paperwork will have been generated by this time, including, where necessary the following:

- Hard-copy prescription
- Label for the bottle, including all auxiliary labels
- Sticker/tag that is adhered to the back of the hard-copy prescription that reflects all information entered in the patient profile and is part of the permanent pharmacy record
- Patient information leaflet
- Any clinical messages that still need to be addressed by a pharmacist (or student with pharmacist supervision)
- Any documents describing insurance/copay information the patient will want to review
- Supplemental marketing pieces that complement the other drug information
- Receipt that indicates copay or other prescription price

At this point, the prescription can be filled. Once the correct drug is selected from the shelf, it is counted and placed in a vial with the correct cap (child-proof unless a snap cap is requested by the patient) and the label is applied. In busy pharmacies, there may be enough technicians involved so that the filling technician double-checks the work of the entry technician. This helps to prevent errors or problems from being passed forward. The more trained eyes that can review a prescription, the less chance errors will be made or key information missed. Oftentimes, students will be placed in the role of secondary checker prior to the pharmacist's final verification.

QUICK TIP

To help ensure that the proper medication is chosen from the shelves, the National Drug Code (NDC) on the prescription label should be matched to the NDC on the stock bottle.

Once everything is assembled, the items (documents, stock bottle, labeled prescription vial, and anything else) are given to a pharmacist for the final check. The final verification encompasses many steps to ensure the right drug gets to the right patient at the right dose and schedule to ensure optimal response. During this process, there are no shortcuts. Pharmacists are the last people in the healthcare system to assess the appropriateness of a prescription before it is dispensed to a patient. We must remain focused and use our training, skills, knowledge, and whatever technology is available to verify that everything about the prescription is perfect. As a student on your community pharmacy APPE rotation, you should ensure that you pay close attention to how your preceptor manages this complex process so that you will be well prepared to complete the tasks yourself once you become a pharmacist.

Managing Drug Utilization Review Messages

One of the first things to address during prescription verification is any DUR messages generated during the entry process. All pharmacy dispensing software systems include an application that screens for numerous clinical issues. This screening process may also be completed by software third-party payers use when claims are filed. The goal of these software programs is to provide pharmacies with information to support the safe dispensing of medications. Resolution of some or all of these problems could be performed by pharmacy students, depending on the student's training and the preceptor's comfort level with student involvement. Typically, you will be involved in addressing the more clinical (versus administrative) issues. Some of the common types of messages are included in **Figure 10-2**.

Figure 10-2. Examples of DUR Messages

- Allergy warnings

- Drug interaction alerts

- Adherence issues (such as refill too soon, refill too late)

- Therapy duplications

- Inability to screen alert (if the new drug is not recognized by the software program, a message is generated stating the screening process did not take place and a manual check is needed)

- Age warnings—often for pediatric and geriatric individuals

- Dosing frequency alerts—the dose prescribed is higher or lower, or the prescription directions called for more doses per day than what is typically prescribed

Source: Courtesy of the Indian Health Service and the U.S. Public Health Service.

There are many ways to manage these messages. If a pharmacist is entering prescriptions, they can be addressed immediately. If technicians are entering prescriptions, the best option is to generate a printed copy of the message and allow the checking pharmacist to manage the issue. Some messages are easily addressed (verifying a dose), although many require additional effort, which normally includes a phone call to the prescriber, conversation with the patient, research using a point-of-care reference database (such as Lexi-Comp Online™), PubMed database search, phone call to a manufacturer, or any combination of these. The ultimate goal is to resolve the issue so the prescribed drug can be dispensed, replace the prescribed drug with a safer option, or seek additional follow-up with a healthcare provider before the medication is dispensed. Regardless of the outcome, it is imperative that the pharmacist (or student) documents all actions either on the prescription and/or the patient's computerized profile. Remember, if it is not documented, it never happened.

QUICK TIP

Getting students involved in addressing DUR messages is an excellent learning exercise. We do this frequently with our APPE students and include a practice exercise with previously generated DUR messages as an introductory activity during the first week of the rotation.

CASE QUESTION

L.B. has addressed a drug-interaction DUR message by calling the prescribing physician and changing a patient's medication. Now that the potential interaction has been addressed, how should L.B. document his intervention?

Patient Counseling

Another important aspect of the dispensing process is patient counseling. There are many ways pharmacists address this issue. Some have a staff member make the offer to counsel patients, others offer counseling to certain patients directly, and some counsel every patient regardless of whether their prescriptions are new or refills. The number of pharmacists providing medication counseling has doubled over the past 30 years, but as a profession, we are still coming up short. Not only can the counseling session be used to review a new prescription, but a quick review of the patient's profile may also uncover additional issues to discuss, such as adherence to chronic medications, response to therapy, or home monitoring.

One of the main barriers to optimizing patient outcomes with drug therapy is adherence. Numerous studies have shown that pharmacists can play a critical role in helping to improve adherence, and one way to do this is through patient counseling. Our experience has shown that counseling at the first fill of a new prescription addresses many issues the patient had not considered nor had been discussed by anyone at the physician's office. Counseling also helps establish the patient–pharmacist relationship and lets the patient know we care about him or her as a person, not just a customer.

One common approach to patient counseling is the "Three Prime Questions."[1] **Figure 10-3** lists the three prime questions to ask when patients are receiving a new drug, along with some additional issues or questions that often arise. A number of other important factors must be considered when providing effective patient counseling, such as those listed in **Figure 10-4**. It is important to remember to focus on the positive attributes of the medication more than the negative. If all you do is mention side effects, the patient is not likely to want to take the drug.

Figure 10-3. Three Prime Questions Asked During a Counseling Session for a New Medication

"WHAT DID YOUR DOCTOR TELL YOU (INSERT MEDICATION NAME HERE) WAS BEING USED TO TREAT?"

Depending on the patient's response, you may have to describe this if the use is obvious (such as an Epi-Pen®) or you may need to ask the patient more questions to better determine his or her condition for a medication with multiple uses (such as lisinopril, which has multiple indications).

"HOW DID YOUR DOCTOR TELL YOU TO TAKE (INSERT MEDICATION NAME HERE)?"

Depending on response, you may need to provide additional details, such as

- Number of times per day
- Time of day
- Amount to use per dose (eye drops, creams, etc.)
- Administration in relation to meals
- Administration in relation to other medications
- How long to use (i.e., cream for 7 days, antibiotic until gone, etc.)

- What to do about a missed dose
- Storage

"WHAT TYPE OF RESPONSE DID YOUR DOCTOR TELL YOU TO EXPECT FROM (INSERT MEDICATION NAME HERE)?"

Depending on response, you may need to provide additional details, such as

- Beneficial effects to expect
- Time frame to expect benefit—when the patient will notice a change, if at all
- What to do if there is no response within the expected time frame
- Side effects that might occur
- What to do if side effects become unbearable or serious
- Who to call with questions
- What to avoid while taking the medication (sun sensitivity, foods to avoid, etc.)
- What to do if feeling better but still have some medication remaining (such as antibiotics)
- Plan for follow-up with patient's primary care provider
- Home monitoring options (for individuals with diabetes, asthma, hypertension)
- When and how to obtain refills

Source: Adapted with permission from The Indian Health Service and the U.S. Public Health Service.

QUICK TIP

It is very easy to initiate counseling by telling the patient everything you know about his or her new medication. DO NOT take this approach. Get in the habit of asking the three prime questions to determine what the patient knows and fill in the blanks.

Figure 10-4. Factors That Affect Optimal Patient Counseling

- Know with whom you are speaking—your approach with a spouse, family member, or neighbor will be much different than when talking directly with the patient.
- Attempt to counsel in an area away from distractions and other patients and customers.
- Don't appear rushed—give the patient your undivided attention.
- Begin by asking the three prime questions reviewed in Figure 10-3.
- Maintain eye contact throughout the session.
- Use patient-appropriate language and visual aids or demonstrations where appropriate.
- Try to establish a caring relationship with the patient; demonstrate empathy; show respect.
- Provide supplemental materials or information (this may just be the patient information leaflet or there could be additional documents and adherence aids, such as a dropper for a liquid antibiotic).
- Ask the patient to do a "teach-back"—have the patient tell you what he or she is going to do when getting home and reinforce key information.
- Do not multitask—the counseling session should be your only priority, not also answering phones, checking prescriptions, answering questions, etc.
- Be prepared for patients with special needs, such as hearing or visual impairments or those for whom English is a second language.

The patient counseling process is one where you can get involved early and often. It is very likely that you will begin your APPE rotations with a wealth of experience in counseling patients throughout your didactic curriculum, IPPE rotations, or paid internships. You will be expected to have a core knowledge base of the most commonly prescribed medications so you can participate in patient counseling activities soon after starting your rotation, although many preceptors will provide some support activities, such as simulated practice sessions and shadowing of pharmacists providing counseling for patients. Once you are comfortable with the process and the preceptor and pharmacists are comfortable with your abilities, you can take the lead with patient counseling. Your preceptor is always a good resource to offer support, answer questions, and ensure the correct information is shared.

CASE QUESTION

L.B. is counseling a patient about his new antibiotic prescription. He explains that the agent may cause stomach cramping, diarrhea, and a rash. How could he improve his counseling session to emphasize the benefits of the medication and improve adherence while still covering these important side effects?

One cannot address all the issues with patient counseling without taking into consideration one of the most important factors—patient confidentiality. The Health Insurance Portability and Accountability Act (HIPAA) of 1996 regulates the use and disclosure of protected health information (PHI), requires those with access to PHI to take appropriate steps to ensure the confidentiality of communications about PHI, and also outlines penalties for violations. In a typical community environment, there are many situations in which confidentiality must be addressed yet could be compromised. It is imperative that attention is paid to where conversations take place, who else might be within earshot, the topics being discussed, with whom you are speaking, and voice volume. When it comes to phone conversations, you may have to find a more secure environment to discuss patient-specific issues. Another area where confidentiality needs to be addressed is in the OTC medication section. This is an area where consumers can congregate, so when discussing patient-sensitive issues, try to have these conversations away from others.

As a student, you should have completed a training session on the HIPAA legislation prior to starting your APPE rotations. You may also be required to complete site-specific training. Regardless, you need to be aware of situations where confidentiality could be breached and prevent that from happening. Talk with your preceptor to ensure you are familiar with the pharmacy's policy on confidentiality and adhere to it.

Extemporaneous Compounding

A certain subset of community pharmacies, primarily those looking to create a unique market niche, will get involved in compounding medications. The profession got its start on the basis of being able to mix various chemicals together to create medicines. With the advent of commercially available drugs from major manufacturers, the need for compounded medications has diminished but not disappeared. There are still many situations where a compounded medication is ideal, such as when a unique dosage form is needed for a particular drug, a specific dose has to be administered, a certain ingredient has to be avoided, or a mixture of multiple medications is best given at once. Some patient groups that typically benefit from compounded medications include infants and children, persons with allergies or sensitivities, women with hormonal issues, and pets without commercially available options.

Pharmacists interested in compounding usually receive additional training, set up an area specific for compounding, and focus specific resources to market and advertise their services. Oftentimes, compounded medications provide another revenue stream, depending on volume and the role of insurance reimbursement. Certain rules and regulations govern the compounding of medications, and you should become familiar with them during your community pharmacy APPE experiences. There is a very important distinction between compounding and manufacturing. Pharmacists preparing medications for individual patients must ensure they document their activities accurately and in a timely manner. Much debate has taken place on the national stage between advocates and opponents of compounding, and more will take place. Those interested or involved in compounding must stay abreast of any proposed or enacted legislation that impacts this area of pharmacy practice.

PATIENT-FOCUSED ACTIVITIES

Pharmacists have a wealth of knowledge and skills that should be utilized beyond the traditional dispensing of medications. The healthcare system is getting more complex and patients are shuffled between providers and systems without an ideal process to ensure seamless care. It has been shown that patients are much more likely to visit their community pharmacist than any other healthcare provider, so it makes sense that we try to maximize these opportunities to help. Many community pharmacists are offering services such as MTM, adherence assessments, wellness and screening programs, and detailed consultations on OTC products. These types of programs not only benefit patients but also provide pharmacists with enhanced job satisfaction, improve patient loyalty, and create opportunities to generate additional revenue.

> "Students in an APPE community pharmacy rotation should be challenged to participate in as many activities as possible that involve direct patient care. This is the future of pharmacy."—Preceptor

Medication Therapy Management Consultations

Patient care programs and pharmaceutical care have been in place for over three decades. These were a preface to what is now known as MTM. The Medicare Modernization Act (MMA) of 2003 was formulated to establish the Part D prescription drug plan. As a component of this plan, Part D programs were designed to provide MTM services to eligible patients. Because the law was very vague, numerous pharmacy organizations came together to develop a definition for MTM. It was defined as a distinct group of services that

> optimize therapeutic outcomes for individual patients. MTM services are independent of, but can occur in conjunction with, the provision of a medication product. MTM encompasses a broad range of professional activities and responsibilities within the licensed pharmacist's or other qualified health care provider's scope of practice.[2(p. 572)]

It is important to note that MTM differs from counseling at the point of dispensing, as it requires more detail than counseling on an individual prescription. MTM is not a brown-bag review as these reviews stop at the end of the session and do not require follow-up. Lastly, MTM is not a disease state management (DSM) program because it looks at the entire patient, not just one disease state.

CASE QUESTION

L.B. has been counseling patients more effectively and has been asked to begin working up patients in the MTM program. How do MTM services differ from traditional counseling?

Why did MTM become necessary in the community setting? For one, the key to sustaining any business is to maintain a profit. Revenue sources for many community sites include prescriptions, OTC products, immunizations, front-end products and specialty services such as MTM consults, DSM programs, compounding, and durable medical equipment. Revenue is continually decreasing on the product side due to declining reimbursement. Therefore, pharmacies must come up with unique ways to increase their revenue sources—MTM being one option. Second, there is a need to decrease the high costs associated with adverse drug events. The high number of medications most Medicare patients take leads to an increased incidence of drug therapy problems. These can be identified by the pharmacist at the MTM visit.

QUICK TIP

MTM in the community pharmacy setting requires perseverance, patience, persistence, and collaboration to do what is necessary to improve patient outcomes.

Most of the patients who present for an MTM visit will be covered by Medicare Part D. The focus of this discussion will be primarily on this patient population, but it is important to remember that there may be other sources of payers for MTM, such as self-pay or private insurers. A typical patient will present with multiple medications, will have multiple disease states, and is likely to spend a significant amount of money on Part D–covered medications. To be eligible, patients have to be taking a minimum number of medications and have a minimum number of chronic diseases. Also, eligible patients must be likely to incur expenses of at least $3,000 for Part D–covered medications annually.

Medicare requires all three of these criteria to be met for patients to be eligible for MTM services. Keep in mind that these are only Medicare-defined criteria. Pharmacists can also offer MTM services to non-Medicare patients and establish a compensation structure to fit a business model. A number of third parties can be employed to connect MTM-eligible patients with pharmacists willing to provide the service, such as Mirixa, Outcomes, or PharmMD. Other insurance providers may have internal MTM programs staffed by pharmacists or nurses who deliver MTM via telephone or in person.

Services provided will vary based on patients' individual needs and pharmacist expertise. The services may also be influenced by third-party requirements. Although there is not one set formula, there are some core components that should be included, such as the medication therapy review (MTR), personal medication record (PMR), and medication action plan (MAP). The MTR is designed to collect patient-specific information and assess medication therapies to identify and prioritize drug therapy problems and create a plan to resolve them. MTRs can either be comprehensive or targeted. In a comprehensive MTR, the patient will bring in all of his or her medications, including prescription, OTC, and herbal products. These will be assessed for potential drug therapy problems, and resolution will follow. A targeted MTR addresses a specific medication problem or can be conducted for ongoing monitoring and is ideal for those patients who have already completed a comprehensive MTR. Most commonly, an MTR will be a face-to-face consultation with the patient. In-person visits are generally preferred, especially if this is the first visit with the patient. In some cases, the pharmacy may have a private room for the pharmacist and the patient to meet and discuss health-related issues. During the interview, the pharmacist will gather such information as demographics, a medical and medication history, social history, family history, immunization status, allergies, and health risk factors. Once these data are collected, the next step is to evaluate the medications for possible drug therapy problems. If laboratory values are available, they should also be assessed at this time. Once drug therapy problems are identified, a plan will need to be developed with the patient and proper education will need to take place. For a full discussion of the identification of drug therapy problems, see Chapter 13.

QUICK TIP

A typical MTM interview may begin with an assessment of the patient's healthcare priorities in relation to his or her medications, specifically the importance of comfort, cost, and convenience. The answer to this question may have an effect on the types of recommendations you make.

The PMR is a comprehensive record of the patient's medications (prescription and nonprescription medications, herbal products, and other dietary supplements). The PMR can be formulated to fit patient-specific needs but should include demographics, allergies, immunizations, and physician name, in addition to the medication list. The PMR should be updated on a regular basis by the pharmacist and should be given to the patient at the end of each MTM visit. It may be advisable to provide a copy to the patient's physician too.

The MAP is a document containing specific information for patients to use to aid them in resolving the drug therapy problems that have been identified. It is a list of instructions the patients need to complete, allowing them to track their progress. This document should be created in collaboration with the patient and written in patient-level language. It is important not to overwhelm the patient with this list and make sure certain problems are prioritized. Lower-priority problems may need to be addressed at future visits. The patient should be able to achieve all of the items on the action plan. To complete the MAP, proper monitoring and follow-up will need to be decided on collaboratively with the patient. Intervention or referral may be required in certain circumstances. This may include obtaining additional laboratory work, consulting with the patient's physician, or referring to another type of specialist, such as a dietician.

At the end of every encounter, proper documentation is required. Documentation can either be done by hand or on a computer system. Some programs will provide a template for the pharmacist to complete, often a variation of a SOAP note, where one collects Subjective and Objective information and then develops an Assessment and Plan. Documentation serves to facilitate communication between providers, protect against professional liability, and justify billing. It also serves as a means to track outcomes and demonstrate the benefit of the MTM service. Good communication between all parties involved and proper documentation are essential to making an MTM visit successful.

To be successful at performing an MTM visit, your therapeutic knowledge must be up to date. Some common disease states you will encounter with typical MTM patients include diabetes, hypertension, hyperlipidemia, asthma, chronic obstructive pulmonary disease (COPD), osteoporosis, pain management, anxiety, depression, and insomnia. You may also be involved in educating a patient on proper device use, immunization status, or smoking cessation programs. Once you have identified the actual or potential drug therapy problems, you will be required to formulate a plan to address these issues.

QUICK TIP

If your site does not have a data collection form, develop your own with your preceptor's assistance so you are efficient when conducting the interview.

Adherence Assessments

As a pharmacist, you are in a critical position to help patients understand the vital role medications play in managing chronic conditions. Nonadherence to medications continues to be a growing concern in this country, with nonadherence rates from the low teens to more than 80%.[3-7] In the community setting, you should be able to recognize patients that are at an increased risk for medication nonadherence, determine the cause, and apply methods to improve medication adherence. Patients who are most prone to nonadherence include those with asymptomatic disease, psychiatric disorders, advanced age, and complicated regimens. Causes of medication nonadherence may be related to a number of factors, including the patient, the condition, the therapy, socioeconomic status, or the health system. The patient may be forgetful, have other priorities, have physical barriers, or a lack of information about his or her medications. Condition-related factors may include asymptomatic diseases for which the patient sees no benefit from treatment or psychiatric conditions such as depression, which have been documented to decrease adherence. Therapy-related factors may include a complex medication regimen or adverse drug effects. Socioeconomic factors may include such things as a low health literacy level, education level, cultural beliefs interfering with taking medication, or financial barriers. All of these factors may make it difficult for the patient to be adherent to medications. For a pharmacist to tackle nonadherence issues, it is important to understand that a "one-size-fits-all" approach will not work. Each patient will present with different issues that need to be addressed to improve adherence.

QUICK TIP

Adherence assessments can be performed at any stage of the community pharmacy practice continuum.

Critical to improving nonadherence is performing a patient interview and truly listening to the patient. During the patient interview, you should be able to ascertain if patients believe the medication is helping them, if they are motivated to improve their current health status, and if they believe the benefits of taking the medication outweigh the risks. It will also be necessary to verify the patient can pay for the medication, understands how to take the medication, and remembers to take the medication at the correct time. Some key questions that will help you conduct the interview are listed in **Figure 10-5**.

Figure 10-5. Key Questions for Assessing Adherence

- How are your medications helping you?
- What are your goals in the next few months?
- How is your health condition keeping you from achieving these goals?
- What have you been told about the benefits of your medication?
- What side effects are you having?
- Medications can be very expensive. How do you manage to pay for your prescriptions?
- Tell me (show me) how you take your medications.
- What system do you use to help you take your medication?

After a thorough interview, there are some ways to improve adherence. If financial reasons are the main barrier, it may be helpful to assess if the patient is eligible for Medicare or Medicaid. If not, there are also numerous patient-assistance programs offered that help to relieve financial burden from particular medications. You can help patients determine if they meet the criteria set forth by such programs. Some organizational systems to help patients remember to take their medications include a pill box, Doc-U-Dose®, or alarm system that can be set to remind the patient to take the medications. Other times, a phone call to the patient after a new medication is dispensed may help to alleviate any confusion the patient may be experiencing or any side effects that may prompt a patient to stop taking the medication. Educating a patient on the benefits of the medication and how to minimize risks may help to alleviate unnecessary fear leading to nonadherence. In some cases, it may be necessary to work with the prescriber for alternative medications. Most importantly, you can work with the patient to construct a regimen that is tailored to address his or her specific nonadherence issues.

Wellness and Screening Programs

A paradigm shift in modern healthcare is underway, from a reactive approach (treating existing disease) to a proactive approach, including preventive health, exploring lifestyle options that foster positive health behaviors, and taking the initiative to educate on these topics. This shift provides pharmacists with opportunities to offer wellness programs. What your APPE site offers will vary depending on a number of factors. Some examples of wellness screenings pharmacies offer include the following:

- Blood pressure checks
- Blood sugar checks
- Hemoglobin A1c (HbA1c) checks
- Osteoporosis evaluation (typically via heel assessment using ultrasound technology)
- Body fat analysis and body mass index (BMI) calculation
- Cholesterol tests (total cholesterol, low-density lipoprotein [LDL], high-density lipoprotein [HDL], triglycerides, or any combination)
- Medication reviews
- Nutrition and dietary reviews (often cooperatively with a dietician or nutritionist)

Our experience suggests patients are very receptive to these programs and appreciate the information and education provided. In addition to providing the screening results, additional activities and opportunities may arise. For example, if someone with diabetes stops in to have his or her blood sugar checked and enters into a discussion about his or her medications, it might be determined that there are opportunities to help optimize insulin therapy, review administration technique, or review other medications to ensure the patient is obtaining the best outcome. Others may be unaware of the services offered by modern community pharmacists until they attend a screening event. Lastly, wellness programs may help uncover undiagnosed disease states and improve patient outcomes. You may provide education about untreated disease, information to the individual's primary care physician, and follow-up to determine if the action steps recommended were completed. All of these activities are prime opportunities for students to get involved.

CASE QUESTION

L.B. has organized a blood glucose screening event for members of the community. One patient mentions that he has a diagnosis of diabetes and has not taken his insulin due to cost concerns. His glucose is 260 mg/dL today. How can L.B. improve this patient's care?

OVER-THE-COUNTER CONSULTS

A recent study by the Consumer Healthcare Products Association (CHPA) assessed the value of OTC medications in the United States. It found that almost 80% of Americans had used at least one OTC product during the 12-month evaluation period and that a majority (92%) stated they would seek another form of medical treatment if OTCs were not available. Considering the cost of OTCs in seven main categories and the cost of other forms of medical care and services if OTCs were not an option, the authors concluded that the total value of OTCs, including direct and indirect costs, is just over $102 billion annually.[8]

From the perspective of a community pharmacist, anyone considering an OTC product is a candidate for a self-care evaluation. Although OTCs may achieve significant savings for a majority of users, others may not be candidates for an OTC medication and should be referred to their physicians. Not only do we have many opportunities to counsel patients about their prescription medications, we also have opportunities to guide individuals in the selection of OTC products. To best determine who is and is not a candidate, there are many assessment techniques that can be used to evaluate individuals for self-care. Regardless of what technique is selected, it is important to remember that not everyone who is interested in making a purchase should do so. There are four potential outcomes from a self-care consultation based on what is in the patient's best interests, including the following:

- *Product recommendation:* an assessment suggests the condition is not serious and can be managed through an OTC product. An example is a college-aged male with a mildly sprained ankle who asks about pain reliever and anti-inflammatory options. The pharmacist determines the individual is a candidate for oral non-steroidal therapy.

- *Referral to primary care provider only:* an assessment suggests the condition is serious enough to warrant a visit to a primary care provider. An example is a middle-aged woman with frequent heartburn who has already tried a 2-week course of a proton pump inhibitor and asks what else she can use. Based on the information provided, the pharmacist tells her the next step needs to be an appointment with her physician.

- *Product recommendation and referral to primary care provider:* an assessment suggests that an OTC product may provide temporary relief until a visit to a primary care provider can be scheduled. An example is a mother whose 3-year-old daughter has had a 104.2-degree fever for a couple of days. The child should see her pediatrician, but in the meantime the use of a children's antipyretic is indicated. The key is to stress to the parent that the medication is temporary and a visit needs to be scheduled.

- *Suggest nonpharmacologic strategies:* an assessment suggests the condition is self-limiting and no medication is warranted at this time. An example is a middle-aged individual with hypertension presenting with some mild congestion, primarily in the early morning, with no other symptoms. He has a humidifier at home, and the pharmacist suggests using this for a couple days and then re-evaluating.

One assessment process used in practice is the QuEST/SCHOLAR-MAC process.[9] Elements of the QuEST/SCHOLAR-MAC process are listed in **Table 10-1**, with an example of a case study using this process.

THE BUSINESS OF COMMUNITY PHARMACY

Financials

This may sound oversimplified, but if a business does not make money, it will not be in business for very long. Again, in very simple terms, the revenue coming into the pharmacy must exceed the expenses going out the door. Controlling that equation on a daily basis, with all the forces and factors in and out

TABLE 10-1. EXAMPLE QUEST/SCHOLAR-MAC CASE STUDY

A young, college-aged male approaches you, the pharmacist, and asks, "What can I take for my headache?"

INFORMATION TO OBTAIN FROM THE PATIENT	WHAT THE PATIENT TELLS YOU
Quickly and accurately assess the patient: Ask about the current problem (SCHOLAR)	
Symptoms What are the main and associated symptoms?	"I have been studying for finals and feel like my head is going to explode."
Characteristics What is the situation like? Is it changing?	"It is better now than it was a couple of hours ago, but I still have this dull pain in my head that won't go away." (When asked about pain on a scale of 1–10, with 10 being the most intense pain, the customer says the pain is 4.)
History What has been done so far?	"I laid down for a couple minutes."
Onset When did it start?	"Early this morning."
Location Where is the problem?	"Mostly my head, but my neck and shoulders are also achy."
Aggravating factors What makes it worse?	"Studying or reading."
Remitting factors What makes it better?	"Lying down."
Ask about other *Medications, Allergies,* and *Conditions* (MAC): Within reason, get as much detail as possible to assist in the decision-making process.	"I take a generic version of Prilosec once a day for a stomach ulcer. My doc told me to use this and he wrote me a prescription, but I buy it over the counter because I don't have insurance." "I don't have any allergies." "All I have is a mild ulcer, mostly when I eat the wrong stuff or have too much to drink, which isn't too often. I'm in the pre-med program and I can't afford to screw up or my dad will stop paying my tuition and I'll end up working at Chipotle."
THE "E.S.T" PIECES OF QUEST: ESTABLISH, SELECT, AND TALK	YOUR ASSESSMENT, RECOMMENDATION, AND COUNSELING
Establish that the patient is an appropriate self-care candidate • Any severe symptoms? • Any symptoms that persist or return repeatedly? • Is the patient self-treating to avoid medical care?	Based on your assessment of the patient's situation, the answers to all three questions are "no," so the patient is a candidate for self-care.
Suggest appropriate self-care strategies	*Medication:* Because this patient has a history of ulcer disease, it is not appropriate to recommend a nonsteroidal anti-inflammatory drug (NSAID) to treat his headache. Suggest acetaminophen at a dose of 325 to 650 mg every 4 to 6 hours (no more than 3 g/day). It can be good for pain relief but has no anti-inflammatory activity. Also recommend general care measures: rest and sleep, use ice pack, try to relax and manage stress, and try to avoid triggers.

Talk with the patient about	Key Counseling Points:
• Medication action, administration, and adverse effects • What to expect from the treatment • Appropriate follow-up	"Acetaminophen (which is generic Tylenol) will help relieve the pain, and you should see some pain relief within 30 to 60 minutes. Only use it when you need it because it works fairly quickly." "Take with a full glass of water." "It is very important that you avoid alcohol while taking this medication." "Side effects are very uncommon. In very rare cases people get a minor rash. Other than that there is very little to worry about." "It's important that you also try to get some time to relax, get a good night's sleep, and find some balance between the intense studying and break times." "If symptoms worsen, do not get any better, or become intolerable, call your doctor. If your symptoms last for more than 10 days, that's another reason for you to call your doctor."

Source: Adapted with permission from the American Pharmacists Association.

of one's control, is much more complicated. The traditional source of revenue in a community pharmacy is through the processing of prescriptions. However, with over 90% of dispensed prescriptions paid for by third parties, it is become more challenging to turn a profit in this area. Some examples of costs pharmacies incur include salaries and benefits for personnel (pharmacists, technicians, others), supplies, medications, and overhead (rent, utilities). Examples of sources of revenue include prescriptions, OTC medications, other front-end merchandise, immunizations, and patient care services (such as MTM). Considerable effort is dedicated to controlling the cost side of the business, whether it is a single-pharmacy independent or a 7,000-plus-store nationwide chain. Very small percentage discounts on supply purchases, such as labels and paper, can save hundreds of thousands of dollars annually. On the dispensing side, negotiating another few cents of reimbursement per prescription from a third party can generate significant dollars in the long run. Many community pharmacies have full-time staff dedicated solely to the financial side of the business. Hopefully, you will have an opportunity to interact with someone in this department to learn firsthand how the financial end of the community pharmacy business operates.

Marketing

Community pharmacies can have the best staff, best products, and best services, but it may all be wasted if the community is unaware of the services offered. Community pharmacies are businesses, and, as such, they need to implement core principles of marketing, advertising, and merchandising. Pharmacies must determine how to best meet their patients' and customers' needs, wants, and demands. Needs and wants are often consumer driven, whereas the demands may be created by the business through unique strategies of offering appealing, reasonably priced products consumers may not have initially considered.

There are five core elements in the traditional "marketing mix," also known as the five "Ps": product, price, placement, promotion, and positioning. Each plays off the other, so if all are addressed collectively, a marketing strategy has a significant chance of succeeding. Many hours are spent determining what products to promote, where to promote, how to price them, and where to position them in the store. Advertising helps with carrying out a marketing strategy, but it is only one aspect of that strategy. Many advertising avenues are available, from bag stuffers and signage in an individual store to a national advertising campaign on television or in print media. Ideally, organizations develop processes and metrics to determine the effectiveness of a particular strategy or campaign, as the return on investment is important for companies that invest considerable resources in this area. Often, however, it comes down to subjective assessments of success. From a pharmacy student's perspective, everyone in an organization is responsible for marketing and advertising through their daily work and interactions, so the messages delivered in a campaign should be consistent with the messages delivered by employees. Talk with your preceptor about the marketing strategies employed by the pharmacy where you are placed and learn how they address this important aspect of community pharmacy.

REFERENCES

1. Gardner M, Boyce RW, Herrier RN. *Pharmacist-Patient Consultation Program: An Interactive Approach to Verifying Patient Understanding.* New York, NY: Pfizer; 1991.

2. Bluml BM. Definition of medication therapy management: Development of profession wide consensus. *J Am Pharm Assoc.* 2005;45:566-572.

3. Coleman CI, Limone B, Sobieraj DM, et al. Dosing frequency and medication adherence in chronic disease. *J Manag Care Pharm.* 2012;18:527-539.

4. Viswanathan M, Golin CE, Jones CD, et al. Interventions to improve adherence to self-administered medications for chronic diseases in the United States: A systematic review. *Ann Intern Med.* Sept. 11, 2012. doi: 10.7326/0003-4819-157-11-201212040-00538. [Epub ahead of print]

5. Gharibian D, Polzin JK, Rho JP. Compliance and persistence of antidepressants versus anticonvulsants in patients with neuropathic pain during the first year of therapy. *Clin J Pain.* Aug. 21, 2012. [Epub ahead of print]

6. Sheehan DV, Keene MS, Eaddy M, et al. Differences in medication adherence and healthcare resource utilization patterns: Older versus newer antidepressant agents in patients with depression and/or anxiety disorders. *CNS Drugs.* 2008;22:963-973.

7. Yeaw J, Benner JS, Walt JG, et al. Comparing adherence and persistence across six chronic medication classes. *J Manag Care Pharm.* 2009;15:728-740.

8. The value of OTC medicine to the United States. http://www.yourhealthathand.org/images/uploads/The_Value_of_OTC_Medicine_to_the_United_States_BoozCo.pdf. Accessed July 22, 2012.

9. Leibowitz K, Ginsburg D. Counseling self-treating patients quickly and effectively. Proceedings of the APhA Inaugural Self-Care Institute; May 17-19, 2002; Chantilly, VA.

SUGGESTED READING

Centers for Medicare & Medicaid Services (CMS). Available at https://www.cms.gov/PrescriptionDrugCov Contra/Downloads/MTMFactSheet.pdf

George J, Elliott RA, Stewart DC. A systematic review of interventions to improve medication taking in elderly patients prescribed multiple medications. *Drugs Aging.* 2008;25:307-324.

Ho PM, Bryson CL, Rumsfeld JS. Medication adherence: Its importance in cardiovascular outcomes. *Circulation.* 2009;119:3028-3035.

Krinsky DL, Berardi RR, Ferreri SP, et al., eds. *Handbook of Nonprescription Drugs: An Interactive Approach to Self-Care.* 17th ed. Washington, DC: American Pharmacists Association; 2012.

Lewis RK, Lasack NL, Lambert BL, et al. Patient counseling: A focus on maintenance therapy. *Am J Health-Syst Pharm.* 1997;54:2084-2098.

MacLaughlin EJ, Raehl CL, Treadway AK, et al. Assessing medication adherence in the elderly: Which tools to use in clinical practice? *Drugs Aging.* 2005;22:231-255.

MTM Central Resource Library: http://www.pharmacist.com/mtm-central-resource-library

Osterberg L, Blaschke T. Adherence to medication. *N Engl J Med.* 2005;353:487-497.

Sabaté E, ed. *Adherence to Long-Term Therapies: Evidence for Action.* Geneva, Switzerland: World Health Organization; 2003. http://apps.who.int/medicinedocs/pdf/s4883e/s4883e.pdf

Shea SC. *Improving Medication Adherence: How to Talk With Patients About Their Medications.* Philadelphia, PA: Lippincott Williams & Wilkins; 2006.

Tietze KJ. *Clinical Skills for Pharmacists: A Patient-Focused Approach.* 2nd ed. St. Louis, MO: Mosby; 2004.

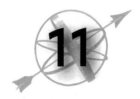

MANAGEMENT AND LEADERSHIP ROTATIONS

Jason Glowczewski, PharmD, MBA

CASE

N.S. is a pharmacy student on week two of his management and leadership APPE rotation. Like many others, the day begins with a meeting. During this meeting, someone wearing a suit asks N.S. how engaged he believes the pharmacy's employees are and how the culture differs from other hospitals that N.S. has experienced. After he answers, the preceptor whispers, "That was the hospital president." Later in the day, N.S. delves into the 10 projects on his prioritized to-do list but gets stuck trying to fix a complex formula in a newly developed spreadsheet looking at the financial impact of adding a new drug to the formulary. N.S. works out a solution, finishes the project, and e-mails the result to his preceptor, who appreciates the hard work and already has two additional projects that need urgent attention.

WHY IT'S ESSENTIAL

Although a management or leadership rotation is often an elective experience, the lessons learned can immediately be applied to other APPE rotations and eventually be helpful in your role as a pharmacist, where you must be comfortable supervising and managing others, regardless of their practice setting or level of experience. When the pharmacy manager is not immediately available, the pharmacist is in charge of all nonlicensed personnel. The ability to supervise and provide guidance to nonlicensed personnel impacts daily workflow as well as patient safety. Knowing how to provide constructive criticism, motivate others, and handle conflict are all skills that pharmacists must command. In many ways, managing others is both science and art. Like clinical information, management styles and techniques can be researched and learned through peer-reviewed published data, although practice is crucial to properly execute these techniques.

The management rotation offers you additional benefits beyond experiencing the daily activities of a management-level preceptor. As a manager or director, your preceptor is often a key decision maker in the organization's hiring process and likely knows others in similar positions within affiliated or competing organizations. With significant experience interviewing candidates for jobs, your preceptor can be an excellent resource for practicing interview skills or even participating in mock interviews. Another important management task is providing feedback and employee evaluations. Once understood, employee evaluation skills can help the practicing pharmacist be prepared for his or her own evaluation and better envision how managers view goals, success, and raises.

....

"Career success often depends on how people manage themselves and interact with others—and possessing these skills is a significant factor in differentiating the good performer from the outstanding performer. A management rotation also helps students understand the 'big picture' view of the environment in which they practice so they can align their contributions to best meet the needs of the department, the organization, and the patients we serve."—Preceptor

....

ARRIVING PREPARED

To take full advantage of all of the opportunities a management rotation can offer, you must arrive prepared. Contact the preceptor a few weeks before the start of the rotation to confirm start time, location, suggested reading, professional attire, and any supplies needed. Although white lab coats are commonly worn on clinical rotations, they may not be appropriate on a management rotation, depending on the management setting. When preparing for the rotation, it is important that you thoroughly understand the practice setting that you are about to enter. An online review of the business, including location, mission statement, financial performance (if publically traded), and services offered, may be helpful. Also, information may be available about the preceptor, such as publications, research interests, awards, or activities in professional organizations. It is further advisable for you to evaluate your own social media to ensure that tech-savvy preceptors do not have an unfavorable first impression before the rotation begins (see Chapter 1). APPE rotations are the gateway to residency and independent pharmacy practice, so it is best to be prepared with the optimal outward online projection of one's experiences.

To cultivate and project a level of confidence in the management and leadership realm, it may be necessary to review terminology commonly used by pharmacy leadership. This terminology is often learned on the rotation, but arriving prepared presents an excellent opportunity to thrive on the rotation, rather than merely survive. Important management concepts that should be reviewed prior to starting the rotation include the following:

- Employee engagement
- Six Sigma
- Full-time equivalent (FTE)
- Productivity
- SWOT (Strengths, Weaknesses, Opportunities, and Threats) analysis
- FMEA (Failure, Mode, and Effects Analysis)
- Root-cause analysis
- Gap analysis
- Culture (as it relates to business)
- Management, leadership, and the difference between the two
- The Joint Commission, Centers for Medicare & Medicaid Services (CMS), and Core Measures (in the hospital setting)
- SCIP (Surgical Care Improvement Project) and HCAHPS (Hospital Consumer Assessment of Healthcare Providers and Systems) (in the hospital setting)

Equally important to arriving prepared for the rotation is learning about your preceptor on day one. Like many clinical preceptors, a manager will be very busy onsite and attending meetings away from the rotation site. You may be asked to join your preceptor for some of these meetings, although this may not always be the case. Learn your preceptor's preferred communication method, such as office phone, cell phone, e-mail, text message, or contacting an administrative assistant. Knowing the best communication method can mean the difference between getting an instant answer and getting no response to an important question.

CASE QUESTION

When N.S. answers the hospital president's question about employee engagement in the department, is he putting the department or preceptor at risk in any way? Is 1 week enough to be able to assess a department's culture or engagement level?

A TYPICAL DAY

Management rotations may vary considerably depending on the practice setting, as well as the experience level and position of the preceptor. Although day-to-day activities can fluctuate greatly, fundamental lessons in leadership and management will help you to develop similar core management and leadership skills. For example, a chief pharmacy officer or vice president may have directors and managers directly reporting to the position, whereas a manager may have staff pharmacists as direct reports. Each of these leaders will likely be responsible for maintaining a budget, evaluating and motivating employees, attending meetings, giving presentations, and contributing to the organization's goals and success.

You must be prepared for significant day-to-day variation in the rotation experience, with rapidly changing priorities and projects. If a typical student day could be constructed, it might look like the following schedule:

- 8 a.m.—Arrive at the hospital and work on quality dashboard
- 9 a.m.—Attend pharmacy and therapeutics committee meeting
- 11 a.m.—Free time to work on projects (finish quality dashboard and begin to analyze end-of-month performance)
- Noon—Eat lunch and work on audit of surgery billing
- 1 p.m.—Attend management meeting with preceptor, focusing on annual hospital goals
- 2 p.m.—Meet with preceptor in preparation for staff meeting
- 3 p.m.—Assist running the department staff meeting and take meeting minutes
- 4 p.m.—Continue working on billing audit and begin reading handout on servant leadership for discussion the next day

Moving from a highly structured academic life to a more practical setting during APPE rotations can be a substantial adjustment. When considering the typical day on a management rotation, be prepared to be flexible and to receive project instruction with limited details. Communicate with the preceptor to confirm expectations, goals, and priorities for projects to help ensure success on the rotation.

MEETINGS

An integral part of management rotations is meeting attendance. Although attendance is important, knowing the intended level of participation in the meeting is even more crucial. Some meetings will require active participation, whereas others will be for observation only. You may even lead meetings, such as small-group staff meetings or brainstorming sessions to solve departmental issues. Strategies for running specific meeting types may be found in a number of reputable sources, including those listed in the Suggested Reading section of this chapter.

General tips for running effective meetings include the following:

- Ensure that all key participants are invited to the meeting.
- Send out a meeting agenda in advance of the meeting.
- Start meetings by discussing the purpose and goals of the meeting.
- Begin and end the meeting on time.
- Take accurate meeting minutes and send them out after the meeting has ended.
- Ensure that everyone in the meeting is an active participant.
- Clearly delineate people responsible for action items as well as a timeline for completion.
- Summarize the meeting and set the next meeting time and location.

Once you have a plan for the level of participation within the meeting, it is important to keep in mind some inappropriate actions that must be avoided. Meetings can be long and, when you do not have a vested interest in the outcome, the experience may seem boring. Falling asleep is never acceptable. Remember that your preceptor not only fills out your evaluation but also could be a critical job reference. If drowsiness occurs, consider that falling asleep on the job for a pharmacist can result in immediate termination. Of a similar nature, you may believe that it is acceptable to check e-mails and send text messages during meetings because preceptors and other managers are doing so. The difference is that the managers are sending work-related e-mails and handling work-related emergencies. You must use extreme discretion with all mobile communication.

CASE QUESTION

N.S. is halfway through the rotation and has lunch with another APPE student, C.C., from a different school. After eating, C.C. asks the management student to wake her up in half an hour. The intent is for C.C. to sleep in the cafeteria during lunchtime. Is this acceptable? What should N.S. do? Could sleeping in the cafeteria create the wrong initial impression at the site?

Prepare for meetings in a way that emulates your preceptor. If the preceptor researches a topic to be discussed and brings a pad of paper for taking notes, it is important that you are similarly primed and equipped. In some organizations, leaders have laptops or tablet devices at meetings and type notes, whereas in other settings a laptop would isolate users from peers and would be culturally unacceptable. In addition to being engaged in the meeting and conveying interest, it is important to exercise caution in any reply you give directly during a meeting. A brief premeeting discussion should take place between you and your preceptor so that expectations are clear for what and how much should be said during the meeting. Further, management-level meetings may contain sensitive information that should not be shared with other employees. Sensitive information may include, but is not limited to, salary information, benefit changes for the next year, confidential employee relation issues, or even information about possible layoffs.

One of the most common meetings that you may be asked to participate in (or even lead) is a staff meeting, which is a regularly scheduled meeting between a department leader and the department staff to share information, implement changes, seek feedback, and build relationships within the department. You can help your preceptor lead staff meetings by identifying recent agenda topics, researching and formatting information for presentation, and taking meeting minutes to document the outcomes of the meeting.

FORMULARY MONOGRAPHS AND THE PHARMACY AND THERAPEUTICS COMMITTEE

In an institutional setting, you may spend time with the pharmacy and therapeutics (P&T) committee. The P&T committee is a multidisciplinary panel that is responsible to the medical staff and has the task of managing a formulary. The P&T committee is typically made up of a physician chairperson and a mix of physicians, pharmacists, nurses, and other clinical members, as defined by an organization's bylaws. Medication-use evaluations (MUEs), adverse drug event monitoring, medication error review and prevention, and development of guidelines such as formulary substitutions are all duties of this committee.[1] The P&T committee may offer the opportunity for you to write up formal formulary monographs or review trends in medication safety for presentation to the group.

As medication experts, pharmacists play the major role in preparing and presenting drug information to the P&T committee for review. The drug information is often formatted as a formulary monograph. Drug reviews presented to the committee may be classified as new, therapeutic class reviews, revisions, or expedited reviews of new medications. Each organization may have a standard template for formulary review, and the acceptable length can vary greatly. It is important to understand expectations before beginning a review.

Critical components of a formulary monograph include the following[1]:

- Drug name (brand and generic)
- Look-alike/sound-alike medications
- Food and Drug Administration (FDA)-approved indications and off-label uses
- Pharmacology and mechanism of action
- Dosage forms and storage requirements/issues
- Dose information for each indication, if different
- Pharmacokinetic data
- Use and dosing in special populations
- Pregnancy and breastfeeding category and considerations
- Comparative efficacy with similar agents—including safety, efficacy, cost, and convenience
- Clinical trial information and analysis
- Other medication safety considerations, such as interactions, monitoring, or storage requirements
- Financial analysis—including annualized impact and reimbursement information in the out-patient setting
- Overall recommendation and any restrictions that will be in place for the drug

Formulary management and monograph preparation are foundational components of a medication safety program and offer you a unique opportunity to gain in-depth knowledge of a drug from both a clinical and financial perspective. To support the development of a complex financial analysis and make the information concise for P&T members, be prepared to use spreadsheet programs such as Microsoft® Excel® to collect, analyze, and prepare graphs for presentation.

Computer Skills

Although electronic systems have become an integral tool in the management of pharmacy departments, managers must deal with an unprecedented quantity of data. The manager must collect the pertinent data, process the information, and package everything in a way that can be shared with others to effect change or validate theories. To do this, managers must possess basic computer software skills, particularly with word processors such as Microsoft® Word®, presentation software such as Microsoft® PowerPoint®, and spreadsheet software such as Microsoft® Excel®.

Pharmacy students are often comfortable with Word® and PowerPoint®, yet many are uncomfortable with Excel®. Ideally, basic Excel® skills should be developed before beginning a management rotation. Many free tutorials exist online, particularly on the Microsoft® website. Below is a list of basic and intermediate Excel® functions that may be helpful on rotations.

Data collection:

♦ Format the cells in Excel® by changing width and height, changing fonts, and adding borders

♦ Data validation tools to ensure consistent entry or to create drop boxes for ease of data entry

Data analysis and formatting:

♦ Pivot tables

♦ How and why to make absolute references using the $ symbol

♦ Formulas

- Sum

- Average

- Count

- Standard deviation

- V-lookup (advanced function)

♦ Conditional formatting—useful for making stoplight charts (intermediate to advanced)

Other important skills for the presentation of data:

♦ Use the "print screen" function to quickly copy any information on your computer screen into Excel®, Word®, or PowerPoint®

♦ Create appealing graphs, modify colors, and add trend lines

♦ Modify a spreadsheet by changing column and row height and width, as well as adding borders to create paper forms or to present raw or summarized data

♦ Add video, sound, graphs, charts, and other external data to presentation slides

---

QUICK TIP

At some point technology will fail. Always have one or two electronic backups and one paper backup for critical presentations.

When using word processors such as Microsoft® Word®, there are several basic to intermediate features that can be of great assistance on a management rotation. The first tool can be enabled under the spelling and grammar tab of the program's preferences, called "readability statistics." When this feature is enabled, it will allow you to get a measure of readability when you run the spelling and grammar check. This tool is helpful when creating patient-directed advertisements, brochures, or other educational materials. Although each organization will have its own standards, a sixth-grade reading level is a great goal if you want to ensure that information is well understood by the general public.

Although creating appealing written materials must be a priority, another challenge you must meet head-on is the ability to communicate information concisely. Inserting a flow chart in Word®, PowerPoint®, or Excel® can be helpful for presenting complex information visually. Tables are another visual tool available in Word® and PowerPoint.® Although it is possible to insert tables in Word®, it may make more sense to enter the information in Excel® and then import the information into Word® or PowerPoint® if dealing with numerical data.

QUICK TIP

Avoid using a calculator to calculate the sum of information in tables in any program. Use a spreadsheet with the proper formulas. This will reduce the risk of a manual calculation error.

MISSION AND GOALS

Even though you will probably find the organization's mission online in advance of the rotation, it will be important to consult with the preceptor to learn about the organization's specific goals. The student's goal on the rotation should be to help the preceptor further the organization's goals and mission. During the rotation, when you encounter projects such as goal setting and strategic planning, you will be at a unique disadvantage to hospital employees, as it takes time to learn the organizational culture and habits and have a full understanding of where the department is on the journey to achieving its goals. The advantage that you have, however, is the available time to assist with collecting, analyzing, and presenting the data.

Goals must be SMART: specific, measurable, attainable, realistic, and timely. This acronym not only applies to goals but also can be used as a guiding principle when taking on projects. The project must be well defined (specific), measurable, attainable (generally within 1 month or less), and realistically completed with high quality.

In addition to contributing to organizational goals, it is important for you to come to the rotation able to explain why you chose a management rotation and what you hope to learn from the rotation. Further, you must be prepared to explain and develop personal career goals during the rotation because the preceptor is likely to be in a key position to help provide feedback and assist with networking. If personal and professional goals are shared with your management preceptor, there is a good chance that the preceptor may help further such goals, possibly becoming a mentor.

BUDGETS, BUSINESS PLANS, AND PRODUCTIVITY

Managers are often pulled in many directions, with employee relations, goal achievement, and managing the department's finances. You are generally not expected to create a budget, yet you may assist in attaining budget goals though cost-saving initiatives. In any pharmacy setting, a fresh set of eyes can have advantages, so it is imperative that you speak up about potential cost savings with your preceptor.

Cost savings in pharmacy departments can typically be divided into two opportunities: supply costs (generally medications) and labor costs (personnel). Borrowing from Six Sigma and Lean methods, you can perform a waste walk to help look for waste. The seven types of waste are the following:

1. Defects
2. Overproduction
3. Inventories
4. Overprocessing
5. Unnecessary motion
6. Unnecessary transport
7. Handling and waiting

Once identified, action and quality improvement plans can be implemented to reduce the targeted waste. Waste walks, Lean Six Sigma, and other quality methods can be helpful tools for students to leverage to make a financial or quality impact on their site.

QUICK TIP

Remember that every rotation is essentially a job interview, either for that site or for a letter of recommendation for another position. Leverage every tool available to contribute to the success of the department and preceptor to make an impact.

Business plans are another tool at a manager's disposal for creating new services and receiving funding to make a new project a reality. Understanding how to write and implement a business plan is a vital skill for pharmacy students with the desire to create and build new clinical services in any setting. It is unlikely that a management preceptor will be writing a new business plan every month, so you must be proactive and ask what business plans have been implemented in the past or how you may contribute to the development of a business plan for a new service. Business plans often require a great deal of research that is well suited to the pharmacy student's skills. Although selling the plan to the senior administration will be the preceptor's focus, the better the plan, quality of the research, and integrity of the data, the easier it will be to justify the new service.

Business plans often reference FTE positions, but FTEs have a broader use in the management of a department. Learn how your preceptor manages productivity, a benchmark used in many organizations to evaluate staffing needs and effectiveness. It can be calculated many different ways, such as by determining how many FTE employees worked during a given period of time, allocating a fixed number of hours for employees per dose dispensed, or evaluating whether the total dollars spent on wages was within budget. Productivity is an extremely important concept to take away from the rotation, as it could be very helpful in the future to justify additional help or retain existing staff.

Personal productivity is another dimension of productivity that is vital for success on a management rotation. Like managers, students on management rotations will often have a great deal of latitude in daily activities. This flexibility can be used to learn site-specific workflow, research questions and problems, or work on short- or long-term projects. To be successful, seek the preceptor's guidance in the priority of projects and then complete projects as quickly as possible with high-quality work. It may be helpful to ask the preceptor if it is acceptable to take home projects and work, thereby demonstrating commitment to the assignments (although highly sensitive or protected information may not be allowed to leave the site). Students that complete projects on or ahead of schedule, ask for additional projects, and still participate in all daily meetings with engagement will be the most successful.

HUMAN RESOURCE MANAGEMENT

Building and maintaining strong relationships with department staff and improving employee engagement is likely to be a goal of both the preceptor and senior leaders in an organization. Make it a goal to do the same at the rotation site. Learn the names of as many people as possible in the institution, including what the individual prefers to be called. Consider what has been learned from researching employee engagement, servant leadership, and culture, as well as how to apply this information to interactions with the pharmacy staff. Further, if you notice that employees lack critical elements for engagement, such as having the necessary materials to do their job, understanding expectations, or feeling recognized, bring this up with the preceptor. Raise these issues in a positive way, describing the problem as an opportunity to get involved, contribute, and improve a situation.

When it comes to learning and experiencing human resource management principles on a management rotation, the medical ethics concept of "first do no harm" is an excellent guiding principle. How could you cause harm on a management rotation? Contributing to or getting caught up in department gossip, sharing confidential information obtained in management meetings, or unknowingly violating the law as it relates to fair labor practices creates significant risk for the student, preceptor, and facility. Even if you are not formally conducting an interview, there may be times when you need to meet a job-seeking candidate, provide a tour, or walk the candidate out. Innocently asking questions about the age, marital status, children, or social group membership of the candidate could violate fair labor practices, especially if you are believed to be working for the organization or share information with someone that has the authority to make hiring decisions. Before involvement in any job interview, make sure that your personal knowledge about illegal interview questions is fully up to date.

CASE QUESTION

One afternoon, N.S. bumps into someone he knows who is a candidate for a job at the rotation site. While on break, N.S. catches up with this acquaintance and asks about plans to get married and have children, what church he attends, and an injury to his leg. Could this be a problem? Does it matter if others are in attendance during this discussion?

To maximize the personal benefit gained from the management rotation, make sure that interview skills are covered as a human resources topic. This topic has a dual benefit of providing exposure to interviewing others, which most pharmacists will need to do at some point, and providing up-to-date interview skills that may be helpful in pursuing a residency or job. Behavior-based interviewing is a commonly used technique that you should familiarize yourself with and hopefully put into practice while on the rotation.

QUICK TIP

Ask the preceptor if it would be possible to schedule a mock interview, even if in a highly abbreviated format. This is a great way to learn how to interview others and practice important skills in a real situation.

Reviewing interview skills with the preceptor is an excellent lead in to present your current curriculum vitae (CV) for feedback. Be prepared for the preceptor to ask questions about specific activities or events and take all feedback as constructive. Ask for honest feedback on how your CV compares to the CVs of other students that the preceptor has interviewed or how the document could be refined to better present unique skills or accomplishments.

AUDITS

Audits have many meanings to the pharmacy leader. Audits may be internal or external. Examples of external auditing bodies include the board of pharmacy, The Joint Commission, Department of Health, Occupational Safety and Health Administration, Drug Enforcement Agency, and Food and Drug Administration. Internal audits can come from an internal audit department, higher-level administration within the company, or quality department or may originate within the department as a self-audit.

Your role in external audits is often to self-audit and implement process improvements to facilitate compliance. It is helpful for students to understand which external organizations are likely to conduct an audit and if the typical audit is scheduled or unscheduled. Many of the auditing organizations offer checklists on their websites to facilitate self-auditing and compliance. As unannounced audits are common, many organizations practice continuous readiness in an effort to be prepared for inspection or audit.

QUICK TIP

Pharmacy students on rotation must be compliant with all accreditation standards, and violations on the part of the student could become violations for the institution. Make sure that proper identification is worn at all times and that rules dictating proper footwear (closed-toe shoes) and restrictions on food and drink are followed.

Pharmacy students involved with internal audits often serve in the role of the auditor. This role begins with forming a basic understanding of the information to be audited, collecting data, analyzing data, and assisting department personnel with implementing an improvement plan. If results from the audit could be helpful to others outside the organization, it may be possible to publish the findings in either poster presentation or written format.

REFERENCE

1.   American Society of Health-System Pharmacists. ASHP guidelines on the pharmacy and therapeutics committee and the formulary system. *Am J Health-Syst Pharm.* 2008;65:1272-1283.

SUGGESTED READING

Agency for Healthcare Research Quality. AHRQ quality indicators toolkit for hospitals: Gap analysis. http://www.ahrq.gov/qual/qitoolkit/d5_gapanalysis.pdf. Accessed October 2, 2012.

Alexander M, Walkenbach J. *Microsoft® Excel® Dashboards & Reports.* Hoboken, NJ: Wiley Publishing; 2010.

ASHP Foundation. Leadership Resource Center. Leader's toolbox. http://www.ashpfoundation.org/leadership-toolkit/. Accessed October 15, 2012.

Buckingham M, Coffman C. *First, Break All the Rules.* New York, NY: Simon & Schuster; 1999.

Covey S. *The 7 Habits of Highly Effective People.* New York, NY: Free Press; 1989.

Hospital Care Quality Information from the Consumer Perspective. HCAHPS fact sheet. http://www.hcahps online.org/Facts.aspx. Accessed September 28, 2012.

Institute for Safe Medication Practices. Failure mode and effects analysis (FMEA). http://www.ismp.org/tools/ FMEA.asp. Accessed September 23, 2012.

Murray A. *The Wall Street Journal Essential Guide to Management*. New York, NY: HarperCollins; 2010.

Pocket Mentor: Running Meetings. Boston, MA: Harvard Business School Press; 2006.

U.S. Department of Health & Human Services Agency for Healthcare Research and Quality. Patient safety primers: Root cause analysis. http://psnet.ahrq.gov/primer.aspx?primerID=10. Accessed October 1, 2012.

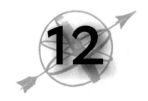

ACADEMIA

Susan P. Bruce, PharmD, BCPS; Dale E. English II, PharmD, FASHP;
Janis J. MacKichan, PharmD, FAPhA; and Timothy R. Ulbrich, PharmD

CASE

L.R. is a pharmacy student beginning an academic APPE. L.R. is interested in exploring teaching further, although her plans after graduation are still unclear. During the first day of the rotation, the preceptor reviewed all rotation activities and informed L.R. that she would be preparing and presenting a 2-hour large-group lecture in the cardiology module at the end of the rotation. L.R. has limited experience preparing for large-group presentations and feels a bit overwhelmed. In addition, L.R. will be facilitating a small-group cardiology case discussion.

WHY IT'S ESSENTIAL

Teaching is an inherent quality of a successful pharmacist. Experiencing an academic pharmacy APPE is an excellent way for you to develop teaching skills, regardless of the practice setting you choose after graduation. Some students may not be interested in an academic APPE because they perceive it will be helpful only in becoming a faculty member. However, during an academic pharmacy APPE, you will likely be involved in a variety of teaching and learning scenarios, including large-group teaching, small-group teaching, one-on-one teaching, and student assessments. Learning about how people learn and developing your own teaching style are helpful skills for any pharmacist. The experiences obtained can be translated to teaching patients, pharmacy students, and other healthcare providers.

ARRIVING PREPARED

Prior to beginning an academic APPE, you should think about what you would like to gain from the experience. What are the audiences a pharmacist teaches? How can the skills obtained in an academic APPE help you in that role? Are there other scenarios where teaching or presenting information to a group of people will be helpful? While building rotation objectives, you should keep your mind open to what will be learned during the rotation. So much goes on behind the scenes to prepare for teaching activities that you are not likely aware of! If you are thinking about a position after graduation that includes a teaching component, you should make sure to take time during the rotation to talk with faculty about their careers. Doing so will help you learn more about what teaching positions entail and perhaps guide you to a position with ideal teaching components.

Because faculty members' day-to-day activities differ depending on their positions, you should learn about the different types of faculty positions before starting the rotation. In addition to reading about the different position types,[1-3] you are encouraged to interview faculty during the rotation to learn about what they like and dislike about their positions. There are three general types of faculty positions in colleges/schools of pharmacy: tenure track, non-tenure track, and voluntary. *Tenure track* positions are typically fully funded by the institution and emphasize scholarly activity (writing grants, conducting research, and publishing in peer-reviewed journals), campus-based teaching, and course administration and possibly involve a percentage of time spent at a practice site precepting students and caring for patients. *Non-tenure track* positions tend to be located primarily in pharmacy practice departments, and the salary may be "shared" between the institution and a practice site (hence the terms *shared* or *co-funded faculty*). The teaching responsibilities of these types of faculty usually focus more on precepting than on didactic teaching, and there tends to be less emphasis on scholarly activity. Non-tenure track positions in PhD-dominated departments or divisions (pharmaceutical sciences, social sciences, and administrative pharmacy) tend also to focus more on teaching than on scholarly activity. Many of the preceptors you have had on IPPE or APPE rotations are voluntary faculty. They are salaried by their practice site but hold faculty appointments at the college. These individuals are especially important given the ever-expanding need for quality rotation experiences.

QUICK TIP

The general descriptions of faculty positions vary from school to school, so it is important that you ask questions about how your school compares to others.

A TYPICAL DAY

There is no typical day in an academic APPE! The rotation schedule will depend on the activities in which you are participating. Faculty members usually work months ahead of the course schedule to determine specific classroom activities and overarching curricular improvements. As a result, many activities in an academic rotation are predetermined and scheduled months in advance. You will be responsible on the first day for reviewing the rotation calendar, understanding your role in each of the activities, and determining how to manage your time to ensure you are adequately prepared for each activity. Like faculty, students completing an academic pharmacy rotation must have excellent organizational and time-management skills.

TEACHING SKILLS

The backbone of an academic pharmacy rotation will help you develop your teaching skills. You may be asked to participate in a number of activities, ranging from development of a teaching philosophy, large-group lectures, small-group activities, to other unique opportunities that will depend on your rotation site.

Writing a Teaching Philosophy

During an academic rotation, you may be asked to begin developing and collecting materials that showcase your teaching experiences, such as a teaching philosophy or a teaching portfolio. A teaching philosophy is an evolving document that serves two purposes. First, the philosophy is a means of providing evidence to learners, peers, and employers of your understanding of the purpose and value of the teaching process. Second, a philosophy serves as means of self-reflection, allowing you to put deep thought into the learning process and how you can improve as a teacher. The teaching philosophy is generally written in a first-person narrative form and is one to two pages in length. When completing an academic rotation, you should consider drafting a philosophy before teaching for the first time and then revisiting and revising the document on a regular basis.

Students and new teachers often find the process of constructing a philosophy to be daunting. A teaching philosophy that focuses heavily on self-reflection can be difficult and uncomfortable to write.

Asking yourself the following questions when drafting a philosophy may be a helpful way to get started:

- What happens to the learner during the learning process?
- What is the ultimate aim of teaching?
- What characteristics are present in "great" teachers?
- What strategies or techniques do "great" teachers use?
- When students are engaged during class, what is happening during that time?
- What factors go into making a learning environment ideal?
- What is the teacher's responsibility and what is the student's responsibility?
- How will the teacher measure effectiveness? How will the teacher know that he or she has been successful?[4]

QUICK TIP

It takes time and significant reflection to articulate your personal approach to teaching. The process of self-reflection is just as important as the product, which will likely be revised many times along the way!

Large-Group Teaching

When starting an academic rotation, you will likely be given a large-group teaching assignment in addition to other small-group opportunities. Similar to L.R.'s reaction to the cardiology topic assignment, this can be overwhelming. The apprehension often comes from the aspect of speaking in front of a large group. Planning and delivering this lecture can require a significant amount of time that consists of writing objectives, developing the presentation, and writing test questions. It is integral to meet with the appropriate course director or other faculty members early to identify the overarching goals for the assigned session and where it fits in with the other content students are learning. Understanding what the students have (or have not) already learned in class will allow you to develop the lecture at the appropriate level and may provide opportunities for building on previous material. Before jumping in, you should also be aware of any course standards with regard to learning objectives (e.g., how many objectives should be written), style of presentation (e.g., PowerPoint® versus discussion or cases), and the number and format of test questions that will be expected from the session. First, identify the session's objectives because they will drive the important content areas that you will cover as well as the test questions that you will write. Well-written objectives will be beneficial to both the teacher and learners.

In pharmacy education, the traditional presentation style for a didactic session is often centered on the content expert delivering a large amount of information via PowerPoint® slides. Use of this technology has potential benefits, such as ease of conveying information, student comfort, and decreased anxiety by the lecturer. However, using presentation software has potential limitations, such as conveying overwhelming amounts of information, asking the learner to simultaneously focus on both the slides and the presenter's narrative, and putting the learner in a passive role. The books *Beyond Bullet Points*, *Presentation Secrets of Steve Jobs*, and *Presentation Zen* highlight key concepts to develop when delivering a presentation.[5-7] These concepts are designed to transform a traditional slide presentation that is overwhelmed by text and bullets to a presentation that minimizes the amount of text and uses more images, allowing the learner to focus on the presenter.

Some of the concepts that can apply to all teachers include:

- *Planning in analog.* Rather than jumping right into filling the slides in on your computer, take a step back to map out and plan the presentation. This will help you avoid putting excessive information on slides and allow for a consistent message throughout.

- *Make it personal.* Rather than just talking about a disease state or treatment regimen, talk about how this will directly apply to the students or the patients they may be treating via use of a patient case.

- *Use the rule of three.* Long-term memory is lost when the brain is inundated with large amounts of information. Breaking the topic into three clearly defined categories or main points may allow for better retention.

- *Create visual slides.* The focus on creating slides should be to supplement the speaker, not replace the speaker. Therefore, slides should be free of clutter (bullets and text) and replaced with relevant images and taglines that are easy to remember. Images used must be relevant to avoid distraction. Unrelated clipart or other images should be avoided unless they directly relate to the text or point being made.

- *Make numbers meaningful.* Large numbers are often lost in long-term memory because they are hard to grasp or relate to. For example, you may supplement "46 million Americans are smokers" by saying "on average, one out of every six students in this room uses tobacco."

- *Practice.* A good lecture should emulate a sales pitch in terms of intentional planning and practice. The practiced presenter will be more enthusiastic, engaging, and adept at facilitating group discussion.

Keeping students engaged can be a challenge with today's learners. Teachers are often competing for students' attention with technology-related distractions such as e-mail, instant messaging, texting, and social media. Therefore, consideration should be given to using an active presentation style (e.g., use of handouts, multimedia, etc.) to grab the learners' attention. If adequately constructed and delivered, active learning provides a change of pace in the classroom and allows the students to actively participate in their own learning rather than passively sitting and listening. A few examples of active learning techniques are outlined in **Table 12-1**.

Although the benefits of engaging students via active learning may be apparent, these techniques may not always be well received if done without much thought and planning. In addition, several challenges exist in changing the dynamic of the traditional lecture-oriented classroom, such as student comfort with traditional didactic lecture, student expectation of the teacher telling them what they need to know, and the expectation for the student to actively participate.

As you get ready to enter into the large classroom, the following items should be considered:

- *There is no "right" way to lecture.* An effective style should be one that is measured by student learning and may vary from one teacher to another, depending on the style of the presenter, the unique characteristics of the learner, and the topic being presented.

TABLE 12-1. EXAMPLES OF ACTIVE LEARNING TECHNIQUES

ACTIVE LEARNING TECHNIQUES	DESCRIPTIONS
Computer-based interaction systems (e.g., audience response system—"clickers")	Students can participate in a class session by responding to questions or statements using computers or technology systems such as audience response devices, commonly known as "clickers."
Concept maps	Creating (as an individual or part of a team) a diagram that shows the mental connections between a major concept presented and other concepts learned.
Mini-cases	Students apply didactic lecture material or readings by working on a clinical scenario.
Muddiest point	Toward the end of class, students write down on a card one item that was most confusing and requires further clarification. These cards are collected, and the instructor uses these to address recurring concerns or themes prior to the next class.
One-minute paper	A short writing assignment where students are asked to write a response to a question about an important term, name, or concept from a lesson.
Think-pair-share	A question is posed to the class, and students are given a period of time to individually reflect or write down their answer. Students then pair up with another student to share their responses, and a larger class discussion follows.

- *Consider varying your methods during the class (e.g., lecture, cases, clicker questions, small-group work, etc.).* This will help to engage students with different learning styles and will keep students attentive by changing the pace.

- *When it comes to content, less is more.* In a 1- or 2-hour lecture, it is easy to try to transfer as much knowledge as possible. However, the retention of that material by an overwhelmed learner will be minimal. Therefore, consider supplementing the lecture with readings or cases to free up some of the lecture time.

- *Consider using active learning techniques (e.g., clicker questions, mini-cases, etc.) strategically to break up the lecture and keep students attentive.* For example, the presenter may consider doing an active learning technique every 15 to 20 minutes rather than presenting all the material at the beginning and then doing cases or some other active learning technique at the end.

- *Use the time at the beginning of class wisely.* Student retention of material covered at the beginning of class is high compared to the end of class. Rather than spend a great deal of time reviewing objectives or logistics related to the course, consider jumping right in to set the tone of the session.

- *Like it or not, teaching has a performance side to it.* Be cognizant of your voice, mannerisms, gestures, movements in the classroom, pace, and other factors. Consider recording your presentation to identify gestures that you may not be aware of. A common mistake is to focus so heavily on the content that the delivery is overlooked.

- *When asking questions, communicate a true interest in receiving input from the class.* Avoid asking a question, glancing at the room, and then providing a response. This approach will not encourage future participation among the learners.

CASE QUESTION

L.R. is getting ready to work on her 2-hour class session. What questions should she ask about her audience?

Small-Group Teaching

You will likely be asked to participate in some small-group teaching experiences, including journal club discussions, physical assessment workshops, or breakout sessions. Although you may be more comfortable with small-group teaching, the amount of planning should not be underestimated for a successful group encounter. The large-group or lecture-type setting may be beneficial to introduce a topic, whereas a small-group or breakout session may be valuable to apply the information learned.

Besides providing an opportunity for application, several other benefits to small-group teaching exist:

- Compared to a lecture environment, students working in groups to solve problems and other tasks tend to learn and retain more information.

- Small-group sessions allow students to understand and experience the importance of working in teams to share ideas and provide feedback. This is essential to mirror what will happen during pharmacy practice experiences and residencies.

- These sessions allow students to express ideas verbally rather than on a multiple-choice exam. For example, a student may have to verbalize how he or she would prioritize, assess, and plan for a series of problems a patient is having rather than answer a multiple-choice question that does not require any rationale or feedback from peers.

- Having a high-functioning group allows the members to ask questions of each other and provide feedback in a welcoming environment that encourages further learning. This environment allows the student the opportunity to receive immediate feedback.

- A small-group setting encourages more self-directed and independent learning that will be experienced on rotation and in practice.

- A small-group setting allows for an intimate discussion where students may be more willing to participate than in a large-group discussion.

As you get ready to start the small-group discussion, it is important to understand group dynamics. For example, has the small group been together before, or is this the first time they are together? If it is the first time, you should consider some type of introduction or "ice-breaker" to allow the group interaction to start. In addition, it is vitally important to change your role from a lecturer in a large-group setting to a facilitator in a small-group setting. It is easy to get into lecture mode; however, this type of approach will not welcome participation among the learners. Lastly, at the beginning of each session, the facilitator should outline the objectives for the session and corresponding expectations for the group.[8]

CASE QUESTION

L.R. is preparing for her teaching assignment in the small-group cardiology case discussion. What are some techniques that L.R. can use during this session to help facilitate discussion rather than lecture?

Managing the Learning Environment

While on an academic rotation, you may engage in discussions about classroom management. *Classroom management* refers to the process of maintaining a controlled, orderly environment that is conducive to learning.[9] The well-managed classroom provides an environment in which teaching and learning can flourish, whereas a mismanaged classroom can be harmful to students and instructors alike.

Robert Boice, professor emeritus at Stony Brook University, systematically researched the experiences of new faculty and showed that the ratings of teachers by students are closely correlated with incivility incidents in the classroom. His research found that the numbers of classroom incivilities are low to moderate during the first few classes with a new instructor when the students are "checking the teacher out." Professors who used positive motivators (showed respect and encouragement) and strong social immediacies (showed verbal and nonverbal signs of warmth, friendliness, and approachability) saw a drop in the number of classroom incivilities after the first few classes. In contrast, professors who were perceived to be aloof, cold, uncaring, and condescending experienced an increase in the number of classroom incivilities.[10]

So what can you do during your academic rotation to minimize your contribution to classroom incivilities?

- *Demonstrate caring.* Get to class early and chat with students. Smile. Verbalize concern for the students' learning and future success, learn as many names as possible, and show empathy for the stresses they may be experiencing. Project the image of an ally, not an adversary.[11]

- *Set the ground rules.* Set high expectations. Describe how everyone's learning is important and what behaviors will contribute to an effective classroom environment. If necessary, state what annoyances will not be tolerated.

- *Recognize and reward positive behaviors.* Examples include complimenting the class on high attendance, expressing appreciation when a noisy class quiets down, or thanking students who contribute to class discussion.

- *Model correct behavior.* It is important to show respect for students by following the rules you set for them. Instructors who appear rude, sarcastic, insensitive, or domineering can incite incivility from students. Avoid putting down students; talking with your back to the class; reading your slides; being unprepared; being disorganized; speaking too quickly, softly, or with a monotone; starting class late; or keeping class over time.

- *Command class attention.* Make steady eye contact to all parts of the classroom. Use an open body posture and broad gestures. Walk around the room if it feels right. Use your voice effectively: enunciate clearly, vary volume and pace, use dramatic pauses, and provide emphasis. Convey enthusiasm and passion for the topic by telling stories and sharing personal experiences with the topic.

Ideally, the course director has already set the ground rules for appropriate behavior in the classroom. Nevertheless, you may encounter incivilities in the classroom that need to be addressed during the class, as shown in **Table 12-2**.

Finally, it is important for you to reflect on your own *classroom persona.* Successful classroom management requires a persona that invites respect and balances authority with approachability. You should strive to project an image of relaxed confidence, good will, and an in-command no-nonsense (but friendly) attitude.[8,12]

TABLE 12-2. HANDLING COMMON CLASSROOM INCIVILITIES

COMMON CLASSROOM INCIVILITIES	SUGGESTED INSTRUCTOR RESPONSES
Talking, chatter	Try pausing until the talking stops. Direct a question to the student next to the talker. Embarrassing the talkers is not recommended.
Use of cellphones, texting, or laptops for nonclass activities	Explain to all students at the beginning of class why such activities are distracting to other students. Walk around the room—maintain a presence.
Student monopolizes class time with questions	Ask the student to talk to you after class or to e-mail the question. Advise the class that you will share your answers with everyone by e-mail or through the classroom management software. If the question is pertinent and time is not constrained, invite other students to answer it.
Argumentative questions or comments that are disrespectful	Calmly acknowledge the student's input during class and move on. By not overreacting or becoming defensive, you may win the sympathy and support of the other students. You or your preceptor should seek guidance from the course director for further follow-up with the student involved.

CASE QUESTION

L.R. is about halfway through presenting the cardiology lecture when she notices two students carrying on a private conversation and giggling during the lecture. How should she handle this?

Using Technology in the Classroom

The use of technology in the classroom has grown significantly since the turn of the millennium. Technology is expected to enhance the students' educational experience. It is important to determine your expectations for technology use in the classroom to adequately prepare yourself for a positive classroom experience.

You should take inventory of the current technology at your disposal. This starts with identifying the classroom in which you will be working and taking a trip to that classroom during off hours to "scope it out." This reconnaissance work should also include a call to the technical support group that oversees the classroom technology so you will be completely informed of the breadth and limitations of available classroom technology. A well-informed use of classroom technology can truly maximize the experience for everyone involved.

You should also take the time to research and assess the use of classroom technology by current faculty members. If current faculty members' use of classroom technology is fairly extensive, this allows you to look at multiple approaches and incorporate the methods that suit you. On the other hand, if the current faculty members' use of classroom technology is minimal, this may allow you to introduce students to new active learning approaches or provide faculty development in the use of classroom technology.

QUICK TIP

Make sure you test the technology before the session in which you plan to use it. In addition, it is a good idea to have a backup plan in case the technology does not work properly on the day you intend to use it.

Most importantly, you must remember that the ultimate purpose of classroom technology is to enhance the educational experience. It is important that the use of classroom technology in no way distracts from the delivery of the educational content. The teacher that does his or her homework and finds the all-essential middle ground between underuse and overuse of classroom technology will ultimately provide the best learning environment. See **Table 12-3** for a summary of technologies commonly utilized in the classroom.

CASE QUESTION

L.R. is very interested in using the "clicker" system to keep students engaged during her lecture. How should she prepare?

TABLE 12-3. BROAD LIST OF TECHNOLOGIES THAT SUPPORT CLASSROOM INSTRUCTION

AUDIENCE RESPONSE SYSTEMS

- TurningPoint—popular audience response system from TurningTechnologies. www.turningtechnologies.com
- Poll Everywhere—(free for up to 40 participants) *basic* audience response system gathers audience responses via mobile devices or Twitter accounts. www.polleverywhere.com

PRESENTATION SOFTWARE

- Microsoft® PowerPoint®—presentation software, part of Microsoft® Office® Suite. http://office.microsoft.com/en-us/powerpoint/
- Prezi—the zooming presentation editor. http://prezi.com

SCREENCASTING

- Jing—records what is on your computer screen (up to 5 minutes) and uploads it to the Web. www.techsmith.com/jing
- Camtasia Studio—advanced version of Jing. Allows you to record, edit, annotate, create interactive content, etc. http://www.techsmith.com/camtasia.html

PODCASTING

- Audacity—easy capture and editing of audio recordings. www.audacity.sourceforge.net

SOCIAL BOOKMARKING

- Delicious—bookmarks to share with others and carry with you. www.delicious.com
- Diigo—social bookmarking/annotation. www.diigo.com

BLOGS

- Blogger—popular free blogging tool; from Google. www.blogger.com
- WordPress—very popular and contains many templates. www.wordpress.com

CREATE A WEBSITE/WIKI

- Google Sites—webpage or wiki creation. http://sites.google.com
- Weebly—choice of several basic templates. www.weebly.com
- Wikispaces—simple Web pages that groups can edit together. www.wikispaces.com

VIDEO UPLOADING/HOSTING

- YouTube—most widely used video site. www.youtube.com
- Vimeo—online video community with higher-quality videos. www.vimeo.com

(CONTINUED ON NEXT PAGE)

(CONTINUED FROM PREVIOUS PAGE)

WEB CONFERENCING

- Adobe® Connect—www.adobe.com/products/adobeconnect.html

- Skype—Instant messaging/VoIP tool. www.skype.com

- GoToMeeting—www.gotomeeting.com

- WebEx—www.webex.com

SOCIAL NETWORKING

- Facebook®—#1 social networking site. www.facebook.com

- Ning—site to create your own social network for a group, class, or organization starting at $25/mo. www.ning.com

- LinkedIn®—site used to connect with other people in your professional network. www.linkedin.com

- Twitter®—micro-sharing site; also great for building a professional learning network. www.twitter.com

COLLABORATIVE TOOLS

- Google Docs—collaboration suite. http://docs.google.com

OTHER TOOLS AND RESOURCES

- Animoto—easy creation of stunning videos. Upload several pictures and pick music, and it automatically makes a video montage (30 seconds or less is free). www.animoto.com

- SlideShare— the world's largest community for sharing presentations. View other presentations, get inspired, and post your own. www.slideshare.net

- Zoomit—ability to zoom in or out on the screen. Just install, launch, and then press Ctrl +1 to zoom in/out from anything on the screen; can also annotate. www.snapfiles.com/get/zoomit.html

ASSESSING STUDENT PERFORMANCE

Once the classroom activities have been planned, you may be asked to help assess student learning. Assessment activities can vary from rotation to rotation, but being able to measure performance and communicate assessments to learners are skills that can be applied to any number of pharmacy careers.

Writing Objectives

When assigned a lecture, you will need to familiarize yourself with how to develop learning objectives. Writing objectives is a task not to be taken lightly and can provide another fundamental learning experience. The process of writing objectives should be grounded in the foundations of Bloom's Taxonomy. Bloom's taxonomy of learning is composed of three domains: cognitive, affective, and psychomotor. The cognitive domain is grounded in the knowledge and development of intellectual skills, sometimes thought of as the *knowing*, and is the domain associated with writing objectives. You are encouraged to research the affective and psychomotor domains, although they are outside of the scope of this text.[13-17]

The verbs used in your objectives describe your expectations for learning and can range from lower-order thinking skills (such as *know*) to higher-order critical thinking skills (such as *evaluate*). The expectations for learning in the cognitive domain are arranged in six key categories. **Table 12-4** provides these six categories, key words, and example wording for objectives that may be used to convey the expectations for your learners.[14,15] The categories can then be divided into lower (categories one through three) and higher (categories four through six). When writing objectives, you should consider the level of knowledge that you expect your audience to gain at completion of your session or course.[14-17]

Once the learning objectives are drafted, it is important to ensure you have connected the activity's objectives to those of the course. Taking this process another step further, all course objectives should fit into the greater overall objectives within the program to meet the accreditation standards for educating

TABLE 12-4. OVERVIEW OF BLOOM'S TAXONOMY—COGNITIVE DOMAIN

Note that some observable verbs appear in multiple categories depending on the meaning of its usage

CATEGORIES AND EXPLANATIONS	OBSERVABLE VERBS	OBJECTIVE WORDING EXAMPLES
Knowledge or Remembering (Recollection of information or data)	Arrange, define, describe, duplicate, identify, know, label, list, match, memorize, name, order, outline, recall, relate, repeat, recognize, reproduce, select, state	Know brand and generic medication names. Outline the U.S. Pharmacopeia's (USP) Chapter <797> procedure for preparing a compounded sterile preparation.
Comprehension or Understanding (Understanding and interpretation of information or a problem in an individual's own terms)	Classify, comprehend, convert, defend, describe, discuss, distinguish, estimate, explain, express, extend, generalize, give an example, identify, indicate, infer, interpret, locate, paraphrase, predict, recognize, report, restate, review, rewrite, select, sort, summarize, tell, translate	Explain the mechanism of action for beta2 selective antihypertensive medications. Interpret significant laboratory data in determining a ST elevation infarction (STEMI).
Application (Using knowledge or a concept in a new situation; applying classroom learning to "real-life" situations)	Apply, choose, change, compute, construct, demonstrate, discover, dramatize, employ, illustrate, interpret, manipulate, modify, operate, practice, predict, prepare, produce, relate, schedule, show, sketch, solve, use	Demonstrate the proper technique for patient use of a metered dose inhaler (MDI). Prepare a business plan for the formation of your own independent pharmacy.
Analysis (Selecting components of knowledge and concepts and identifying the relationships among its parts)	Analyze, appraise, break down, calculate, categorize, compare, contrast, criticize, diagram, deconstruct, differentiate, discriminate, distinguish, examine, experiment, identify, illustrate, infer, inventory, outline, question, relate, select, separate, test	Analyze medication treatment options for omission and/or duplication of appropriate medications. Select the best medication treatment option given a specific patient case.
Synthesis or Creating (Building structure from parts of knowledge creates a whole and emphasizes the creation of relationships for new situations)	Arrange, assemble, categorize, collect, combine, compile, compose, construct, create, devise, design, explain, formulate, generate, manage, modify, organize, plan, prepare, propose, rearrange, reconstruct, relate, reorganize, revise, rewrite, set up, summarize, synthesize, tell, write	Design patient care plans. Write a policy and procedure for the daily cleaning of a USP Chapter <797> compliant cleanroom.
Evaluation (Making conclusions based on given criteria, ideas, and/or materials)	Appraise, argue, assess, attack, choose, compare, conclude, contrast, criticize, critique, defend, describe, discriminate, estimate, evaluate, explain, interpret, judge, justify, predict, rate, relate, score, select, summarize, support, value	Compare the differences in current insulin treatments. Explain and justify a medication treatment plan.

future pharmacists. Taking a step back to examine the bigger picture in this manner is a process known as *curricular mapping*. If you are unfamiliar with this concept, you should speak with the course director or the individual in charge of curriculum at your institution to gain greater understanding.

Writing Test Items

Writing test items is key to ensuring that your audience has mastered the information you presented. Writing test items is another critical aspect of the academician's role in ensuring the success and competency of future pharmacists. Writing test items should follow similar rules to writing objectives. The information that is tested should be mapped back to a classroom session objective, which is mapped back to a course objective and, ultimately, to a core curriculum objective. Remembering this concept will assist you in determining the level of competence expected by all students enrolled in any specific course. It is important to map your questions back to your learning objectives in order for the students to be clearly aware of your expectations for examination.

Many universities employ individuals who are highly educated in test item writing. Typically employed by the assessment department, you should take full advantage of these individuals and their services. They may be able to identify ineffective test item structure and ensure you are testing the knowledge and skills that you intend to evaluate.

A generally accepted rule of thumb is that each multiple-choice question should take about 20 to 30 minutes to write. Although it is vital to include only one correct answer, careful consideration should be paid to the reasonable distractors. A *distractor* is an answer that is plausible but incorrect. For instance, consider the following question and its distractors:

Which of the following is an antihistamine medication?

a. apple

b. diphenhydramine

c. metformin

d. turnip

The individual taking this examination can begin by quickly eliminating the first and last answer if they know their fruits and vegetables. Are you testing their true knowledge of medications if you do not even list four medications? If you are unable to come up with three reasonably plausible distractors, you need to consider the value of placing this question in your examination bank.

It is also important that you create "lead-ins" to your questions that are relevant and align with the delivery of your classroom instruction. For example, if you presented a lecture on aseptic technique and provided examples of where in practice this is of key importance, you would want to frame the scenario for the learner so the importance of the test item and its correct answer can be seen as relevant and meaningful to the future pharmacist. The following lead-in provides you with a specific example of this concept:

You are the responsible pharmacist in your institution's fully compliant USP Chapter <797> sterile preparations room and are instructing the new pharmacy intern on the proper procedures for donning all required garb. Which of the following are the correct procedures?

Although the question may be one of simple recall, the lead-in sentence provides the examination taker with a relevant and meaningful example of why this information is important to a future pharmacist. Lead-ins that do not provide relevance and meaning are simply time consuming and of no benefit to those involved.

CASE QUESTION

L.R. is asked to develop five multiple-choice questions related to her cardiology lecture. How should she proceed?

Giving Student Feedback

One critical skill of a successful educator is the ability to give feedback to others in a constructive, professional manner. While you are completing your academic rotation, you should pay close attention to how students in each learning situation are being evaluated. Are there specific criteria for each activity? Are the criteria objective? Are they open to interpretation by the grader (which may be acceptable in some scenarios and unacceptable in others)? How will the feedback be provided to the learner—verbally or in writing? All of the variables above must be considered when evaluating learners. For individual classroom activities, it is important for the instructor to set the expectations regarding the specific activity. It is the students' responsibility to review the expectations and ask any clarifying questions. For example, if a classroom activity involves counseling patients and the students will receive feedback based on a rubric, the rubric should be shared prior to the counseling session. Sharing the evaluation criteria with students prior to the assessment does not weaken the assessment nor give students an unfair advantage; in fact, it strengthens the activity. Informing students how they will be evaluated on a specific activity allows them to prepare accordingly and helps the instructor to determine if the activity achieved its intended outcome. See Chapter 17 for additional information on student evaluation.

Learning to provide feedback in a constructive and professional manner can be difficult and may take some time to develop. The skills, however, are transferrable to many situations a pharmacist will face—interacting with a patient who is incorrectly administering a medication, educating a technician who mishandled an encounter with a patient, or critiquing pharmacy students learning at the site.

The Teaching Portfolio

Throughout your academic rotation, you will start to compile several items that will make up the beginnings of a teaching portfolio. The primary goal of the teaching portfolio is to document progress, achievements, and reflections in teaching, scholarship, and service. The portfolio serves as a collection of evidence of your teaching activities and showcases the process and tools used to document student learning. This portfolio will be used by faculty members during their promotion or tenure process but also serves as a guiding document for the creator in terms of self-reflection and planning. The portfolio is a dynamic document and should be reviewed and updated on a regular basis. It is important to distinguish a teaching portfolio from a professional or other portfolio that you may have developed during coursework or rotations. For example, your professional portfolio may contain a wide array of items, including rotation projects, presentations, and a copy of your curriculum vitae. In contrast, a teaching portfolio contains teaching beliefs, experiences, evaluations, and reflections at its core. There is no "right" way to construct a teaching portfolio, and a wide variety of formats are possible based on personal preference and opinion. However, some general principles to consider include the following:

- The portfolio should contain a reflection of teaching philosophy and goals (see the section on teaching philosophy).
- The portfolio should focus on the quality of the activities rather than the quantity. You should be selective in choosing a wide array of activities that provide evidence of broad experiences (e.g., lecture development, objective writing, test-item writing, etc.).
- The process of creating the portfolio may be just as important as the product. During the creation of a portfolio, reflection on experiences will occur in addition to identifying areas for improvement and focus moving forward.
- Start early and capture items along the way. It will be hard to go back and get materials.
- Highlight both the positives and negatives. The portfolio should showcase certain experiences but should not selectively contain good evaluations. Use negative evaluations to highlight personal growth and improvement.[18,19]

As you get started in developing a teaching portfolio, you should consider talking to faculty members to see various examples. In addition, a faculty mentor will be helpful in providing feedback and suggestions during the portfolio development process. One of the first steps should be to determine what sections the portfolio will contain. Then you should draft a teaching philosophy, as this is the backbone of the portfolio. As you collect materials, gaps should be identified and opportunities to fill those gaps should be sought out (e.g., faculty development workshop, evaluating another lecture, etc.). If it is early enough in the academic rotation, you may be able to seek out additional opportunities to complete various experiences.

Although the structure of a portfolio may be very different from one person to another, an example list and description of items to consider in a teaching portfolio can be found in **Table 12-5**.

TABLE 12-5. EXAMPLE ITEMS FOR A TEACHING PORTFOLIO

PORTFOLIO COMPONENTS	DESCRIPTIONS
Title page and table of contents	A brief title page orienting the reader to the portfolio and a table of contents that will guide the reader to different sections.
Teaching philosophy	The philosophy (described previously in this chapter) placed at the beginning of the portfolio will help give the reader some context of who you are as a teacher and what your philosophy is for enhancing student learning.
Academic curriculum vitae (CV)	The academic CV will highlight experiences in teaching, scholarship, and service, several of which will be included in the portfolio.
Teaching experience log	The focus should be on the number of hours, type of teaching (e.g., large group versus small group), number of students, and synopsis of evaluations.
Roles and activities related to academic advising	Examples include a brief description of any student advising and/or mentoring (e.g., role, frequency of meetings, types of activities conducted with the advisee/mentee).
Examples of teaching materials	Examples include learning objectives, lecture handouts or slides, assignments, and test questions.
Evaluations of teaching	Examples include student evaluations, faculty evaluations, and self-evaluations.
Contributions to the profession	Examples include published articles in teaching journals, participation in organizations related to teaching, etc.
Honors and awards	Examples include teaching awards, invitation to teaching workshops, etc.
Professional development activities	Examples include attendance at teaching workshops and conferences attended.
Summary narrative	The narrative should include what has been learned and plans for further developing teaching skills. This document should reflect on the experiences to date, note strengths and areas of improvement, and define a plan of action. Information for this document can come from self-evaluations, peer evaluations, and student evaluations.

If you are completing an academic rotation, it is likely that you have a strong interest in an academic position. If applying for a residency program that has a teaching component (either experiential or didactic), you should bring your portfolio to interviews. In addition, after residency, you may pursue a position as a faculty member and the portfolio will be important during the interview and subsequent promotion and tenure process. The portfolio will show potential employers that meaningful thought and attention has been given to your teaching experiences.

Networking with Faculty and Staff

Networking is a vital component to any professional's development and future growth. It is something that we do every day, often subconsciously. If you have been actively involved in professional student organizations, you probably observed networking occurring locally. Pharmacy is a small world! As you progress through your career, you will be continually amazed by just how small it can be. When you begin your academic rotation, you will be taken into the depths of the mystical world of faculty members who were instructing you in the not-so-distant past. You should always remember that you are still a pharmacy student, but in many respects, you will be considered a colleague during this rotation. Although expectations may be more in line with the expectations of a junior faculty member, these opportunities can be some of the most rewarding experiences of your APPE rotations.

Effectively networking with faculty members and staff will be a vital component to making the academic rotation a successful and worthwhile experience. You should begin your rotation by working with your primary preceptor and other key faculty members to identify specific areas of scholarship that faculty members may be working on. You can use this information as a way to start a conversation and explore potential areas for personal scholarship. For instance, if you connect with a particular faculty member about a specific area of research, that faculty member may be aware of other academicians or pharmacy practitioners outside of his or her institution that share this area of interest. This can lead to opportunities to immediately expand your network.

Another facet of an academic practice involves attendance at local, regional, or national meetings. Consider asking about the possibility of accompanying faculty members to meetings with outside colleagues, if appropriate. You should take every opportunity to spend time with your preceptors as they meet with other individuals at professional meetings and conferences. These types of opportunities can provide you with wonderful experiences to meet new colleagues who may be a part of your future plans for employment or collaboration.

Scholarship of Teaching and Learning

As described previously, scholarly activity is expected from all faculty to varying degrees, depending on the type of position. *Scholarship* is generally defined as faculty work that is made public, reviewed by peers, and reproducible by other scholars.[20] Until recently, the term *faculty scholarship* was synonymous with research—which brought forth the image of laboratories and a "publish or perish" mentality. Ernest Boyer, an influential American educator, challenged the view that research was the only type of scholarship that was worthy of faculty engagement. He created a broader definition of scholarship that recognized the different missions of universities and colleges. In his model, the scholarship of discovery (what we heretofore referred to as *research*) is only one of four types of scholarship. The other three include scholarship of integration, scholarship of application (service), and scholarship of teaching and learning. His report created debates around the country and influenced many colleges and universities to reconsider how they evaluate their faculty.[21]

The *scholarship of teaching and learning* refers to the formalization of a process that faculties use on a routine basis: trying new teaching methods, studying the learning outcomes, and sharing the results with peers. It has been defined as "the published work on teaching and learning authored by college faculty."[22] Many faculty members in colleges of pharmacy embrace this type of scholarship and publish their findings in a range of journals, including *The American Journal of Pharmaceutical Education* and *Currents in Pharmacy Teaching and Learning*. You will find these resources to be useful if you'd like to investigate different approaches and techniques during your academic rotation.

REFERENCES

1. Zgarrick DP. *Getting Started as a Pharmacy Faculty Member*. Washington, DC: American Pharmacists Association; 2010.

2. Brooks AD. Considering academic pharmacy as a career: Opportunities and resources for students, residents and fellows. *Curr Pharm Teach Learn*. 2009;1:2-9.

3. Raehl CL. Changes in pharmacy practice faculty 1995-2001: Implications for junior faculty development. *Pharmacotherapy*. 2002;22:445-462.

4. Faculty Focus Special Report. Philosophy of teaching statements: Examples and tips on how to write a teaching philosophy statement. http://www.facultyfocus.com/free-reports/philosophy-of-teaching-statements-examples-and-tips-on-how-to-write-a-teaching-philosophy-statement/. Accessed February 2, 2012.

5. Atkinson C. *Beyond Bullet Points: Using Microsoft® Office PowerPoint® 2007 to Create Presentations That Inform, Motivate, and Inspire*. Redmond, WA: Microsoft Press; 2007.

6. Gallo C. *The Presentation Secrets of Steve Jobs*. New York, NY: McGraw-Hill; 2009.

7. Reynolds G. *Presentation Zen: Simple Ideas on Presentation Design & Delivery*. Berkeley, CA: New Riders Press; 2008.

8. Lang J. *On Course: A Week-by-Week Guide to Your First Semester of College Teaching*. Cambridge, MA: Harvard University Press; 2008.

9. Nilson LB. *Teaching at its Best*. 3rd ed. San Francisco, CA: John Wiley and Sons; 2010.

10. Boice R. *Advice for New Faculty Members: Nihil Nimus*. Needham Heights, MA: Allyn & Bacon; 2000.

11. Carroll J. Constructing your in-class persona. *The Chronicle of Higher Education*. http://chronicle.com/article/Constructing-Your-In-Class/45186/. Accessed February 2, 2012.

12. McKinney M. What's your name again? *Inside Higher Education*. Feb. 13, 2006. http://www.insidehighered.com/workplace/2006/02/13/mckinney. Accessed February 2, 2012.

13. Bloom BS. *Taxonomy of Educational Objectives, Handbook I: The Cognitive Domain*. New York, NY: David McKay; 1956.

14. Bloom's Taxonomy of Learning Domains. http://www.nwlink.com/~donclark/hrd/bloom.html. Accessed September 6, 2012.

15. Krathwohl DR, Bloom BS, Masia BB. *Taxonomy of Educational Objectives, the Classification of Educational Goals. Handbook II: Affective Domain*. New York, NY: David McKay; 1973.

16. Simpson EJ. *The Classification of Educational Objectives in the Psychomotor Domain*. Washington, DC: Gryphon House; 1972.

17. Observable verbs for cognitive domain instructional objectives. http://www2.gsu.edu/~mstmbs/CrsTools/cogverbs.html. Accessed on September 11, 2012.

18. The Center for Educational Excellence in Pharmacy: UNC Eshelman School of Pharmacy. The teaching portfolio. http://pharmacy.unc.edu/research/centers/center-for-educational-excellence-in-pharmacy/forms-guidelines/forms-and-guides-folder/preparing-a-teaching-portfolio.pdf. Accessed September 13, 2012.

19. Ohio State University Center for the Advancement of Teaching. Developing a teaching portfolio. www.ucat.osu.edu/portfolio. Accessed September 13, 2012.

20. Glassick CE. Boyer's expanded definitions of scholarship, the standards for assessing scholarship, and the elusiveness of the scholarship of teaching. *Acad Med*. 2000;75:877-880.

21. Boyer EL. *Scholarship Reconsidered: Priorities of the Professoriate*. Princeton, NJ: Carnegie Foundation for the Advancement of Teaching; 1990.

22. Weimer ME. *Enhancing Scholarly Work on Teaching and Learning: Professional Literature that Makes a Difference*. San Francisco, CA: Jossey-Bass; 2006.

SUGGESTED READING

Angelo TA, Cross KP. *Classroom Assessment Techniques: A Handbook for College Teachers*. 2nd ed. San Francisco, CA: Jossey-Bass; 1993.

Bain K. *What the Best College Teachers Do*. Cambridge, MA: Harvard University Press; 2004.

Barkley EF. *Student Engagement Techniques: A Handbook for College Faculty*. San Francisco, CA: Jossey-Bass; 2010.

Leamnson R. *Thinking About Teaching and Learning: Developing Habits of Learning with First Year College and University Students*. Sterling, VA: Stylus; 1999.

Stevens DD, Levi AJ, Walvoord BE. *Introduction to Rubrics: An Assessment Tool to Save Grading Time, Convey Effective Feedback and Promote Student Learning.* 2nd ed. Sterling, VA: Stylus; 2012

Svinicki M, McKeachie WJ. *McKeachie's Teaching Tips: Strategies, Research and Theory for College and University Teachers.* 13th ed. Belmont, CA: Wadsworth Publishing; 2011.

The IDEA Center. IDEA papers. http://www.theideacenter.org/research-and-papers/idea-papers. Accessed September 10, 2012.

Weimer M. *Learner-Centered Teaching: Five Key Changes to Practice.* San Francisco, CA: Jossey-Bass; 2002.

Weimer M, Neff RA. *Teaching College: Collected Readings for the New Instructor.* Madison, WI: Atwood Publishing; 1998.

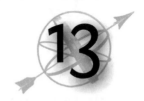

AMBULATORY CARE

Megan Kaun, PharmD, BCPS, BCACP, and Michelle Serres, PharmD, BC-ADM, BCACP

CASE

K.C. is a student preparing to start her ambulatory care rotation in an internal medicine outpatient clinic. She is asked to work up the patients that will be seen that day using the chart in the electronic medical record. She writes down most of the information for each patient using a form to organize the information. She feels confident and is able to present the patient information to the preceptor before the patient arrives. The preceptor notifies K.C. that he is running behind and would like her to begin talking with the first patient about his medications and measure his blood pressure. K.C. suddenly becomes very nervous and is uncertain how to talk with the patient or what to discuss.

WHY IT'S ESSENTIAL

Ambulatory care rotations are one of the four rotation types required by the Accreditation Council for Pharmacy Education (ACPE). Ambulatory care rotations may include a variety of experiences and settings, but all have the common goal of direct patient care in an outpatient environment. Common examples of ambulatory care rotations include physician's offices, anticoagulation clinics, and medication therapy management (MTM) clinics. Ambulatory care rotations may also take place in community pharmacy settings. In this situation, the focus of the rotation is not the dispensing services but rather the clinical interventions made. Skills developed during an ambulatory care rotation emphasize drug knowledge, pharmacotherapeutic plan development, and communication skills with patients and other healthcare team members.

ARRIVING PREPARED

As with all rotations, the preceptor should be contacted well in advance of the rotation to inquire about expectations and preparations. Ambulatory care settings may vary greatly from one rotation to the next, so it is advisable to not make assumptions about how to prepare, what to bring, hours, and expectations of the rotation.

You should ask the preceptor the following questions in your initial communication:

- When and where should I arrive on the first day?
- Are there any restrictions regarding parking?
- How can I best prepare for this rotation?
- Is there anything specific you would like me to bring?

In addition, it is safe to assume the following apply to all ambulatory care rotations:

- Dress professionally, wearing a white coat and nametag identification.
- Bring your favorite drug information reference.
- Bring a notebook, pens, and calculator.
- Bring your lunch on the first day, as you may not have options to obtain lunch throughout the day.
- Review guidelines or references specific to that rotation (for examples, see the Suggested Reading section at the end of this chapter).

Ambulatory care has a primary focus on patient interactions. On this type of rotation, you will be expected to communicate directly with patients, either in person or on the phone. This process can be quite intimidating the first time you try it. You will encounter patients with diverse backgrounds, diverse personalities, and differing levels of health literacy. You must enter the rotation with an open mind and expect that you will need to call on your highest level of communication skills.

QUICK TIP

If patient communication is new or uncomfortable to you, consider practicing with friends or family as if they were your patients. Ask them for feedback on how they felt you were able to ask and answer different questions and provide information.

Depending on the type of rotation, you will likely be asked to work up the patient prior to his or her arrival. Having a systematic process for this workup will help efficiency and accuracy. Areas to consider when working up a patient of any type include the following:

- Is this a new or returning patient to pharmacy services?
  - Identify what service the referring practitioner would like you to provide, such as
    - Diabetes management
    - Medication reconciliation
    - Hypertension management
  - If returning, what was accomplished at the last visit or interaction?
  - If new, what was discussed at the last practitioner appointment or what led to the referral?
- Gather basic information, such as
  - Patient age, height, and weight
  - Past medical history
  - Current medication list
  - Applicable laboratory work (and dates of laboratory work)
- Review common medication administration techniques you may need to teach to patients, such as
  - Insulin or low-molecular-weight heparin injection technique
  - Inhaler use
  - Glucometer use
  - Home blood pressure monitor use
- Identify information important to standards of care

Having a patient workup form can be very helpful in this process. **Figure 13-1** is an example of a workup form that could be used in a diabetes clinic. Your preceptor may provide a workup form for his or her specific clinic, or you may develop a form of your own.

CASE QUESTION

K.C. was very uncomfortable for her first direct patient care experience. Name one technique that she could have used before seeing her first patient that may have improved her comfort level.

As previously mentioned, each ambulatory care rotation is quite different. You should prepare accordingly for each specialty type, including reviewing class notes, textbook chapters, and guidelines for the most common disease states you expect to encounter. Some settings may be family based or internal medicine based, whereas others specialize in one particular disease state. The family medicine-based specialty areas you may encounter include diabetes, anticoagulation, lipids, hypertension, and smoking cessation. In an internal medicine or family medicine setting, you may be able to focus on the following disease states:

- Outpatient infectious disease
  - □ Urinary tract infections
  - □ Upper respiratory infections, sinusitis, and otitis media
- Diabetes
- Hypertension
- Dyslipidemia
- Thyroid dysfunction
- Depression and anxiety
- Pain management
- Asthma
- Chronic obstructive pulmonary disease (COPD)
- Tobacco addiction/smoking cessation
- Anticoagulation
- Gastroesophageal reflux disease

For a specialized clinic, you should read textbook chapters, notes, and guidelines for that particular disease state. Guidelines are listed in the Suggested Reading section at the end of this chapter.

A TYPICAL DAY

A typical day in an ambulatory care rotation will vary greatly depending on the specific rotation you are completing. At some sites you may see patients every day of the week, whereas at others you may see patients less frequently but have more time to perform patient workups, documentation, and presentations or projects. Below is an example of a typical day you may face when on this type of rotation.

The morning may start with working up patients prior to their arrival. At some sites, you may do this ahead of time for all patients, whereas at others you may work up each patient just before he or she

Figure 13-1. Diabetes Patient Workup Form

PATIENT NAME:

DOB:

PCP:

MEDICATIONS: PMH:

Previous visit (changes made/discussed):

Blood sugars:

LAB	VALUE	DATE
A1c		
TC		
LDL		
HDL		
TG		
SCr		
Microalbumin		
Vision Exam		
Blood Pressure		
Weight		
Vaccines		

Plan for today:

Notes:

arrives. Usually your preceptor will have you verbally present the patient's workup at some point prior to meeting with or calling to speak to the patient. Successful presentation of a patient should usually include the following:

- Patient's name
- Age
- Reason for appointment
- Pertinent medical history
- Pertinent social history
- Complete medication list
- Actions completed at last patient visit
- Any recommendations you have regarding the patient's therapy

Additionally, your preceptor may want you to come up with a plan for the appointment. For this, you should discuss the areas you think need to be addressed with the patient and all of the points you would like to see covered. See Chapter 6 for a full discussion of case presentations.

After presenting the case, it is time to meet with the patient. At some sites, this may be face to face, whereas at others, it may be over the phone. The purpose of the visit is both to gather additional information from the patient and to provide the patient with information. Exactly what is discussed and how it is done varies among sites. Typically, you or your preceptor will begin by asking questions to gather information and create a plan that will be delivered to the patient. It is important to keep accurate notes of what patients and practitioners say during the visit so that it can be included in the documentation.

After the patient's appointment concludes, it is time to document. Documentation is vital to create continuity of patient care and also may be required to justify pharmacist billing. Although this is most commonly completed using some type of SOAP (subjective, objective, assessment, and plan) note, documentation can take many forms. Typically, you will write up your note and the preceptor will review it. Once finalized, the documentation is usually added to the patient's record.

In addition to the core areas of direct patient care just discussed, your day may also include a variety of activities, including topic discussions, responses to drug information questions, creating patient or healthcare team education materials, presentations, or spending time with other members of the healthcare team, such as physicians, nurses, social workers, educators, and psychologists.

Identifying Drug-Related Problems

Drug-related problems (DRPs) are the undesirable events that occur outside of the desirable pharmacological response to a medication (or the potential for such events). Identification of DRPs is an essential skill on most rotation types and is put to particularly good use at ambulatory care sites. Identifying DRPs is a challenging skill that takes many years to refine. Having a systematic process will be very helpful, especially early in your career. DRPs are traditionally broken down into nine major categories (see **Tables 13-1** and **13-2**). Using these lists will help you to maximize your ability to properly identify DRPs when applied consistently to each patient situation. All of these DRPs are used throughout the ambulatory care setting and must be evaluated for each patient seen.

TABLE 13-1. TYPES OF DRUG-RELATED PROBLEMS

TYPE OF DRP	EXAMPLE
A problem of the patient is not being treated or is not maximally being treated. a. Missed medical problem b. Suboptimal therapeutic approach c. Suboptimal drug selection d. Medication duplication	Hyperlipidemia is noted by lab data, but the patient is not receiving a lipid-lowering drug. A patient with heart failure is taking furosemide and digoxin but not an ACE-I. A patient is taking HTN medications and BP is better than before but still elevated, yet no additional adjustment in therapy is being made. A patient with diabetes and HTN is taking a beta-blocker instead of an ACE-I. A patient with normal renal function is receiving furosemide for HTN rather than HCTZ. A patient with HTN is taking HCTZ and chlorthalidone.
A drug a patient is receiving is a. Not indicated b. Contraindicated	A patient diagnosed with anemia due to chronic illness is being treated with iron sulfate. A patient is receiving digoxin for no apparent reason. A patient with heart failure is prescribed cilostazol.
A problem of the patient is being caused by one of the patient's medications.	A patient develops symptomatic bradycardia related to the use of his beta-blocker eye drops for glaucoma. A patient develops a rash due to penicillin.
The patient is not being properly monitored in relation to the therapy he or she is receiving. a. Efficacy b. Toxicity c. Pharmacokinetics	A patient initiated on levothyroxine does not have her thyroid function tested after 2 months of therapy. A patient receiving amiodarone does not have pulmonary function tests. A patient with compromised renal function does not have aminoglycoside concentrations measured.
A drug interaction exists or the potential for one exists. a. Adding a medication b. Removing a medication c. Food–drug interaction	A patient taking digoxin is started on amiodarone. Carbamazepine is discontinued in a patient receiving warfarin. A patient on felodipine goes on a grapefruit juice "binge."
A drug dosage is inappropriate. a. Dose too much or too little b. Renal disease c. Liver disease d. Duration of therapy	A patient with iron deficiency is receiving iron sulfate 325 mg daily. A patient is receiving ceftriaxone 2 gm BID IV for pneumonia. A patient with renal failure is receiving ciprofloxacin 500 mg twice daily. Despite the cause being corrected, a patient is still receiving iron sulfate 325 mg TID after 3 years.
A drug is interfering or masking a manifestation of a disease or altering the interpretation of a lab test.	A patient suspected to be infected is given ibuprofen for bursitis. A patient has a PSA test while taking finasteride.

A medication is being administered utilizing an inefficient a. Route of administration b. Dosage form c. Schedule d. Technique	A patient is being given ranitidine intravenously while all other medications are being given orally. A patient with dysphagia is given Bactrim DS tablets. Patient is receiving isosorbide dinitrate every 8 hours. Misuse of a metered dose inhaler.

Patient is not receiving medication.
 	
a. Noncompliance
 	
b. Medical regimen is complicated
 	
c. Costs
 	
d. Patient cannot obtain medication
 	
  (1) Pharmacy ran out
 	
  (2) Not on formulary
 	
  (3) Health professional error
	A patient does not take his atenolol any more because he feels fine and figures he does not need it anymore.
	
	A patient is receiving allopurinol 100 mg TID.
	
	A patient does not take atorvastatin because of its expense.
	
	Medication is not available because it is not on formulary.
	
	Nurse forgets to administer medication.
	
	Physician does not list as discharge medication.

Abbreviations: ACE-I = angiotensin-converting enzyme inhibitor; BID = twice daily; BP = blood pressure; HCTZ = hydrochloro-thiazide; HTN = hypertension; IV = intravenously; PSA = prostate-specific antigen; TID = three times daily.

Source: Courtesy of Dr. Vincent Mauro, PharmD

TABLE 13-2. POCKET DRUG-RELATED PROBLEM LIST

TYPE OF DRP

A problem of the patient is not being treated or is not maximally being treated.
  a. Missed medical problem
  b. Suboptimal therapeutic approach
  c. Suboptimal drug selection
  d. Medication duplication

A drug a patient is receiving is
  a. Not indicated
  b. Contraindicated

A problem of the patient is being caused by one of the patient's medications.

The patient is not being properly monitored in relation to the therapy he/she is receiving.
  a. Efficacy
  b. Toxicity
  c. Pharmacokinetics

A drug interaction exists or the potential for one exists.
  a. Adding a medication
  b. Removing a medication
  c. Food–drug interaction

A drug dosage is inappropriate.
  a. Dose is too much/too little
  b. Renal disease
  c. Liver disease
  d. Duration of therapy

A drug is interfering or masking a manifestation of a disease or altering the interpretation of a lab test.

A medication is being administered inefficiently.
  a. Route of administration
  b. Dosage form
  c. Wrong schedule
  d. Technique

Patient is not receiving medication.
  a. Noncompliance
  b. Medical regimen is complicated
  c. Costs
  d. Patient cannot obtain medication
    1) Pharmacy ran out
    2) Not on formulary
    3) Health professional error

Source: Courtesy of Dr. Vincent Mauro, PharmD.

Physical Assessment Skills

The ambulatory care setting is where physical assessment may be utilized to its fullest in pharmacy practice. Some ambulatory care rotations may require little or no physical assessment, whereas others may require utilizing these skills for each patient encountered. The most common physical assessment skills include the following:

- Blood pressure
- Pulse
- Point-of-care lab assessments
- Foot exam and visual inspection

Blood Pressure and Pulse

The basics of taking blood pressure and pulse should be reviewed prior to the start of the rotation. You should practice on your preceptor, another student, or a colleague before trying it on your first patient to gain comfort and confidence in your skills. Proper measurement of blood pressure starts with selecting the correct cuff size. Choosing a cuff that is too small or too large for the patient will result in a falsely elevated or reduced blood pressure. It is important to ask the patient about recent exercise, nicotine use, and caffeine consumption, as these may affect the accuracy of the reading. Instruct the patient to sit up straight with his or her legs uncrossed. Patients should be seated for approximately 5 minutes before measurement to ensure they are truly at rest. Pulse is typically measured on the patient's wrist by counting the number of beats that occur within 6 seconds and multiplying this number by 10. The cuff should be placed on the upper arm, just above the elbow. Proper placement of the cuff starts with finding the marking on the cuff that is an indicator for the brachial artery. Once this is identified, place this marking on the brachial artery and proceed to wrap the cuff firmly around the arm. The cuff should be inflated to 20 mmHg above the patient's normal systolic blood pressure or to about 180 mmHg if you do not know the patient's usual systolic number. The stethoscope should be placed on the brachial artery under the cuff. You may then release the air from the cuff slowly at a rate of approximately 2 mmHg/second. This will allow you to accurately identify the systolic pressure (the number at which sound is first heard) and diastolic pressure (the number at which sound disappears again). Immediately after the sound disappears, you should release the remaining air from the cuff to ensure patient comfort. It is also important to tell the patient what you found after the reading. Specifically, tell the patient what the reading is and what it means. This is an important step in involving the patient in his or her own care.

QUICK TIP

Some common mistakes encountered when measuring blood pressure include improper placement of the cuff or stethoscope (resulting in an inability to hear the readings), releasing the air too quickly, forgetting to write the reading down right after measurement (resulting in having to remeasure), and leaving the cuff inflated too long before you begin to release air (resulting in patient discomfort and falsely elevated values).

As with most physical assessments, practice makes perfect, so it will be important to practice at least once before trying it on a real patient. Also worth mentioning, white coat hypertension is a very real phenomenon and must be considered when making an assessment of blood pressure. The more nervous or uncomfortable a patient feels, the more likely he or she is to experience white coat hypertension.

Ways to limit this include being as relaxed as possible with the patient, smiling, and avoiding anxiety-inducing conversation before the reading.

Point-of-Care Laboratory Tests

Ambulatory care rotations may also allow you to participate in the collection of small amounts of a patient's blood for point-of-care laboratory tests. Commonly used tests include blood glucose, hemoglobin A1c, cholesterol panels, international normalized ratio (INR), and serum iron levels. Each blood test may need to be completed differently. It is important that you understand the instructions for the particular machine or collection device being used and have a good understanding of how much blood the machine will require before getting started. If you know this ahead of time, it will hopefully prevent you from having to stick the patient twice to obtain the required amount of blood.

QUICK TIP

If you are someone who does not like the sight of blood, consider ways you will handle this situation ahead of time so that you can ensure successful completion of all rotation activities.

Blood Glucose

Blood glucose is the most common measurement you may encounter. Each glucometer is slightly different, so it is important that you are familiar with the glucometer you are using. The first step in the process will be to inform the patient of what you will be doing. Then you will need to sanitize your hands using alcohol or soap and water and put on gloves. At this time, you can prepare the patient and the meter for the test. You should set out all of the equipment you will need for this process. This should generally include a glucometer, test strip, lancet, alcohol swab, and a tissue, cotton ball, or bandage. As a general rule, when you insert the testing strip, the meter will turn on and prepare to accept a blood sample. Some older machines may require entering a code at this step. The code is found on the test strip container. Note that the machine will only stay on for a few minutes and in the event that it turns off before you place the blood sample, the strip will need to be removed and reinserted. The next step is to wipe the area to be lanced with an alcohol swab.

QUICK TIP

When using a lancet device to obtain a blood glucose measurement, avoid using the pads of your patient's finger. This site is quite painful when lanced. Instead, use the outside edges of the finger.

Regulations require that single-use lancing devices be used for each patient to avoid contamination, although they rarely allow you to adjust the depth of the lancet. To minimize discomfort, ask the patient which finger he or she would like to use for testing.

QUICK TIP

To ensure enough blood is obtained from one lance, you may want to prepare the patient's finger by having the patient hold his or her hand out and squeeze the finger from the base up to the tip. This will bring more blood to the tip of the finger.

You should now lance the patient's finger. Bring the test strip to the drop of blood forming on the finger. When enough blood is obtained, you will typically hear a beep or see the screen change. Immediately, hand your patient a tissue or cotton ball to stop the bleeding.

Foot Examination

In ambulatory clinics that care for patients with diabetes, the foot exam is an important tool to help avoid the dire consequences of neuropathy. The examination usually consists of visual inspection for cuts, sores, and risks for infection as well as performing a monofilament test. The most important part of this assessment is the correct positioning and pressure of the monofilament. Review this technique and practice on someone before completing it on a patient.

To conduct a foot examination, you begin by having the patient remove his or her socks and shoes. It is recommended that you wear gloves. Begin by visually inspecting the foot for any abnormalities, including cracks, cuts, wounds, dryness, and swelling. Note any areas of discoloration, which may suggest poor circulation. To conduct a monofilament examination, begin by instructing the patient to alert you anytime he or she feels the monofilament on his or her foot.

QUICK TIP

It may be helpful to demonstrate what the monofilament will feel like by testing it out on the patient's arm.

Next, place the tip of the monofilament on the foot with just enough pressure to cause a slight bend in the monofilament. This should be performed on each area of the foot. Document any areas where the monofilament is placed and the patient does not note sensation.

MANAGING PATIENT VISITS

Patient visits, whether in an office or over the phone, are the major component of any ambulatory care rotation. The skills involved in obtaining medication histories, conducting effective patient interviews, communicating a care plan, and writing effective documentation are essential for success in this rotation type. Preparing for a patient appointment should typically start before the patient arrives by gathering any information you may already have available on the patient. The more prepared you are when starting out with a patient appointment, the more smoothly things will generally go and the more easily you will be able to cover all of the necessary items. Using a patient workup sheet, such as the example shown in Figure 13-1, will aid in this process.

The next important step is the patient interview, a vital skill necessary to gather an accurate medication history. At a minimum, it is important to review all of the medications with the patient to get an up-to-date list of what is being taken and also to investigate adherence. Depending on the rotation, you may get more involved in this area, including asking what each medication is for and the patient's expectations. In addition to discussing medications, the patient interview should include any questions necessary to gather the information needed to make your therapeutic plan or decisions. It helps if you prepare a list of questions beforehand so that nothing is missed. Patient appointments can change focus rapidly, and it is important to maintain control of the encounter. Patients may have a different agenda of items to be discussed, so be prepared to politely steer the conversation back on track.

Once you have all of the necessary information, it will be time to communicate your plan to the patient. At many sites, you may leave the room or telephone call after gathering information to discuss it with your preceptor and formulate your plan. You will then return to communicate the plan to the patient. This is a particularly essential part of the patient's appointment. It is important that you communicate the plan in such a way that the patient will understand best—a process that should be individualized for each patient. Typically, both written and verbal communication of the plan is ideal. If the visit is conducted over the phone, this will often mean mailing the patient some information. Having a written plan in addition to having heard it verbally serves as both a reminder and a resource for patients in case they forget or misunderstand any information. It is vital that patients do not receive too much information because they can become overwhelmed. It is helpful to conclude by summarizing the major two to four bullet-point items you would like the patient to take away from the encounter. For example, if you were talking about a plan for diabetes management, it may be summarized as, "So, the plan is to start taking Metformin 500 mg twice daily, check your blood sugar at least once daily at differing times, and start walking 10 minutes per day."

The final step in the patient visit process is documentation for the healthcare team. The individuals that may utilize or view the documentation will vary among sites, but thorough documentation is essential in the patient care process. The most common documentation type in the ambulatory care setting is the SOAP note. Specifics on writing SOAP notes can be found in Chapter 6. The biggest difference you may notice in writing SOAP notes for an ambulatory care rotation versus other rotation types is the inclusion of subjective information you obtained personally during the patient's visit. All major points should be included; however, succinctness is incredibly important whenever sharing information among healthcare professionals. Although other members of the healthcare team typically look at the SOAP notes in this setting, they also serve as a resource for pharmacy services to recall what has previously been completed with a particular patient. The SOAP notes become an important aspect in continuity of care for patients in the ambulatory care setting.

PHONE-BASED PHARMACEUTICAL CARE SERVICES

As discussed throughout this chapter, your ambulatory care site may incorporate and utilize phone conversations to provide patient care. Phone management may be used in addition to or in place of face-to-face visits. Care may be provided this way to gather information before a patient comes to an appointment, to follow up with a patient, or to complete entire patient interviews and plans. Much like speaking with patients face to face, phone management requires a particular skill set to be executed successfully. It is extremely important to speak clearly, slowly, and politely.

QUICK TIP

Telephone visits may be simulated before beginning your rotation by speaking with friends or family about their medications over the phone.

One of the most difficult elements of a phone interview is the lack of nonverbal communication. This may make it a bit more difficult to gauge a patient's interest and understanding of provided information, requiring additional open-ended questions and repetition of information. Consider some ways in which you will assess these items and overcome this difficulty when speaking with a patient over the phone.

SPECIAL POPULATIONS

One of the unique aspects of ambulatory care services is the need for alteration of information delivery and design of therapeutic plans for different patient populations. Each patient encounter will be slightly different from others; however, there are certain general population types that may be encountered that require a different approach to care. It is helpful to be aware of some of these patient types so that you can become familiar with individualized plan development and the resources at your disposal.

The Complex Patient

One of the most common types of patients you may face will be ones with multiple health conditions and medications. It is not uncommon for some patients to be taking more than 10 medications. This patient population tends to benefit greatly from the help of a pharmacist in the ambulatory care setting. Pharmacists are able to assist in chronic disease state management, assess medication regimens for drug-related problems, rectify issues that arise from polypharmacy, assess medication lists for optimal treatment, assist in cost savings, and educate patients about disease states and medication therapy. Taking a holistic approach to the assessment of the patient's medication regimen and conditions can assist in improving adherence and maintaining the best treatment approach. Systematically using the DRP list (provided in Tables 13-1 and 13-2) is a great way to capture the largest number of interventions possible, particularly when polypharmacy is a factor.

The Underserved Patient

At some point during your ambulatory care rotation, you may come across patients who are considered underserved. This is typically defined as patients with low income, low education, or decreased access to medical care. Patients in this category may have insurance but find it difficult to afford copays for appointments, laboratory tests, or medications, whereas others may not have any coverage. This can affect the ability of patients to care for themselves. You can play a key role in designing affordable regimens for these patients, including pharmacological and nonpharmacological treatments. One the best ways this can be accomplished is by having a good understanding of the costs of common therapies for different disease states and ways care can be made affordable for patients. This may include becoming familiar with discounted generic medication availability, patient assistance programs (PAPs), local or regional programs in place to assist patients, and alternative medication regimens that may be used for chronic disease states. Many community pharmacies have affordable generic lists, and branded agents can be obtained through patient assistance websites such as NeedyMeds.org. At some point during the rotation, you may be asked to complete or assist a patient in completing a PAP application form.

QUICK TIP

You may want to spend some time familiarizing yourself with local pharmacy discount generic medication lists and prices prior to the start of your ambulatory care rotation.

Additionally, underserved patients may face other challenges that may complicate their care. The most common issue faced is a lack of continuity. This may occur because of a lack of follow-up with physicians, absence of a primary care physician, discharge from medical practices, moving homes, homelessness, incarceration, loss of transportation, or loss of phone service. Any of these individual factors can prevent the continuity necessary for appropriate outpatient care and follow-up. These factors often alter the treatment and monitoring recommendations made to the patient.

Education Level, Health Literacy, and English Proficiency

Health literacy and patients' native languages are other factors that must be considered when providing care in the ambulatory care setting. This includes ability of a patient to read, write, speak, and understand English. There are many resources available to assist with the care of patients who may be at a lower literacy level or do not speak English. All health systems are required to provide translation services for patients with communication barriers, such as non-English speakers or patients with hearing or visual impairments. You may need to be creative when providing information to this population of patients. For example, if you are trying to improve adherence in a patient who cannot read or write in English, you may consider using pictures to illustrate what you are describing so that he or she may still have a written reference to take home.

Belief Systems

Other patients who you will likely encounter during your ambulatory care rotation are those with different belief systems. Patients come from a variety of backgrounds and may have beliefs that are at odds with yours or those of the general population. This may affect the care the patient wishes to receive or partake in, particularly when caring for medical issues. It is important to ask patients about their beliefs and assess how it will affect the care plan being developed. For example, you may have a patient who would like to quit smoking but does not believe in Western medicine. In this scenario, the patient may be better served by being recommended behavioral or alternative medicine techniques, such as hypnotherapy or acupuncture. Keeping an open mind, assessing for different patient beliefs, and including the patient in the therapeutic plan development are important and can make an enormous difference in adherence to and efficacy of recommendations.

Caring for Those Who Do Not Care for Themselves

This concept is one of the hardest to accept and overcome in ambulatory care practice. At some point during your ambulatory care rotation, you will likely encounter a patient who has a manageable illness but simply does not seem to want to put forth the effort to manage it, despite his or her healthcare team's best efforts to assist. Unfortunately, as healthcare professionals, we can only advise patients about what to do; we cannot force them to carry out our plan. At the end of the day, it is up to the patients to cope with and complete the day-to-day management of chronic disease states by taking their medications, performing appropriate monitoring, and making important lifestyle modifications. It is important to keep this concept in mind as therapy plans are developed. Continuing to develop and implement different motivation techniques can be helpful in getting patients to take more interest in their care. The psychological aspect of chronic disease is not a point that should be overlooked. Speaking with patients about the changes and effects their condition may have on their daily lives, connecting them with support groups, and referring them to mental or behavioral health services may be incredibly beneficial in helping them to take action.

LAWS AND RULES GOVERNING OUTPATIENT SCOPE OF PRACTICE

Like all aspects of pharmacy practice, ambulatory care comes with its own set of laws and rules that govern the scope of practice in this setting. It is important you are familiar with the laws and rules that oversee ambulatory care or outpatient practice in the state in which you will complete your ambulatory care rotation. State rules can vary greatly in what pharmacists are allowed to do and what documentation has to be in place to do so. Some states allow for pharmacists to meet certain criteria to gain prescriptive authority, whereas others allow for consult agreements between physicians and pharmacists to assist in the management of medication therapy. Government institutions, such as the Department of Veterans Affairs, the Bureau of Prisons, or the Indian Health Services, may operate under unique regulations that act outside the state's authority. Familiarity with the local regulations is absolutely essential as you begin and complete your ambulatory care rotation. The website of the State Board of Pharmacy for the state you are practicing in is the best source of this type of information.

SUGGESTED READING

Anticoagulation

American College of Chest Physicians Antithrombotic Therapy and Prevention of Thrombosis Panel. Antithrombotic therapy and prevention of thrombosis, 9th ed: American College of Chest Physicians Evidence-Based Clinical Practice Guidelines. *Chest.* 2012;141(suppl 2).

Diabetes

American Diabetes Association. Standards of medical care in diabetes—2012. *Diabetes Care.* 2012;35 (suppl 1):S11-S63.

Hyperlipidemia

Expert Panel on Detection, Evaluation, and Treatment of High Blood Cholesterol in Adults. Executive summary of the third report of the National Cholesterol Education Program (NCEP) Expert Panel on Detection, Evaluation, and Treatment of High Blood Cholesterol in Adults (Adult Treatment Panel III). *JAMA.* 2001;285:2486-2497.

Hypertension

Chobanian AV, Bakris GL, Black HR, et al. The seventh report of the Joint National Committee on Prevention, Detection, Evaluation, and Treatment of High Blood Pressure. *JAMA.* 2003;289:2560-2572.

COPD

Rabe KF, Hurd S, Anzueto A, et al. Global strategy for the diagnosis, management, and prevention of chronic obstructive pulmonary disease: GOLD executive summary. Global Initiative for Chronic Obstructive Lung Disease. *Am J Respir Crit Care Med.* 2007;176:(6):532–555.

Tobacco Abuse and Smoking Cessation

2008 PHS Guideline Update Panel, Liaisons, and Staff. Treating tobacco use and dependence: 2008 update U.S. Public Health Service Clinical Practice Guideline executive summary. *Respir Care.* 2008;53:1217-1222.

Asthma

National Heart Lung and Blood Institute. Expert Panel report 3: Guidelines for the diagnosis and management of asthma summary report 2007. 2007:1–74. http://www.nhlbi.nih.gov/guidelines/asthma/asthsumm.pdf

Physical Assessment Skills

Tietze KJ. *Clinical Skills for Pharmacists: A Patient-Focused Approach.* St. Louis, MO: Mosby; 2012.

GERIATRICS

Carla Bouwmeester, PharmD, BCPS, and Michael R. Brodeur, PharmD, CGP, FASCP

CASE

N.W. recently started a geriatric-specialty APPE rotation at a program of all-inclusive care for the elderly. She is assigned to an interdisciplinary team and reports to the daily morning meeting. The team reviews the on-call report that includes a patient who fell and broke her hip, abnormal laboratory values for a patient in a rehabilitation facility, a patient who received his roommate's medications last night at an assisted living facility, and a refill request for acetaminophen. After the morning meeting, the pharmacy resident reviews with N.W. the list of patients who need international normalized ratios (INRs) taken today at the adult day health center and a nearby assisted living facility. While they are talking, a nurse practitioner inquires about the use of medications to prevent intractable skin itching in patients with dementia.

WHY IT'S ESSENTIAL

The number of people in the United States age 65 years and older is now more than 40.4 million.[1] Over the past 20 years, there has been an increase in life expectancy due to decreasing death rates in children and in those over the age of 65. Combined with the historically elevated birth rates of the baby boomer generation, a 31% increase in the number of Americans who will turn 65 is expected over the next few decades.[1] As this generation ages, there will be a significant shift in the number of elderly persons. Not only will there be more persons over the age of 65, but there will also be an increase in the oldest old. Even now, there is an increase in the number of the oldest old who live alone, particularly women, racial minorities with no living children, and unmarried persons with no living children or siblings.[2] This raises concerns over the demand for support systems and healthcare services for this vulnerable population.

Currently, the percentage of people over the age of 65 who consider themselves to be in fair or poor health is 24%.[3] It is estimated that the number of elderly people with poor health will parallel the population increase and rise sharply by the year 2030.[2] As of 2010, 90% of Medicare beneficiaries reported having one or more chronic medical conditions and 46% had three or more.[4]

- The leading causes of death in patients older than 65 years continue to be heart disease, cancer, stroke, chronic lower respiratory diseases, Alzheimer's disease, diabetes, and pneumonia or influenza (see **Figure 14-1**).

- Although the overall incidence of heart disease and stroke decreased over the past decade, the prevalence of these conditions increases with age.

- It is estimated that 67% of men and 80% of women over the age of 75 have hypertension, compared with only 33% to 34% of men and women aged 45 to 54.[3]

- The latest data reveal that 27% of noninstitutionalized people over the age of 65 have diabetes.[3]

- Compared to the other leading causes of death, Alzheimer's disease–related deaths increased by 66% between 2000 and 2008, and it is now estimated that one in eight people aged 65 or older have Alzheimer's disease[5] (and over 89% of the residents in long-term care facilities have some form of cognitive or mental impairment).[4]

As the disease burden increases in the elderly, so does the percentage of prescription medication use. More than 90% of people over the age of 65 take at least one prescription medication, and two out of three people take three or more prescription medications.[3] The number of people in this age group taking multiple medications has risen from 35.3% in 1994 to 65% in 2008, increasing the potential for medication-related problems.[3] It is estimated that more than 17% of hospital admissions for the elderly are a direct result of adverse drug reactions (ADRs).[6] In 2008, the Institute of Medicine report *Retooling for an Aging America* recommended increased recruitment and retention of geriatric specialists in all health professions.[7]

Pharmacists can play a crucial role in the prevention of medication incidents by preventing drug interactions, monitoring medication therapy, and educating patients on safe medication use. Based on the estimated growth of the elderly population, you will encounter these patients in nearly every area of pharmacy practice. During a geriatrics rotation, you will observe how pharmacists interact with this population through dispensing medications, providing patient counseling, managing drug therapy, and contributing to interdisciplinary care teams. The rotation will allow you to gain confidence and apply your knowledge to caring for patients with sensory impairment, physical disabilities, cognitive limitations, psychological challenges, and renal and hepatic deficiencies and those nearing the end of life. Completing a geriatric rotation will familiarize you with the important issues affecting seniors and expand your understanding of the substantial impact a pharmacist can make while serving this patient population.

Figure 14-1. Death Rates Among Persons 65 Years of Age and Over

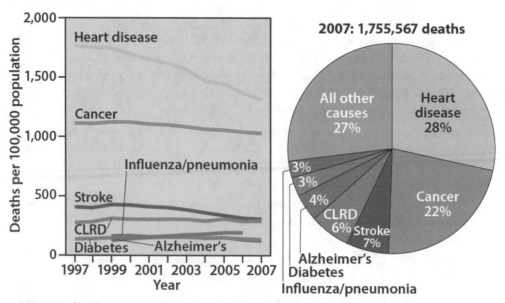

NOTE: CLRD is chronic lower respiratory diseases.
SOURCE: CDC/NCHS, *Health, United States, 2010*, Figure 31. Data from the National Vital Statistics System.

Source: Reprinted with permission from *Health, United States, 2010: With Special Feature on Death and Dying.* Hyattsville, MD: National Center for Health Statistics; 2011.

Arriving Prepared

Contact the preceptor prior to the rotation to discuss logistics (parking, arrival time, meeting place, etc.), dress code, required readings, and disease states to review. The comorbidities of your patient population will vary depending on the setting of the rotation; however, you will encounter most of the common chronic medical conditions. A detailed list of disease states and geriatric syndromes can be found in the *Geriatric Pharmacy Curriculum Guide* (second edition) (available on the American Society of Consultant Pharmacists [ASCP]) website. The most common disease states and conditions encountered in geriatric rotations include the following:

- Cardiovascular
    - Arrhythmias
    - Heart failure
    - Hyperlipidemia
    - Hypertension
- Endocrine
    - Diabetes mellitus
    - Erectile or sexual dysfunction
    - Thyroid disease
- Gastrointestinal
    - Constipation
    - Diarrhea
    - Gastroesophageal reflux disease (GERD)
- Hematologic
    - Anemia
- Infectious disease
    - Nosocomial infections
    - Pneumonia
    - Vaccine-preventable diseases (influenza, herpes zoster, pertussis)
- Musculoskeletal
    - Gout
    - Osteoarthritis
    - Osteoporosis
    - Rheumatoid arthritis
- Neurologic
    - Alzheimer's disease and other dementias
    - Cerebrovascular accident (CVA) and transient ischemic attack (TIA)
    - Pain and neuropathy
    - Parkinson disease
    - Seizures

- Ophthalmology
  - ☐ Cataracts
  - ☐ Glaucoma
  - ☐ Macular degeneration
- Psychiatry
  - ☐ Anxiety
  - ☐ Bipolar disorder
  - ☐ Depression
  - ☐ Schizophrenia
  - ☐ Sleep disorders
- Nephrology and urology
  - ☐ Benign prostatic hyperplasia
  - ☐ Chronic kidney disease
  - ☐ Urinary incontinence
- Respiratory
  - ☐ Asthma
  - ☐ Chronic obstructive pulmonary disease (COPD)
- Syndromes and special problems in the elderly
  - ☐ Falls and gait disorders
  - ☐ Frailty syndrome
  - ☐ Functional decline

It will also be helpful to familiarize yourself with the terminology associated with long-term care and geriatric APPE rotations (see **Table 14-1**), pharmacokinetic and pharmacodynamic changes in the elderly, medications to avoid in the elderly, and any state or federal regulations specific to your practice site.

CASE QUESTION

The pharmacy resident and N.W. are responsible for identifying and tracking medication incidents. These incidents include any medication-related events from prescribing to administration, including order entry, dispensing, delivery, dosing frequency and timing, forgotten or refused doses, duplication of therapy, and adverse events. Identify the potential medication incidents and geriatric syndromes discussed during the morning meeting.

A TYPICAL DAY

Programs of All-Inclusive Care for the Elderly

Programs of All-inclusive Care for the Elderly (PACE) are based on the medical home model and are often described as "nursing homes without walls." These programs are designed to care for medically complex and frail seniors in the comfort of their homes for as long as safely possible. Participants must be at least 55 years old, live within a defined geographic area, and be eligible for nursing home

TABLE 14-1. GERIATRICS TERMINOLOGY

ADHC	Adult day health center	A program that allows older adults opportunities for socialization, supervision, and varying levels of care during the day. This allows respite for caregivers so they can work or care for their own needs during the day. The level of care ranges from socialization and basic support to specialized services for people with dementia or other advanced medical needs.
ADLs	Activities of daily living	Activities needed for self-care: bathing, dressing, mobility, toileting, eating, and transferring.
AIMS	Abnormal involuntary movement scale	Assessment tool used to identify abnormal movement indicative of extrapyramidal side-effects associated with antipsychotic medications.
ALF	Assisted living facility	A type of living arrangement that provides personal care services such as meals, housekeeping, transportation, and assistance with ADLs. Residents pay a regular monthly rent and additional fees for extra services, such as help with medications.
CAM	Confusion assessment method	A tool designed to improve the identification and recognition of delirium.
CCRC	Continuing care retirement center	A housing community that provides different levels of care based on what each resident needs over time. This can range from independent living in an apartment, to assisted living, to full-time care in an SNF. Residents move from one setting to another based on their needs but continue to live as part of the same community.
CMS	Centers for Medicare & Medicaid Services	The agency responsible for Medicare and parts of Medicaid. Responsible for maintaining, updating, and enforcing the regulations and guidelines in the State Operations Manual (SOM).
DNH	Do not hospitalize	Order placed on a patient's chart or record, with the patient's or surrogate's consent, that direct healthcare personnel should not hospitalize the patient. This is usually in place when the patient is receiving end-of-life care and the goal of care is palliation.
DNR	Do not resuscitate	Order placed on a patient's chart or record, with the patient or surrogate's consent, that direct healthcare personnel should not revive the patient if cardiac or respiratory activities cease.

F-tag		Numerical designation for criteria reviewed during the nursing facility survey.
GDR	Gradual dose reduction	Slowly reducing a resident's psychotropic medication(s) over a period of time with the end goal being the resident's attainment of the highest functional status and quality of life while incurring the fewest side effects.
HCP	Healthcare proxy	A person authorized to make healthcare decisions for another person.
IADLs	Instrumental activities of daily living	Activities such as shopping, paying bills, and managing medications.
IDT	Interdisciplinary team	Healthcare team made up of multiple health professionals, which may include physicians, nurses, pharmacists, physical therapists, occupational therapists, speech therapists, dieticians, social workers, case managers, psychologists, and others.
LTC	Long-term care	The provision of medical, social, and personal care services on a recurring or continuing basis to persons with chronic physical or mental disorders. The care may be provided in environments ranging from institutions to private homes. LTC services usually include symptomatic treatment, maintenance, and rehabilitation for patients of all age groups.
MCI	Mild cognitive impairment	MCI is an intermediate stage between the expected cognitive decline of normal aging and the more pronounced decline of dementia.
MDS	Minimum data set	Core set of screening and assessment elements of the Resident Assessment Instrument (RAI), which provides a comprehensive, accurate, standardized, reproducible assessment of each LTC facility resident's functional capabilities and helps staff to identify health problems. This assessment is performed on every resident in a Medicare- and/or Medicaid-certified LTC facility including private pay.
MINI-COG	N/A	Assessment instrument that measures cognitive function, such as impairment associated with dementia, and includes a recall and clock-drawing test.
MMSE	Mini Mental State Exam	Assessment instrument that measures cognitive function by testing memory, orientation, attention, and constructional ability.

MRP	Medication-related problem	An event involving medication therapy that actually or potentially interferes with an optimum outcome for a specific patient.
MRR	Medication regimen review	A systematic approach to ensuring that a patient's medication therapy maximizes desired outcomes while minimizing risks. The goal is to reduce medication-related problems. In nursing facilities, this activity is performed by the consultant pharmacist.
OASIS	Outcome and Assessment Information Set	Represents core items of a comprehensive assessment for an adult home care patient and forms the basis for measuring patient outcomes for outcome-based quality improvement (OBQI).
PACE	Programs of All-Inclusive Care for the Elderly	PACE combines medical, social, and LTC services for frail older adults. PACE is available only in states that have chosen to offer it under Medicaid. The goals of PACE are to help people stay independent and live in their community as long as possible, while getting the high-quality care they need.
POA	Power of attorney	A legal document authorizing someone to act as another person's agent.
QI	Quality indicator	Developed by CMS to represent common conditions and important aspects of care. QI reports reflect a measure of the prevalence or incidence of health conditions based on MDS assessment data.
QM	Quality measure	Information derived from MDS data that are available to the public as part of the Nursing Facility Quality Initiative. The QMs are designed to provide consumers with additional information to make informed decisions about the quality of care in nursing facilities.
QOL	Quality of life	The patient's ability to enjoy normal life activities. Some medical treatments can seriously impair QOL without providing appreciable benefit, whereas others can greatly enhance QOL.
RAI	Resident assessment instrument	The designation for the complete resident assessment process mandated by CMS, including the comprehensive MDS, RAPS, and care planning decisions. The RAI helps facility staff gather information on a resident's strengths and needs that must be addressed in an individual care plan.

RAP	Resident assessment protocol	A problem-oriented framework for organizing MDS information and additional clinically relevant information about an individual's health problems or functional status.
SNF	Skilled nursing facility	A nursing facility with the staff and equipment to provide skilled nursing care and/or skilled rehabilitation services and other related health services.
SOM	State Operations Manual	A manual provided by CMS that contains the regulations and guidelines governing nursing facilities. It is used by surveyors during the survey process as a basis for investigation and evaluation of compliance with CMS standards.

Source: Adapted from Centers for Medicare & Medicaid Services. Glossary. Accessed December 18, 2012. www.cms.hhs.gov/apps/glossary.

care although still living safely in the community. The PACE program provides all services covered by Medicare and Medicaid and assumes full financial responsibility for the patient's medical care. This may include physical and occupational therapy, social work, medications (both prescription and over-the-counter [OTC]), medical specialists, transportation to medical appointments, adult day healthcare, hospital stays, and nursing home placement if necessary in the future. Each PACE program also functions as a Medicare Part D company and provides medications through affiliated or independent pharmacies.

Pharmacy services in PACE programs vary by location but generally include involvement in the interdisciplinary team morning meetings, patient counseling and education, medication regimen reviews, and committee meetings. Every 6 months, each PACE participant is involved in the care planning process to assess progress and establish clinical goals for the next 6 months. Prior to the care plan meeting, each discipline conducts a thorough review of the patient's current health status, interventions made by the team, and progress toward established goals of therapy. This is an ideal time for you to review the patient's medication use over the past 6 months and make recommendations regarding drug interactions, adverse events, side effects, monitoring, duplicate therapy, and untreated conditions. You may also provide medication counseling directly to patients in the PACE clinic or in the patients' homes. Some PACE programs also rely on pharmacists to manage anticoagulation and chronic disease states, giving you the opportunity to get involved in INR point-of-care testing, insulin teaching, or education on the proper use of inhalers. Finally, pharmacists are often involved in committees such as quality assurance, performance improvement, compliance, infection control, hospice services, pharmacy and therapeutics (formulary), and fall prevention. You may be asked to attend committee meetings, assist in preparing reports, present in-service learning programs, or perform medication use evaluations for other healthcare professionals.

• •

"My experience at the PACE program enhanced my understanding of caring for older adults and taught me to consider each patient as a whole rather than managing each disease state separately. I now have a better understanding of the role and significance of the pharmacist on the healthcare team in counseling patients, providing information and recommendations to prescribers and caregivers, performing medication reviews, medication therapy management, presenting in-service educational programs, and ultimately reducing medication-related problems."—Student

• •

Assisted Living

Another potential setting for a geriatric APPE rotation is an assisted living facility (ALF). The exact definition, terminology, and regulations governing ALFs vary widely from state to state. ALFs generally provide community living arrangements for seniors and other individuals who require some level of assistance with basic medical needs, such as medication administration, or activities of daily living (ADLs), such as bathing, toileting, and dressing. Care is usually provided by trained staff but not necessarily nursing staff. ALFs provide 24-hour supervision and security should an emergency arise. The facilities typically provide services such as meal preparation, housekeeping, laundry, transportation, and social programs. Residents usually have their own rooms or shared apartments with a small kitchenette, private bathroom, and common living space. Each resident has a contract with the ALF that determines which services they receive based on their level of independence and need.

Pharmacists provide a range of services in the assisted living environment depending on state regulations and contractual agreements with the facilities or residents. Approximately two thirds of the states require medication regimen reviews (MRRs) for residents in assisted living facilities.[8] An MRR includes an evaluation of the resident's medication regimen to determine appropriate indication, dosage, and administration technique, monitoring of side effects and therapeutic endpoints, identification of drug interactions, and adherence. After completing a MRR, you may be asked to communicate any recommendations directly to the resident, caregivers, physicians, or healthcare professionals at the ALF. Pharmacists may also be involved in assessing the proper acquisition, storage, and labeling of medications in the facility. You may assist in the development or revision of medication-related policies and procedures, provide in-service programs on proper medication administration for residents or ALF staff members, or facilitate the return and destruction of unused or expired medications. Dispensing pharmacies often provide specialized packaging for residents of ALFs to comply with state regulations. You may be involved in preparing medications in the dispensing pharmacy, receiving medications at the ALF, or assisting in other points of the medication distribution system.

Adult Daycare

Adult daycare offers seniors socialization, supervision, and varying levels of care during the day. This allows respite for caregivers so they can work or care for their own needs during the day. The level of care in adult day health centers (ADHCs) ranges from socialization and basic support to specialized services for people with dementia or other advanced medical care. Attendees participate in social activities designed to stimulate cognition and engage them in the community. Most programs offer assistance with transportation, meals, emotional support, education, recreation, and exercise. Medical services at ADHCs may include physical and occupational therapy, nursing, wound care, tube feeding, and administration of medications. Attendees come to the ADHC on a scheduled basis and then return to the comfort of their own homes in the evening.

Pharmacists may be directly employed by an ADHC or have contractual agreements to provide periodic services for the center. One of the most common services pharmacists provide in this setting is the "brown bag" event. The pharmacist schedules a time when he or she will be available to review medications and make suggestions to improve adherence and ease of administration. Attendees are instructed to bring all of their prescription medications, OTC products, and dietary supplements to the event in a "brown bag." You will meet with each person individually to assess adherence, identify potential interactions, and review the indication and instructions for each medication. During the interview, you should attempt to understand how the person is actually taking the medication rather than assuming he or she is taking it as prescribed. You may also be involved in assisting attendees to select the most cost-effective Medicare Part D plan, providing blood glucose or cholesterol tests, or conducting in-service programs.

QUICK TIP

Before preparing for an in-service program, determine the needs of your audience. The content and delivery of a diabetes program will look very different if the audience is a group of elderly seniors or a group of healthcare providers. Remember to use language that is appropriate for your audience.

....

"I got to experience a lot of patient contact, which I thoroughly enjoyed. We socialized with the patients in the day center, which made them feel more at ease when we discussed medication-related concerns. I became close to several patients and enjoyed visiting them on a daily basis."—Student

....

Home Care

Home care is provided by home healthcare agencies, home care aide organizations, and hospice programs to help people who require ongoing clinical and social services.[9] Patients with disabilities, terminal illness, or chronic diseases utilize home care services when they need medical care, nursing, therapeutic treatment, or assistance with ADLs or instrumental ADLs (IADLs) in the home setting. Services are typically provided by nursing staff, occupational and physical therapists, social workers, speech therapists, infusion pharmacists, home care aides, and companions. Hospice is a specialized form of home care that provides comprehensive medical, social, and spiritual care for people who are terminally ill and their families. These services are often provided in the home to enable families to remain together near the end of life. Hospice services provide medications related to the terminal illness, medical supplies and equipment, spiritual support, and 24-hour medical assistance for the family to care for its loved one. The goals of hospice care are to ensure the patient's end-of-life wishes are honored and the patient is kept as comfortable as possible.

Pharmacists care for patients in their homes through involvement in home health agencies, through infusion services, and as part of interdisciplinary hospice care teams. You may have the opportunity to visit patients in their homes to provide medication counseling, education about home infusions, or work with a team to assess home safety. Home visits are an ideal time to assess actual versus reported adherence to medications.

QUICK TIP

When making home visits, always be aware of your surroundings and personal safety. During the home visit, you can also provide visual inspection of medication storage, record use of dietary supplements and OTC medications, and offer to remove unused or expired medications, if allowed by state regulations and standard operating procedures.

"Recently, I was able to participate in a home visit. I went into the experience thinking we would go in, ask some questions, and then teach the patient how to use her inhaler. Instead, the patient expressed extreme gratefulness for our visit and immediately started asking questions about her medications, which might have gone unanswered if we had not physically visited her at home. The patient expressed confusion about how to take one of her medications because it was sent in a separate package and there were only a few pills in it; therefore, she had not been taking it. We were able to explain what the medication was and how to use it, thus avoiding a potential adverse outcome. We were also able to help her organize her medications and remove any old or unused medications, preventing potential medication errors and inappropriate use. This experience really opened my eyes to what it means to have patient contact."—Student

Continuing Care Retirement Community

Continuing care retirement communities (CCRCs) offer several levels of care within the same community. People typically enter CCRCs when they are still independent in performing ADLs and IADLs but anticipate increasing needs as they age. The CCRC provides independent living, assisted living, nursing home care, and hospice services. As a residents' needs evolve, they will move from one area of the community to another to receive the care they require while remaining in familiar surroundings. These communities often require very high initial down payments and monthly service fees. CCRCs can provide a means for a married couple to remain in the same community, despite differing levels of care. The facilities tend to be large in size to accommodate the different care settings.

Pharmacists are involved in both dispensing and consulting services within CCRCs. Pharmacies may contract with CCRCs to provide compliance packaging for medications, automated refills, and delivery. You may be involved in verifying orders, creating custom labeling and packaging, or creating quality improvement projects related to the medication distribution system. Some pharmacies also provide durable medical equipment (DME), and you may be involved in educating customers about the proper use of the devices, measuring for compression stockings, or determining heights for walkers and canes. You may also have the opportunity to provide in-service programs to residents on safe medication use, disease prevention, or wellness activities. Consultant pharmacists also provide medication regimen reviews for residents in the assisted living or nursing home areas of the CCRC. You may review medical charts and laboratory data to make recommendations to other healthcare providers.

Long-Term Care

Around 1.3 million elderly Americans are currently living in nursing homes.[1] These individuals are commonly referred to as residents and not patients because these facilities are where they may ultimately live for the rest of their lives. As of 1974, federal regulations require that a pharmacist conduct an MRR for each resident in a skilled nursing facility (SNF) at least once a month. Therefore, each nursing facility must obtain both consulting and dispensing pharmacy services to fulfill state and federal regulations.[10] The federal regulations are provided in the State Operations Manual that can be accessed online through the Centers for Medicare & Medicaid Services. These regulations provide guidance for medication use in nursing facilities and focus on assessing efficacy, safety, and appropriate use of each medication. There are specific regulations pertaining to the use of unnecessary medications and the gradual dose reduction and tapering of antipsychotics, sedatives, hypnotics, and other psychopharmacologic medications.

QUICK TIP

When entering the room of a LTC resident, you should knock and determine if it is a convenient time to meet. You should display the same degree of respect as you would if you were visiting the person at his or her home.

Consultant pharmacists provide individual MRRs as well as facility-level reports regarding residents at risk for falls, infection control, and policies and procedures for medication use. You may be expected to perform MRRs by obtaining information from the patient chart, medication administration record, laboratory data, and patient observation and interaction. The MRR should be a succinct summary for other healthcare providers and provide both supporting documentation and rationale for the recommendation. You may also be invited to attend committee meetings, provide in-service programs to nursing staff, or answer drug information requests. Pharmacists may also assist in "med pass" audits where they provide feedback on the medication administration process. You may find it beneficial to observe a "med pass" to understand the complexities of administering medications in a nursing facility.

GERIATRICS

Heterogeneous Population

Older adults, regardless of their living situation, have unique and complex healthcare needs, so it is essential that you have a good general pharmacotherapeutic database to manage the variety of disease states that are encountered. There is great deal of heterogeneity in the geriatric population, and chronologic age does not always equate with physiologic age. For example, it is not uncommon to encounter two 85-year-old patients who are vastly different; one may be very frail and bedbound while the other is physically fit and actively walking many miles a day. The pharmacotherapeutic goals will be very different for these patients. The frail patient will likely be managed less aggressively, with a focus on palliation, whereas more focus on disease prevention will occur in the physically fit older adult. This change in mindset can be a difficult transition for pharmacy students because the didactic curriculum focuses on treatment guidelines and standardized outcomes that may not be appropriate for some older adults and, in some cases, may be harmful. A balance is required between overutilization and underutilization of medications in clinically complex older adults. That balance should look at the patient holistically and assess patient preference, remaining life expectancy, treatment goals, and time until medication benefit.[11] Older adults have been underrepresented in clinical trials and, when included, are usually relatively healthy.

CASE QUESTION

N.W. reviews the patient with the elevated blood glucose discussed at morning report. She discovers that, prior to admission for a hip fracture, the patient had an A1C of 7.1 and that her diabetes was managed with diet and exercise. Since admission, however, her blood glucose has been averaging 220 mg/dL. N.W. recommends to the pharmacy resident that the patient should be started on glyburide 5 mg daily. Do you agree with the recommendation made by N.W.? Why or why not?

Adverse Drug Reactions

There are a number of factors that increase the risk for ADRs in older adults. Polypharmacy is one of the major reasons for increased ADRs in the elderly. Older adults use more prescription drugs than any other age group, which increases the probability of ADRs. Becoming aware of the risk for ADRs and maintaining a high index of suspicion for manifestations of toxicity in the chronically ill, frail elderly is an important challenge for healthcare practitioners. You should adopt the philosophy that any symptom in an older adult is an ADR until proven otherwise.

ADRs in older adults can cause, aggravate, or contribute to common problems, including the following:

- Agitation/confusion
- Delirium
- Depression
- Dizziness
- Drowsiness
- Dysphagia
- Falls
- Malnutrition/dehydration/weight loss
- Incontinence
- Memory loss
- Other psychiatric problems
- Pressure ulcers

Lack of proper indication, inappropriate dosage, and subclinical toxicities of medications are common observations. As described in **Figure 14-2**, the *prescribing cascade* is a known problem, where a medication results in an adverse drug event that is mistaken as a separate diagnosis and treated with more medications, putting the patient at risk for additional ADEs.[12] As the patients gets older, they accumulate multiple medications for a variety of indications, including some that may have been the result of the prescribing cascade. You must reassess the validity of use for each medication and discontinue or consolidate medications whenever possible.

Figure 14-2. Prescribing Cascade

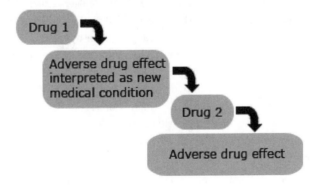

Source: Adapted with permission from Rochon PA, Gurwitz JH. Optimizing drug treatment for elderly people: The prescribing cascade. *BMJ.* 1997;315:1097.

Pharmacokinetics and Pharmacodynamics

Older adults' response to medications differs from that of younger adults. Age-related changes in physiology result in a number of pharmacokinetic and pharmacodynamic changes. Pharmacokinetic changes include changes in absorption, distribution, metabolism, and excretion. **Table 14-2** summarizes a number of physiologic changes in the elderly and their impact on medication regimens.

QUICK TIP

When assessing total phenytoin levels in an older adult, correction should be made for decreased albumin with the following equation:
C adj = C reported /(0.2 x serum albumin) + 0.1.

Kidney function declines with age as a result of a decrease in the number of nephrons, glomerular filtration rate (GFR), and decreased renal blood flow. A common cause of dose-related adverse events in older adults is failure to properly adjust doses for renal insufficiency. Creatinine clearance should be estimated using an equation that accounts for age, such as the Cockcroft–Gault formula. The Cockcroft–Gault is the most widely used and acceptable method for medication dosage adjustment, according to the Food and Drug Administration.[13] You should check dosing based on creatinine clearance using an appropriate resource, such as the *Geriatric Dosage Handbook.*[14]

There are several limitations to GFR-estimating equations that must be considered. They require that serum creatinine be at steady state and are therefore inaccurate in the presence of rapidly changing renal function. In addition, these equations may overestimate GFR in elderly patients with reduced muscle mass, who may have a low creatinine despite declining kidney function. Rounding serum creatinine to 1 mg/dL has been advocated for frail elderly patients with serum creatinine less than 1 mg/dL due to decreased muscle mass but is not supported by the medical literature. The results of creatinine clearance–estimating equations should be interpreted cautiously for elderly patients. When using potentially toxic or renally eliminated medications, appropriately timed medication levels and patient response should be monitored closely.

Appropriate Medication Use in the Elderly

There are a variety of implicit and explicit medication use criteria that can be helpful tools as you work with older adults. Explicit criteria provide a list of medications, medication classes, and other prescribing indicators that enable consistent medication reviews. The most widely utilized explicit criteria is the Beers Criteria, which has recently undergone its fourth revision.[15] The Beers Criteria consists of three lists of potentially inappropriate medications (PIMs) to be avoided in older adults. One list is independent of diagnosis, and medications are categorized by organ system or therapeutic category. The second list considers the diagnosis and is categorized by drug-disease and drug-syndrome interactions. The third list contains PIMs to be used with caution in older adults. The criteria include the rationale for including the medication, recommendation, quality of evidence, and strength of recommendation. The original criteria were designed for use with patients in nursing homes, but they have been adapted and subsequently revised for use in a variety of settings. Although the Beers Criteria does not address underprescribing, drug–drug interactions, or drug class duplications, it is a useful tool to identify medications that require additional scrutiny.

The STOPP (Screening Tool of Older Persons' Potentially Inappropriate Prescriptions) criteria are arranged according to physiological system for ease of use, are broad in scope, and focus on drug–disease interactions.[16] The STOPP criteria are designed to be utilized in conjunction with the START

TABLE 14-2. AGE-RELATED PHYSIOLOGIC AND PHARMACOKINETIC CHANGES

	PHYSIOLOGIC CHANGE	IMPACT	COMMENTS
Absorption	↓ Gastrointestinal motility	Has minimal impact on medication absorption.	
	↓ Gastric emptying	May decrease the rate of absorption.	
	↓ Intestinal blood flow	May decrease the rate of absorption.	
	↓ Muscle mass	IM administration may be problematic and should be avoided when possible.	
	↓ Peripheral blood flow	Medication absorption via the subcutaneous and transdermal routes may be hindered.	Thinning of skin, senile purpura
Distribution	↓ Lean body mass ↑ Fat content	Decreased Vd of medications that are NOT fat soluble (e.g., digoxin) result in higher blood levels. Increased Vd of medications that are fat soluble (e.g., benzodiazepines) result in accumulation in adipose tissue and longer duration of action.	
	Albumin and protein binding	Protein binding may be of limited clinical importance, with the exception of narrow therapeutic index medications (e.g., phenytoin, warfarin), because the transient effects are rapidly counterbalanced by clearance.	Much clinical controversy exists as to whether albumin decreases in "normal" aging. When comorbidities such as infections, cancer, and malnutrition are present, albumin decreases, and this may have an impact on highly protein-bound medications such as phenytoin.

| Metabolism | ↓ Liver mass | Decreased first-pass metabolism | Labetalol and propranolol may have increased bioavailability.

ACE inhibitors enalapril and perindopril are prodrugs that need to be activated in the liver; therefore, they may exhibit slow or reduced metabolism. |
| --- | --- | --- | --- |
| | ↓ Liver blood flow | Medications that are dependent on hepatic blood flow (high extraction ratio agents) have decreased clearance. | |
| | ↓ Phase I (oxidative) metabolism | Decreased metabolism of phase I substrates | Medications that do not undergo phase I metabolism are preferable in older adults (e.g., when selecting a benzodiazepine, lorazepam, oxazepam, and temazepam are preferred). |
| | Phase II (conjugation) metabolism | Aging has little to no impact. | |
| Elimination | ↓ Nephrons | Decreased renal clearance of medications | In general, Cockcroft–Gault underestimates renal function in older adults and MDRD overestimates renal function. |
| | ↓ Renal blood flow | Decreased renal clearance of medications | |
| | ↓ Glomerular filtration rate | Decreased renal clearance of medications | |

Abbreviations: ACE = angiotensin-converting enzyme; IM = intramuscular; MDRD = modified diet in renal disease; Vd = volume of distribution.

(Screening Tool to Alert doctors to the Right Treatment) criteria, which highlight underprescribing or omission of clinically indicated medications.[17] The STOPP and START indicators have been designed for use by clinicians to screen medication regimens in clinical practice.

CASE QUESTION

N.W. reviews the Beers Criteria and sees that sulfonylureas with long durations of action, such as chlorpropamide and glyburide, should be avoided in the elderly. She also notes that sliding-scale insulin should be avoided in older adults due to a higher risk of hypoglycemia without improvement in hyperglycemia management. What tool can N.W. use to identify alternatives to the glyburide and other potentially necessary medications?

The Medication Appropriateness Index (MAI) described in **Figure 14-3** is a tool that measures prescribing appropriateness according to 10 criteria, including indication, effectiveness, dose, administration, interactions, and cost.[18] The MAI is an implicit (judgment-based) set of criteria that can lead to variability in results based on the user's level of experience. You will find the MAI useful in assessing medication regimens in older adults because it provides a systematic framework for evaluation. By working through the 10 questions in the MAI, you will be prepared to present a patient to your preceptor.

Figure 14-3. Medication Appropriateness Index

To assess the appropriateness of the drug, please answer the following questions and circle the applicable score:

* Is there an indication for the drug?

* Is the medication effective for the condition?

* Is the dosage correct?

* Are the directions correct?

* Are the directions practical?

* Are there clinically significant drug–drug interactions?

* Are there clinically significant drug/disease/condition interactions?

* Is there unnecessary duplication with other drug(s)?

* Is the duration of therapy acceptable?

* Is the drug the least expensive alternative compared to others of equal utility?

(Reprinted with permission from Hanlon JT, Schmader KE, Samsa GP, et al. A method for assessing drug therapy appropriateness. *J Clin Epidemiol.* 1992;45:1045-1051.)

Skilled Nursing Facility Regulations

Consultant pharmacists provide MRRs to all SNF residents on at least a monthly basis. Regulations for MRRs in SNFs are published by the Centers for Medicare & Medicaid Services. The latest revision of these regulations contains a number of provisions related to pharmacy services, such as unnecessary medications, pharmacy services, MMRs, and labeling of drugs and biologicals. Although it is important for you to be cognizant that regulations exist, providing good pharmacotherapeutic care with a holistic approach to the nursing home resident will ensure not only compliance with these regulations but also optimal patient outcomes.

The regulations specifically focus on antipsychotic medications due to the history of inappropriate use in nursing homes. Atypical antipsychotic medications used for the behavioral and psychological symptoms of dementia are among the drugs most frequently associated with adverse events in SNFs, especially falls. The Food and Drug Administration (FDA) warned of fatal adverse events in patients with dementia treated with atypical antipsychotics.[19,20] Similar concerns have been raised for haloperidol and other conventional antipsychotics.[21] The regulations stipulate that antipsychotics should only be started to treat specific conditions, and these conditions need to be documented in the resident's chart. If antipsychotics are prescribed, a gradual dose reduction and behavioral intervention should be attempted, unless clinically contraindicated, in an effort to discontinue these medications.

Resources

The American Society of Consultant Pharmacists (ASCP) is a professional organization that represents pharmacists from a variety of practice settings. ASCP provides a wealth of resources and services for its members in the areas of pharmacotherapy, regulations, education, advocacy, and leadership.[22] A free, virtual membership is available to students that allows access to these resources, as well as the peer-reviewed journal *The Consultant Pharmacist,* which publishes research, reviews, and clinical cases. It is recommended that you take advantage of the free ASCP membership before starting a rotation in any geriatric care setting and become familiar with the resources the association offers. Joining ASCP will also allow you to develop your professional network of contacts.

Once you graduate and practice for 2 years as a licensed pharmacist, you may wish to pursue certification in geriatric pharmacy. The Commission for Certification in Geriatric Pharmacy (CGP) was established in 1997, and today there are over 1,000 certified geriatric pharmacists throughout the world.[23] The CGP credential identifies and recognizes those pharmacists who have expertise and knowledge of drug therapy principles for older adults.

SUMMARY

Geriatric APPE rotations provide the opportunity for you to apply your pharmacotherapy knowledge to patient care in a variety of care settings. Older adults are living longer with chronic diseases and taking more medications than in the past. Physiological and pharmacokinetic changes that occur in older adults also increase the risk for ADRs, making the contributions of a pharmacist to the interdisciplinary team extremely important. It is important for you to develop competencies in caring for older adults as the aging population continues to expand. Regardless of where you practice in the future, you are likely to encounter older adults who will benefit from the experience and knowledge you gained during your geriatric APPE rotation.

REFERENCES

1. Administration on Aging. A profile of older Americans: 2011. http://www.aoa.gov/AoARoot/Aging_Statistics/Profile/index.aspx. Accessed March 1, 2012.

2. Administration on Aging. Aging into the 21st century. http://www.aoa.gov/AoARoot/Aging_Statistics/future_growth/aging21/health.aspx. Accessed February 26, 2012.

3. National Center for Health Statistics. Health, United States, 2010: With special feature on death and dying. http://www.cdc.gov/nchs/data/hus/hus10.pdf. Accessed February 26, 2012.

4. The Henry J. Kaiser Family Foundation. Medicare chartbook, 2010. http://kff.org/medicare/8103.cfm. Accessed March 1, 2012.

5. Alzheimer's Association. *2011 Alzheimer's Disease Facts and Figures*. 7th ed. Chicago, IL: Alzheimer's Association; 2011.

6. Kongkaew C, Noyce PR, Ashcroft DM. Hospital admissions associated with adverse drug reactions: A systematic review of prospective observational studies. *Ann Pharmacother*. 2008;42:1017-1025.

7. Institute of Medicine. *Retooling for an Aging America: Building the Health Care Workforce*. Washington, DC: National Academies Press; 2008.

8. American Society of Consultant Pharmacists. Assisted living. https://www.ascp.com/articles/professional-development/assisted-living-members-only-content. Accessed March 11, 2012.

9. Bouwmeester C. The PACE program: Home-based long-term care. *Consult Pharm*. 2012;27:24-29.

10. American Society of Consultant Pharmacists. *Consultant Pharmacist Handbook: A Guide for Consulting to Nursing Facilities*. Alexandria, VA: American Society of Consultant Pharmacists; 2007.

11. Holmes HM. Rational prescribing for patients with reduced life expectancy. *Clin Pharmacol Ther*. 2009;85:103-107.

12. Rochon PA, Gurwitz JH. Optimizing drug treatment for elderly people: The prescribing cascade. *BMJ*. 1997;315:1096-1099.

13. Food and Drug Administration. Guidance for industry: Pharmacokinetics in patients with impaired renal function—study design, data analysis, and impact on dosing and labeling. www.fda.gov/downloads/Drugs/ Guidance Compliance Regulatory Information/Guidances/ UCM072127.pdf. 1998. Accessed July 16, 2012.

14. Semla TP, Beizer JL, Higbee MD, eds. *Geriatric Dosage Handbook 2012: Including Clinical Recommendations and Monitoring Guidelines (Lexi-Comp's Geriatric Handbook)*. Hudson, OH: Lexi-Comp; 2012.

15. Fick D, Semla T, Beizer J, et al. American Geriatric Society updated Beers Criteria for potentially inappropriate medication use in older adults. http://www.americangeriatrics.org/health_care_professionals/clinical_practice/clinical_guidelines_recommendations/2012. Accessed March 8, 2012.

16. O'Mahony D, Gallagehr PF. Inappropriate prescribing in the older population: Need for new criteria. *Age Ageing*. 2007;37:138-141.

17. Barry PJ, Gallagher P, Ryan C, et al. START (screening tool to alert doctors to the right treatment): An evidence-based screening tool to detect prescribing omissions in elderly patients. *Age Ageing*. 2007;36:632-638.

18. Hanlon JT, Schmader KE, Samsa GP, et al. A method for assessing drug therapy appropriateness. *J Clin Epidemiol*. 1992;45:1045-1051.

19. Lenzer J. FDA warns about using antipsychotic drugs for dementia. *BMJ*. 2005;330:922.

20. Schneider LS, Dagerman KS, Insel P. Risk of death with atypical antipsychotic drug treatment for dementia: Meta-analysis of randomized placebo-controlled trials. *JAMA*. 2005;294:1934-1943.

21. Wang PS, Schneeweiss S, Avorn J, et al. Risk of death in elderly users of conventional vs. atypical antipsychotic medications. *N Engl J Med*. 2005;353:2335-2341.

22. The American Society of Consultant Pharmacist. About us. https://www.ascp.com/about-us. Accessed March 12, 2012.

23. Commission for Certification in Geriatric Pharmacy. Pharmacist center. https://www.ascp.com/about-us. Accessed March 12, 2012.

Suggested Reading

American Geriatrics Society. www.americangeriatrics.com.

American Geriatrics Society 2012 Beers Criteria Update Expert Panel. American Geriatrics Society updated Beers Criteria for potentially inappropriate medication use in older adults. *J Am Geriatr Soc.* 2012;60:616-631.

American Society of Consultant Pharmacists. *Consultant Pharmacist Handbook: A Guide for Consulting to Nursing Facilities.* Alexandria, VA: American Society of Consultant Pharmacists; 2007.

American Society of Consultant Pharmacists. www.ascp.com

Barry PJ, Gallagher P, Ryan C, et al. START (screening tool to alert doctors to the right treatment): An evidence-based screening tool to detect prescribing omissions in elderly patients. *Age Ageing.* 2007;36:632-638.

Hutchinson LC, Sleeper RB. *Fundamentals of Geriatric Pharmacotherapy: An Evidence-Based Approach.* Bethesda, MD: American Society of Health-System Pharmacists; 2010.

O'Mahony D, Gallagher PF. Inappropriate prescribing in the older population: Need for new criteria. *Age Ageing.* 2007;37:138-141.

PART III: LIFE AFTER ROTATIONS

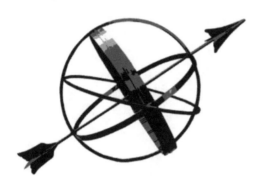

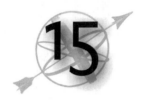

Starting Your Career

Timothy R. Ulbrich, PharmD

CASE

D.W. is a pharmacy student beginning his APPEs. He has decided that he would like to pursue a postgraduate year one (PGY1) pharmacy residency in a health system. He is also considering completing a postgraduate year two (PGY2) residency or fellowship at a later date to fulfill his career goal of becoming a critical care specialist with various teaching opportunities at a nearby college of pharmacy. However, he is overwhelmed at the moment by the process and has decided to focus on the task at hand. He has asked his preceptors to help him to prepare for the residency process and has received several suggestions, including getting his curriculum vitae (CV) up to date, attending local and national meetings, practicing for interviews, and narrowing down his list of potential sites.

Why It's Essential

....

"With all of the unknowns that surround the transition from student pharmacist to new practitioner, many approach graduation with a significant degree of uncertainty and doubt. Fortunately, there may not be another time in one's career where the opportunities are so exciting and diverse, so these reservations quickly fade in the enthusiasm of discovering and exploring the world of pharmacy."—Preceptor

....

The transition from student to practitioner can be rewarding and daunting at the same time. Regardless of the career goals you have in mind, several core skills are necessary to achieve a smooth transition into becoming a new practitioner. An early start on developing these skills will better position you during the job or postgraduate training interview process. During this critical junction, you will begin to define your career, contemplate areas of expertise, and continue to build your professional network.

Advanced Pharmacy Practice Experiences as a Career Stepping Stone

As you get ready to start your APPEs, it is important to recognize that these experiences should be viewed as a month-long (or longer) interview for a job or postgraduate training program, such as a residency or fellowship. Whether or not you are placed at a site of interest, having a positive learning experience and leaving with a good recommendation is essential. The APPEs are a chance to network with various practitioners and to receive feedback on practice and professional skills. As you navigate the residency or job market, having positive experiential rotations will make the choice easier for the employer and you. A student who has a successful rotation after a thorough review from the site will have a leg up on other candidates without similar exposure. In addition, a rotation experience allows you to identify the culture of the program and to determine if you would be a good fit. For example, if you are interested in a residency, you may not have thought about the impact the number of coresidents can have. However, after completing a rotation at a large teaching hospital, you may determine that you would prefer to work in a group environment and, therefore, pursue a program with more than one resident.

Making the most out of the experiential rotations is a must and should be driven by the student. A site will likely have a set of core objectives and activities to be completed, but you may wish to seek out additional opportunities. For example, if you have an interest in research, pairing up with a resident or pharmacist working on a project may allow you to get extra experiences. However, these experiences will rarely be handed out, and motivated students will have to seek them out. Informing your preceptor of your goals at the beginning of the rotation will help to identify available opportunities. Therefore, seeking rotation sites that will allow for these opportunities is important. If possible, you should be strategic about choosing rotations and sites that may interest you for a job or residency. In addition, the timing of these can be key. For example, if you are considering a managed care residency program, having a managed care rotation before the American Society of Health-System Pharmacists (ASHP) meeting in December should be a top priority. During the interview process, you will be able to speak to this experience and any associated projects.

DEFINING CAREER GOALS

If you have not already done so, you should spend some time writing down short- and long-term personal and professional goals. This will help to streamline your job or postgraduate training search process. In this chapter, the focus will be on professional goals. Short-term goals can be defined as the rotations you would like to complete, settings in which you would like to practice, and postgraduate opportunities you would like to pursue. Long-term goals should focus on a 5-year and 10-year plan. It may be helpful to consider the short- and long-term goals together, as they often inform one another.

CASE QUESTION

Thinking of D.W., how would his long-term goal of becoming a critical care specialist with teaching opportunities inform his short-term goals?

In the example of D.W., setting the long-term goal first allows corresponding short-term goals to be set, such as achieving an "A" in the critical care module, taking a critical care elective, or obtaining a critical care APPE rotation. This method of working backward can be very effective in setting short-term goals and steps to help achieve a bigger, and sometimes seemingly distant, goal. For D.W., working back from a long-term goal of obtaining a position as a critical care pharmacist may reveal that several steps need to be taken first (e.g., updating his CV) to obtain a PGY1 residency that will ultimately lead to an opportunity to complete a PGY2. This, in turn, will allow D.W. to complete a CV gap analysis to determine areas that he needs to work on to make himself more marketable for a PGY1 position.

CURRICULUM VITAE AND RESUME

It is likely that you have had experience constructing both a CV and a resume. It is important to distinguish between the two. A *CV*, meaning "life story" or "course of life," is much longer, comprehensive, and detailed than a resume. A *resume* is typically one or two pages in length and summarizes the skills, experiences, and education of the writer. The CV, in contrast, usually contains more detailed information on the skills and experiences of the candidate, as well as a more thorough listing of teaching and research experiences, publications, presentations, awards, and professional involvement, among other items. CVs are most commonly used during the application process for academic, scientific, or research positions. Students applying for residencies, fellowships, or other postgraduate opportunities will likely be expected to submit a CV with their application materials. However, some positions may not be keen on a detailed CV as part of the application process. In those cases, it is prudent to develop a one- to two-page resume using the CV as the framework. Several example CVs and pearls for creating a CV can be found at http://www.accp.com/stunet/cv.aspx.

As you are constructing your CV, some important tips should be considered:

- The CV should be continuously updated, with the last date of update noted in the footer or another identifiable place in the document. Continuous updating will ensure that you have captured all of your activities while decreasing the stress and burden if you are required to produce a CV on short notice.

- You should be careful of the appearance of "fluff" or "padding" that gives the impression that you are trying to make your CV longer or more impressive than it really is. Therefore, the following should be avoided:

  □ abnormally wide margins or large font types

  □ describing high school accomplishments in detail

  □ duplicating items—for example, avoid putting a presentation that you completed during a rotation both underneath the rotation description and in a separate presentations section.

- Be as concise as possible. Use bullets where appropriate and avoid full sentences and paragraphs.

- Be ready to speak about any item on the CV. For example, if you list your name on a publication, you should be prepared to talk about that project as a whole, even if your role was minimal. It may be helpful to identify your role on each project (e.g., data collection for a research project) to avoid the impression of being more involved than you actually were.

- Items should be listed in reverse chronological order, with the most important entries listed first within that chronological order. For example, if you were constructing a leadership section and had two roles (president of the Student Society of Health-System Pharmacists and treasurer of Student Council) that began at the same time, it would be prudent to put the more prestigious and active role (society president) first.

- Avoid having categories that include only one item (e.g., one presentation), as it may have a weaker appearance. Try to find a way to incorporate these items into another section of the CV.

- Consistently format fonts, font sizes, and placement of dates.

- Leave sufficient white space to allow for easy reading, but do not leave so much white space that the document appears to be padded.

BUILDING A PORTFOLIO

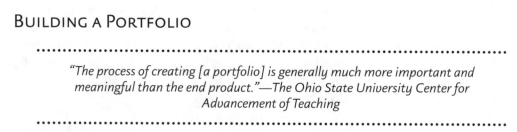

"The process of creating [a portfolio] is generally much more important and meaningful than the end product."—The Ohio State University Center for Advancement of Teaching

Some universities may require students to construct a portfolio during the experiential rotations. Generally, a portfolio is intended to document learning and experience. A portfolio can be constructed as a documentation of evidence to be evaluated (e.g., by a preceptor or potential employer) and a tool for self-growth and reflection. A portfolio should be unique to the creator, and it may be significantly different from one student to the next. For example, a student applying for a fellowship may have a heavy focus on the research section, whereas a student applying for a hospital-based residency may highlight more of the practice-related projects completed during experiential rotations. In addition to documenting achievements and providing a means of self-reflection, a portfolio may help to set you apart from your peers by showing thought, organization, and reflection on completed work.

Prior to putting together a portfolio, make sure your CV is up to date. Having a current CV will allow you to identify what sections may or may not be included in the portfolio. Although a portfolio may look different from one student to another, some sections to consider include the following:

- Title page
- Table of Contents
- CV
- Personal Statement of Goals and Objectives
- Licensure or Certifications
- Experiential Rotations
    - ☐ Project Examples
    - ☐ Rotation Evaluations
- Teaching Experiences
- Research Experiences
- Recognition and Awards
- References

After putting together a portfolio, you should receive feedback from various preceptors and mentors. You will likely receive several different opinions, and it is up to you to ultimately decide what will suit you best. After receiving feedback and making the appropriate adjustments, it is time to showcase the portfolio during postgraduate training or job interviews. Some sites may be more interested in the portfolio than others, but feel free to offer it without being pushy. Creating the portfolio will also familiarize you with the details of your work, which will be of great benefit during the interview.

LETTER OF INTENT

A letter of intent for a job, residency, or other position should represent a thoughtful reflection of how your experiences, strengths, and goals match up with the position of interest. A general structure for letters of intent may be recommended and the same letter will likely suit several different positions, but each position may require you to highlight a different section of the letter. Therefore, it is very important to avoid drafting one letter and simply changing the position information. In general, the letter of intent should begin with a paragraph that briefly introduces you, why you are interested in the position, and how you learned about the position. The body of the letter speaks to your experiences, your strengths, and why you should be offered the position or interview. Within this section of the letter, it is important to have a balance between showcasing strengths and the appearance of bragging. Lastly, the concluding paragraph succinctly reiterates your interest in the program.

CASE QUESTION

What items should D.W. consider highlighting in his letter of intent?

In general, the more specific you can be regarding the position, the better. For example, give specific examples of why you are interested in the program instead of broad generalities. For the example of D.W., it would be important for him to identify that the residency site offers rotations in critical care as well as a PGY2 in critical care. Therefore, the program aligns with his long-term goal of obtaining a position as a critical care specialist. This shows that the candidate has done his research on the program and put sincere thought into why that program may be a good fit. In addition, if the program has a long track record of successful research projects and emphasizes this experience during the residency, it would benefit D.W. to speak to his research experiences during pharmacy school in his letter of intent. A sample letter of intent can be found in **Figure 15-1**.

QUICK TIP

A letter of intent can be used as an easy screening tool for an employer. Therefore, this letter should not be taken lightly. Minor grammatical errors and not following instructions may be an easy way for a program to decide to throw the application into the "do not interview" pile.

INTERVIEW SKILLS

Although the interview process may appear daunting, it should be viewed as a chance to showcase your strengths and experiences. Having the ability to effectively communicate, especially within interdisciplinary teams, is a skill that will be evaluated seriously. Therefore, finding ways to overcome your nerves is essential to give you a chance to hit a homerun on the interview (in other words: practice, practice, practice!). Having a good CV is important, but if you are not able to communicate your experi-

Figure 15-1. Example of a Letter of Intent

LETTER OF INTENT

Student Name
Address
City, State, Zip

Date

Program Director
Program
Address
City, State, Zip

Dear _____:

I am writing this letter to express my interest in the PGY1/PGY2 Masters in Healthcare Administration program at Hilbert Health-System. After speaking with several of the residents at the American Society of Health-System Pharmacists (ASHP) Midyear Clinical Meeting, I firmly believe that this program incorporates many components that will prepare me to achieve my long-term goal of obtaining a leadership position in an integrated health system.

Throughout my academic career at Schuyler University, I have been actively involved. Understanding that I was entering a new program, the opportunity for change was always engrained by my faculty, mentors, and preceptors. I have pioneered several new organizations and led many projects that not only have made a positive impact on the institution and the student body but also have improved my ability to practice pharmacy. In developing several organizations and projects from their infancy, I have been an integral part of the planning, execution, assessment, and evaluation processes. For example, I was responsible for establishing the Schuyler chapter of the Student Society of Health-System Pharmacists (SSHP). I have also been highly involved in interprofessional activities throughout my academic career, and my involvement in the Institute for Healthcare Improvement (IHI) has allowed me to be influential in implementing several quality improvement and patient safety projects in a health system.

As an advocate of change, I am involved in the Pharmacy Practice Model Initiative (PPMI) at my university as well as at my place of employment. One of my career goals is to allow pharmacists to move away from distributive functions to nondistributive, direct patient care roles that will allow patients to have highly individualized and exceptional pharmaceutical care. As professional development chair of the Schuyler SSHP chapter, I was instrumental in organizing Health-System Pharmacy Week and am currently establishing programming for a PPMI week during the spring of 2012.

In summary, this program is directly aligned with my career goals. Upon completion of this residency, I will have the tools necessary to build a strong foundation in health system management. As a resident at your institution, I can assure you that I will work hard to have a positive impact on patient care.

Thank you for your time and consideration.

Sincerely,

ences effectively, their effect will be diminished. As you begin the interview process, some things to keep in mind include the following:

- **Research.** Knowing what a position or program is all about is essential during the interview process and will allow for meaningful conversations throughout the process. For D.W., if he knows that the program has a track record of graduating residents that go on to shared faculty positions at a college of pharmacy, this will allow him to talk specifically about experiences that may be attractive to the program. Doing adequate research will enable you to have thoughtful questions ready when you are asked the expected question, "What questions do you have for us?"

- **Practice, practice, practice.** As nerves kick in during the interview, it can be comforting to the candidate to rely on practiced responses. For example, sitting down with a peer to ask each other mock interview questions will allow you to be prepared for tough questions in advance. In addition, you should spend time studying your CV. This will allow you to know your experiences well and fall back on those experiences during a jam in the interview.

- **Plan for a meal (and mealtime etiquette).** During the interview, a meal may or may not be offered. Therefore, it is important to be prepared for this part of the interview and to brush up on mealtime etiquette. Many sites will use the meal to put you in a more relaxed setting in hopes of getting a glimpse of "less-rehearsed" responses.

- **Group versus individual.** Although individual interviews are most common, a group interview is not out of the question. Therefore, you should determine what type of interview will be encountered and prepare accordingly. If you find yourself in a group interview, you should be prepared to be assertive enough to stand out from the other candidates while not appearing to be overbearing. Again, practice makes perfect. Even if a group interview is not on the schedule, other group interactions (such as meals) may be present.

- **Presentation or cases?** Several residency and fellowship programs are now requesting that candidates deliver a live presentation or complete a case on-site during the interview. Knowing this in advance is essential to being prepared and avoiding unnecessary anxiety on the interview day.

QUICK TIP

The interview is your time to shine. For many residency programs, grade point averages and other factors will take a back seat when the interview occurs. Therefore, adequate time and practice should be spent in this area.

POSTGRADUATE TRAINING OPTIONS

Residencies, Fellowships, Masters Programs, and More!

On completing the doctor of pharmacy curriculum, you have the option of completing additional training, such as a residency, fellowship, or doctoral programs. You should spend adequate time researching these programs and speaking to current participants to determine if they are appropriate options to pursue. The decision to pursue postgraduate training is an individual one. Family situations, career aspirations, and other factors will determine if you pursue additional training. Talking with peers, practitioners, and faculty helps to work through the thought process.

Because residency programs are the most common postgraduate training option pursued by pharmacy students, they will be discussed in detail below. Fellowships are typically 1 or more years of advanced education and training in a specific area of interest that has a heavy research component. Additional options include master's degrees (e.g., MPH, MBA), doctorate degrees, and law degrees, among others.

Postgraduate Year One and Postgraduate Year Two Residencies

Residency training is the most common form of postgraduate training in the United States. Approximately 30% of graduates applied for and 20% of graduates obtained a residency in 2012. In recent years, two prominent pharmacy organizations, the American College of Clinical Pharmacy (ACCP) and ASHP, have released a shared vision for postgraduate residency training as a prerequisite for direct patient care. This, among other factors, such as the rapid expansion of pharmacy schools in the United States contributing to a more competitive job market, has resulted in a significant rise in the number of students pursuing residency training. However, the site development to accommodate the increase in applicants has not kept pace, and there is a significant shortage of available sites in relation to the number of applicants. At the conclusion of the 2012 residency match process, over 1,400 pharmacy graduates (39% of residency applicants) remained unmatched to residency programs.

Residency training is divided into the PGY1 and PGY2 categories, with a PGY1 serving as a prerequisite for completing a PGY2. Accreditation for these programs is provided by ASHP. The accreditation standards for both PGY1 and PGY2 residencies have specific outcomes, goals, and objectives that are important for the resident to achieve through various experiences defined by the site.

PGY1 residencies are yearlong intensive training programs that primarily focus on developing and enhancing practice knowledge and skills. Most PGY1 programs take place in a hospital or health system where the resident is exposed to several inpatient pharmacy services. However, a smaller percentage of residency programs place the resident in a community, ambulatory, or managed care setting. The PGY1 is completed under the guidance of qualified preceptors and is most often geared toward gaining a wide variety of experiences. For example, a health-system resident may participate in practice experiences in the areas of internal medicine, critical care, pediatrics, and so on. Generally, 1 year of residency training is equated to approximately 2 to 3 years of professional practice. In addition to the practice component, PGY1 residents will be expected to develop leadership skills, participate in education and training (e.g., precepting or teaching certificate programs), develop project management skills, and engage in research.

In contrast, PGY2 residencies are yearlong intensive training programs that allow the resident to specialize in one area, such as cardiology, pediatrics, or ambulatory care. This year of training is intended to allow the practitioner to begin focusing on one area to develop an expertise for that specialty.

PGY1 Programs: Pharmacy, Community Care, Managed Care

A PGY1 residency can fall under one of three categories: pharmacy, community care, or managed care. As previously mentioned, the focus of the PGY1 health-system residency is to expose the resident to several different experiences. Most often, this occurs by having the resident participate in a rotational sequence. For example, the resident may have six required rotations (such as internal medicine, intensive care, family medicine, and others). In addition, the resident may have a couple of months available for electives that can be tailored to the resident's areas of interest.

In contrast to general pharmacy residencies, community residencies are relatively new. In 1986, community pharmacy residency programs (CPRPs) were established by the American Pharmacists Association (APhA) to formalize residency training in community pharmacy practice. Thirteen years later, APhA and ASHP partnered to accredit CPRPs. As of July 2012, there were 92 PGY1 CPRPs employing more than 150 residents, with the practice site most commonly being a chain, supermarket, independent, or health system pharmacy. A large number of the programs are affiliated with colleges of pharmacy and include a significant teaching component. Community residencies are most often longitudinal in nature, allowing the resident to have several experiences over the course of the year rather than for one month at a time. Community pharmacy residencies focus heavily on the process of developing patient care services. For example, the resident may be charged with developing an immunization or medication therapy management service.

Managed care residencies are also relatively new compared to health-system residencies. In its simplest form, managed care focuses on delivering healthcare services in a way that efficiently uses resources to achieve optimal patient care. Although the outcomes established for a PGY1 resident in managed care mirror some of the outcomes of the general pharmacy residency, there are some unique outcomes specific to managed care. For example, managed care residents may participate in conducting medication therapy management services, conducting drug utilization reviews, and designing benefit structures, such as a formulary. Most managed care residencies take place within health plans, pharmacy benefit managers, and health maintenance organizations that may or may not be affiliated with a college of pharmacy. Students interested in learning more about managed care residencies should download *The Student Pharmacist's Guide to Managed Care Pharmacy Residency Programs* available at http://www.amcp.org/WorkArea/DownloadAsset.aspx?id=9567.

Factors to Consider When Choosing a Residency

Choosing a residency program can be overwhelming. Therefore, it is important to consider and prioritize several factors when considering programs. Although not all-inclusive, the following questions should be considered when evaluating a residency program:

- *Is the program accredited?* If not, what is the program's plan for obtaining accreditation?
- *What is the reputation of the program locally and nationally?* What do the faculty, preceptors, and current residents have to say about the program?
- *How many residents per year does the program have?* You should consider whether you would work better in a small or large residency class.
- *What type of rotations will be offered during the residency?* In addition, what type of flexibility is there with elective rotations? For example, is a resident allowed to change a rotation later in the year if he or she identifies a practice area of interest and accepts a job in that area?
- *What types of precepting opportunities are available?* How many student-months are expected of the resident, and is there flexibility to take more, if interested? How soon will the resident be expected to take students? What type of preceptor training is available?
- *What is the patient population like?* Does this match your practice areas of interest?
- *What is the staffing component for the residency (e.g., every other weekend versus every third weekend)?* What are the on-call requirements? Are there opportunities to staff for additional pay if the resident chooses to do so?
- *Is a teaching component offered?* Is there a teaching certificate program associated with the residency? If yes, what are the requirements of the program, and how many hours will the resident be expected to teach? Will there be both large-group and small-group opportunities available?
- *What is the culture of the institution?*
- *What are the residents who completed the program doing now?*

- *What is the history of the residency research projects?* How many have been published or presented? What type of research support or mentorship is available for the resident?

If you are interested in a PGY2 program, you may explore various PGY1 programs based on the availability of PGY2 programs at the same site. Although this strategy may be effective, basing your selection of a PGY1 site primarily on the availability of PGY2s is not recommended. You should base your selection on the factors previously described, and one of those factors may be the availability of PGY2 programs. If you select a PGY1 program with the hopes of also completing a PGY2 program at that site, you should be aware of the early commitment process. This process is an agreement made in December of the PGY1 year between the resident and the site, allowing both parties to forego the match process. Although this may be beneficial for some, caution should be exercised, considering that you will be only a few months into your clinical rotations when required to make the decision.

QUICK TIP

As you are considering many different residency programs, the process can become overwhelming. Therefore, you should consider developing a spreadsheet or other type of tracking system to allow for an efficient search process. The spreadsheet should contain some of the factors mentioned above (e.g., number of coresidents, type of institution) to allow you to organize and prioritize the search process, including time spent at the ASHP Midyear Meeting and Personnel Placement Services.

The Match

As residency opportunities continue to become increasingly competitive, the match process, coordinated by the National Matching Service (http://www.natmatch.com/), has received a great deal of attention and should be closely studied. In short, this is an orderly process that matches residency applicants with residency sites based on their respective rank lists. For example, after D.W. completes five residency interviews, he decides that he is interested in four of the sites and will now rank the sites from one to four, with number one being the site in which he is most interested. The sites will then do the same and the match program will sync up the two lists. The match is only for ASHP-accredited or ASHP-eligible programs (e.g., precandidate or candidate status). Therefore, programs that have not applied for precandidate or candidate status will not show up in the match process. It is important to emphasize that you should rank only sites in which you are truly interested. Results of the match signify a contractual agreement between the applicant and the site and are legally binding.

The Scramble

The scramble process works to bring together unmatched residents and programs with available positions. Following the match results, the National Matching Service provides a list of unfilled positions to applicants and programs. This open process occurs instantly after the match results are released, and, therefore, you should be prepared to jump in right away. Considering the competitive nature of the residency market, waiting around may cost you a position. Because the scramble process happens quickly, it is important to plan for this option in advance. For example, before match day it would be helpful to have a conversation with family members about their willingness to move to another city or state. Having a faculty mentor or support from the college or university during this time can also invaluable. Faculty members may be familiar with other programs (or individuals at those programs) and may get conversations started during the scramble process. Because this day is so hectic, you may consider taking time off from your rotation site, if possible, to navigate this process.

Utilizing Personnel Placement Services

Personnel Placement Services (PPS) coordinates employers and applicants for on-site interviews at the ASHP Midyear Clinical Meeting. PPS includes interviews for a variety of positions, including pharmacist positions, fellowships, and PGY1 and PGY2 residencies. Depending on the year, site participation may vary; therefore, you should identify who is participating in PPS before registering. PPS typically allows you to have approximately 30 minutes to sit down face to face with program representatives. Some programs use PPS as an interview or screening tool, whereas others use it for informational purposes. You should be prepared for both situations. PPS requires a separate registration fee. More information about PPS can be found at http://www.careerpharm.com/basicppsinfo.aspx.

Timeline for Residency Search

Establishing a timeline for a residency search is important due to the number of factors that need to be considered throughout the year. An example of a timeline for the residency search can be found in **Figure 15-2**. It is important to start early. In addition, while shooting for a matched position, it is essential to consider an alternative plan. For example, you should consider whether or not you are willing to move to a different area if a position in the scramble is available. Thinking in advance about an alternative plan will allow for a quicker turnaround in securing a job or different residency position.

CASE QUESTION

Considering D.W. is just starting his APPE rotations, what should be the primary focus of his residency search process?

FINDING WORK-LIFE BALANCE

As you begin your career, the inevitable topic of work-life balance will come up. It takes work to achieve work-life balance, although this balance looks different for each pharmacist. It should be viewed on a spectrum that, for some, may look like a 50-50 split but, for others, is shifted in one direction or another. Family situations, job satisfaction, and enjoying time (or lack thereof) with coworkers are just a few factors that may determine where the balance point lies. For many starting a career, it is a goal to achieve some work-life balance. However, it can be difficult to know what that means if it has not been modeled by others. Therefore, it is very important to observe mentors and preceptors in this area. Finding out what allows them to achieve a balance and how they have made it a priority can be very helpful.

Transitioning from student to practitioner likely means you will no longer have those long fall, winter, spring, and summer breaks. Vacation time provided by employers varies. You may assume that more vacation time makes a given position sound attractive when applying to jobs, but the real question is whether the employer will encourage the employee to take the time or whether the employee will feel pressured to work through it. If vacation time is a top priority for you to avoid burnout, finding a position that will encourage and support this is important.

Working toward a work-life balance also involves setting aside time for hobbies and passions outside of work. It is important to identify one or two of these hobbies and allocate time accordingly. Whether it is time with family, a hobby, or volunteer work, it will take effort and work to create adequate time. Investments in those activities are likely what have gotten you to this point, making you a well-rounded individual. Therefore, maintaining these activities will only make you a stronger employee on the job. Pharmacy is fun, but pharmacy is not everything. Although achieving work-life balance can be

Figure 15-2. Example of a Residency Search Timeline

RESIDENCY SEARCH TIMELINE

Pharmacy School

- Identify areas of interest through experiential rotations and internships
- Identify geographical areas of interest to complete a residency
- Participate in shadowing opportunities for areas of interest
- Review the residency information on the ASHP website (www.ashp.org)
- Build a CV and conduct a gap analysis to identify areas where further work is needed
- Plan final-year rotations considering sites of interest

Summer Before Final Professional Year

- Formalize the CV and continue to update
- Identify gaps in the CV and seek out opportunities during rotations to fill those gaps
- Determine (and make plans for) the meetings to attend to learn more about programs of interest (e.g., ASHP and local showcases)

Fall (September–November) of Final Professional Year

- Register for the matching program (http://www.natmatch.com/ashprmp/)
- Identify and secure writers for letters of recommendation
- Participate in mock interviews
- Research the programs attending the ASHP Midyear Clinical Meeting (booth locations and times)
- Develop questions to ask programs during local showcases or the ASHP Midyear Clinical Meeting
- Develop an "elevator speech" to use during encounters at showcases or the ASHP Midyear Clinical Meeting

Winter (December–January) of Final Professional Year

- Attend the ASHP Midyear Clinical Meeting
- Send thank-you notes after the ASHP meeting
- Review application requirements for programs of interest
- Draft letters of intent
- Submit requests for transcripts
- Submit applications (usually due in early January)
- Attend on-site interviews (usually end of January into February or March)
- Write thank-you notes after interviews
- Develop rank list
- Match day! (Mid-to-late March)

work, stressing over it will defeat the purpose. However, be aware of it. Discuss it with family, friends, and coworkers to identify the desired level of balance and set goals to achieve that balance.

Suggested Reading

Askew JP. *From Student to Pharmacist: Making the Transition*. Washington, DC: American Pharmacists Association; 2010.

Crouch MA, ed. *Securing and Excelling in a Pharmacy Residency*. Burlington, MA: Jones & Bartlett Learning; 2013.

Murphy JE, ed. *Resident Survival Guide*. Lenexa, KS: American College of Clinical Pharmacy; 2011.

Reinders TP. *The Pharmacy Professional's Guide to Resumes, CVs, & Interviewing*. 3rd ed. Washington, DC: American Pharmacists Association; 2011.

STAYING INFORMED

Steven R. Smith, MS, RPh, BCACP

CASE

R.L. is a newly graduated pharmacist. Since finishing his APPE rotations, he is worried about maintaining all of the knowledge he has gained. After attending some continuing pharmacy education (CPE) presentations, he feels that the content was not really as helpful as he had hoped.

Why It's Essential

••

"A pharmacist maintains professional competence."—Code of Ethics for Pharmacists, APhA[1]

••

••

"I just got done with 6 years of pharmacy school. Why do I have to keep learning?"—Student

••

Keeping up with new pharmacy knowledge is essential to offering the best care to patients. The Food and Drug Administration (FDA) approved an average of 23.5 new molecular entities each year over the past 6 years. In addition to approving new agents, the FDA approves generic medications and adds new formulations, indications, adverse reactions, and black-box warnings to product package inserts more often than can be counted. At the same time, keeping up with changes to state and federal laws is vital to practicing pharmacy safely. While you must stay current on laws that apply directly to pharmacists and pharmacy technicians, you must also keep up on laws that pertain to physicians, nurses, physician assistants, advance practice nurses, and all other healthcare professionals if the laws have implications on the drug use process. To add to the challenge, advances in diagnostic testing and medical treatments are ever present, published by many healthcare professional organizations and government agencies each year. Thus, becoming a pharmacist is a commitment to lifelong learning through continuing professional development.[2]

QUICK TIP

Laws and regulations are always changing. In Ohio, for example, one-fifth of State Board of Pharmacy regulations are reviewed each year and are modified, removed, or replaced with new regulations written to keep current with the practice of pharmacy.

Lifelong Learning and Continuing Pharmacy Education

CPE required to maintain your license is a small part of what it takes to maintain competence to practice pharmacy. Competence encompasses knowledge, skills, attributes, behaviors, and attitudes. You must incorporate these competencies into the activities of your professional practice. Although it is the responsibility of the provider of CPE to ensure the quality of the program, it is the responsibility of each pharmacist to seek knowledge, build skills, and achieve the competence necessary for your pharmacy practice. Each pharmacist must select CPE programs and other activities to enhance the quality of care being provided to patients in his or her practice setting. Accreditation Council for Pharmacy Education (ACPE) states that, as a pharmacist or pharmacy technician, you should[3]

- Identify your individual educational needs

- Pursue educational activities that will produce and sustain more effective professional practice to improve practice, patient, and population healthcare outcomes

- Link learned or acquired knowledge, skills, and attitudes to opportunities for application in practice

- Continue self-directed learning throughout the progression of your career

CASE QUESTION

R.L. feels that he is particularly weak in his ability to precept pharmacy students effectively, but his counseling skills are quite sharp. What kinds of CPE activities should R.L. focus on at this time?

Reporting CPE

Each state sets the requirements for licensure for pharmacists. Both the number of contact hours of CPE and the frequency of reporting vary from state to state. The best source to get this information, as well as the process of reporting, is the state board of pharmacy website for the state in which you will be licensed.

In 2011, a system for tracking and reporting CPE, called the CPE Monitor, was developed as a collaborative effort of ACPE and the National Association of Boards of Pharmacy (NABP). The system authenticates and stores completed CPE units for pharmacists and pharmacy technicians from ACPE-accredited providers. Pharmacists and pharmacy technicians should register and obtain an e-Profile ID from www.MyCPEmonitor.net. CPE providers will request your ID and will enter the Universal Activity Number, a unique number assigned to the CPE program you attended. This will be verified by ACPE and linked to NABP, making it possible for boards of pharmacy to download your CPE log for license renewal.[4]

CASE QUESTION

R.L. is unsure about the requirements for CPE in his state. Where can he go to find out how many continuing education units (CEUs) are required to renew his license?

QUICK TIP

Some states require you to obtain a certain number of CPE credits from live programs, whereas other states require CPE on law, human immunodeficiency virus (HIV), or other specific categories.

Identifying Quality CPE

What are the characteristics of a quality CPE program? From the ACPE guide for providers of CPE, a quality CPE program is a structured activity that promotes problem solving skills and critical thinking. Programs should be developed based on a needs assessment of practicing pharmacists and be designed to increase knowledge and skills to enhance your practice. It must be planned independent of commercial interest or bias with specific and measurable objectives to be accomplished during the program. Too often, objectives and content of the program are left to the speaker. However, developers of a quality CPE should communicate desired goals and objectives, information about the intended audience and the expectation for active audience participation and assessment to the presenters. Educational materials should enhance learning rather than just be a copy of the speaker's slides. Finally, a quality CPE must allow for evaluation of the program and achievement of the program goals and objectives. Just because a CPE program is free does not mean you should accept anything less than the quality as defined by ACPE.[5]

The advantage of ACPE-approved CPE is that all states accept these credits toward relicensure. For those licensed in more than one state, ACPE credit can be used for relicensure in each state. Some states also approve providers of CPE. This CPE is usually only accepted toward relicensure by the state that approved the provider.

· ·

"No one really ever talked about the best way to go about getting CPE."
—Student

· ·

Formats and Sources of CPE

CPE is available as

- Live programs such as organization meetings, teleconferences, webinars, and dinners
- Printed programs such as journals, newsletters, and monographs
- Digital programs in e-journals, webinars, and e-mails

Live programs have the advantage that participants are able to interact with the program faculty. Local, state, and national pharmacy organization meetings are a common source of live CPE. Local organization meetings are typically held monthly, often as a dinner meeting. State organization meetings may be held once or twice a year, are held in a convention center venue, and last 2 or more days. National pharmacy organizations also hold one or two meetings per year in a city with convention facilities to handle the large numbers of attendees. Although more costly to attend, state and national meetings offer more contact hours of CPE during the course of the meeting and may offer application-based programming leading to certificates.

Many journals are delivered to your home and some are moving to digital versions via the Internet. Professional journals, whether in a hardcopy or digital format, are part of the membership in many professional organizations. Some of these journals offer CPE with a separate CPE subscription fee or a per-CPE processing fee. In all cases, CPE from articles or monographs is contingent on passing a post-test. Printed formats offer the convenience of completing programs whenever and wherever you would like. Internet and digital formats are also convenient and can be timely, with a short publication cycle.

QUICK TIP

Be careful to avoid biased CPE presentations. A skewed presentation can provide only one side of a story and negatively impacts patient care.

CERTIFICATIONS

Certification is another voluntary step for pharmacists to increase their knowledge and skills in a particular practice area while earning recognition. Currently, three main bodies offer pharmacy-specific certifications: the Board of Pharmaceutical Specialties (BPS), American Pharmacists Association (APhA), and Commission for Certification in Geriatric Pharmacy. Other certifications exist but are utilized to a much lesser extent among pharmacists.

The BPS tests and recognizes six practice areas. Requirements to sit for the tests are based on years of experience as a licensed pharmacist and residency training.[6]

BPS areas include the following:

- Ambulatory Care Pharmacy
- Nuclear Pharmacy
- Nutrition Support Pharmacy
- Oncology Pharmacy
- Pharmacotherapy (with the option of including added qualifications in Cardiology and Infectious Disease)
- Psychiatric Pharmacy

APhA offers structured programs as a means to gain knowledge and skills in three specific areas. These programs are available to all licensed pharmacists.[7]

APhA certificate training programs include the following:

- Pharmacy-Based Immunization Delivery (self-study, live courses, final examination, live technique assessment)
- Pharmaceutical Care for Patients with Diabetes (self-study, online activities and case studies, live interactive seminar, final examination)
- Delivering Medication Therapy Management Services in the Community (self-study, live seminar, postseminar exercise)

More information about APhA certifications can be found at http://www.pharmacist.com/Content/NavigationMenu3/ContinuingEducation/CertificateTrainingProgram/CTP.htm.

The American Society of Consultant Pharmacists (ASCP) created the Commission for Certification in Geriatric Pharmacy to oversee an exam-based certification available to any pharmacist licensed for at least 2 years. It demonstrates knowledge in medication therapy management issues common to older patients.[8] Pharmacists that pass the examination earn the title of Certified Geriatric Pharmacist (CGP).

PROFESSIONAL ORGANIZATIONS

How do you select a pharmacy organization to join? Joining and being active in state and national pharmacy organizations allows you to

- Support efforts to monitor and influence the political and legislative arenas that impact pharmacy practice
- Support efforts for the voice of pharmacy to be heard regarding healthcare policies in the United States
- Keep current with healthcare accrediting bodies' standards
- Influence and support efforts to advance the practice of pharmacy
- Network with pharmacists throughout your state, across the United States, and internationally
- Obtain quality CPE

Table 16-1 lists several national pharmacy organizations. When selecting which organizations(s) to join, think first of your practice setting. Look at the mission of each organization to see if it matches your needs. Because it is nearly impossible for an individual to track everything going on in Washington, DC, you may think of your membership as an insurance policy for our profession. These organizations are more likely to have the resources to act on our behalf on a national level. Ask what the organization is doing to influence federal laws that may affect pharmacy, the drug use system, the drug approval process, and the role of pharmacy in the healthcare system. Is the organization active politically to get pharmacy's message to legislators? Is the organization working with other national pharmacy organizations to send one message for all of pharmacy? Other benefits of national organizations include quality CPE, networking, and access to activities to advance your practice. If you enjoy organizational work, there is a great need for volunteers to work on the organization's missions. It is extremely satisfying to work on a committee of pharmacists from across the country on a project that moves the profession forward.

Many of the reasons to join and volunteer for a state-level pharmacy organization are the same as at the national level. State organizations offer quality CPE, legislative oversight at the state level, and networking closer to home. Laws at the state level have a more direct impact on your practice, and it is through these organizations that you can have a voice. State-level organizations may also be more visible to citizens in your state as a resource for public health issues, a resource for the media to gain objective information on medications, and, through service projects, a resource to improve understanding of medications.

Local pharmacy organizations may offer CPE via monthly meetings, create speaker's bureaus for other local organizations, and provide networking and public service opportunities, such as health screenings and medication brown bags. Members who are active at the state and national level can share information on activities and issues for discussion at the local level, creating a clearing house for information from the state and national pharmacy organizations. Local pharmacy organizations are dependent on volunteers to run for offices, coordinate CPE activities, and run community service projects. Volunteering is a great source of satisfaction, fosters career development, and helps pharmacists give back to their profession.

CASE QUESTION

R.L.'s first position as a pharmacist is in a nursing home, working as a consultant. Which pharmacy organization would be the best fit for him to join? What certification should he consider pursuing?

Table 16-1. Selected National Pharmacy Organizations

ORGANIZATION	WEBSITE	STUDENT MEMBERSHIP
Academy of Managed Care Pharmacy	www.amcp.org	$35
American Association of Pharmaceutical Scientists	www.aaps.org	MS and PhD students: $40
American College of Apothecaries	www.acainfo.org	$20
American College of Clinical Pharmacy	www.accp.com	$35
American Pharmacist Association - Practitioners: APhA-APPM - Scientists: APhA-APRS - Students: APhA-ASP	www.pharmacist.com	$40
American Society for Clinical Pharmacology & Therapeutics	www.ascpt.org	$55
American Society for Parenteral and Enteral Nutrition	www.nutritioncare.org	$45
American Society for Pharmacy Law	www.aspl.org	$40
American Society of Consultant Pharmacists	www.ascp.com	E-membership is free
American Society of Health-System Pharmacists	www.ashp.org	SSHP: $42
College of Psychiatric & Neurologic Pharmacists	www.cpnp.org	$20
Hematology Oncology Pharmacist Association	www.hoparx.org	$30
International Pharmaceutical Federation	www.fip.org	$47
National Community Pharmacists Association	www.ncpanet.org	$35
National Home Infusion Association	www.nhia.org	$50
National Pharmaceutical Association	www.npha.net www.snapha.net	$35
Pediatric Pharmacy Advocacy Group	www.ppag.org	$40
Society of Critical Care Medicine	www.sccm.org	$30

Conclusion

Pharmacy, like other healthcare professions, requires lifelong learning for us to give the best care to our patients. A subset of this learning plan is obtaining CPE to meet legal requirements to maintain licensure. Selecting quality CPE programs will aid you in maintaining your competencies and gaining new skills needed for a successful pharmacy career. Pharmacy organizations, national, state, and local, are a source of CPE and provide opportunities to serve our profession. In addition, our organizations help advance pharmacy practice, expand our role in the healthcare system, and increase recognition of our ability to ensure safe medication use.

References

1. American Pharmacists Association. Code of ethics for pharmacists. http://www.pharmacist.com/code-ethics. Accessed October 15, 2012.

2. Accreditation Council for Pharmacy Education. Continuing professional development. http://www.acpe-accredit.org/ceproviders/CPD.asp. Accessed October 15, 2012.

3. Accreditation Council for Pharmacy Education. Definition of continuing education for the practice of pharmacy. http://www.acpe-accredit.org/pdf/CE_Definition_Pharmacy_Final_1006-2007.pdf. Accessed October 15, 2012.

4. National Association of Boards of Pharmacy. CPE monitor service. http://www.nabp.net/programs/cpe-monitor/cpe-monitor-service/. Accessed October 15, 2012.

5. Accreditation Council for Pharmacy Education. Accreditation standards for continuing pharmacy education. http://www.acpe-accredit.org/ceproviders/standards.asp. Accessed October 15, 2012.

6. Board of Pharmaceutical Specialties. http://www.bpsweb.org. Accessed February 16, 2012.

7. American Pharmacists Association. Certificate training programs. www.pharmacist.com/apha-certificate-training-programs. Accessed February 16, 2012.

8. Commission for Certification in Geriatric Pharmacy. http://www.ccgp.org/. Accessed February 16, 2012.

Suggested Reading

ACCP White Paper. Clinical pharmacist competencies. *Pharmacotherapy*. 2008;28:806-815.

American Pharmacists Association. The pharmacist's continuing education resource. http://apha.imirus.com/pdf/2008/Dec_CE_resources.pdf. Accessed February 16, 2012.

Council on Credentialing in Pharmacy. Scope of contemporary pharmacy practice: Roles, responsibilities, and functions of pharmacists and pharmacy technicians. http://www.pharmacycredentialing.org/Contemporary_Pharmacy_Practice.pdf. Accessed February 16, 2012.

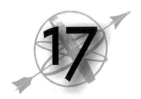

Giving Back: Becoming a Preceptor

Mate M. Soric, PharmD, BCPS

CASE

T.H. is a newly licensed pharmacist with an interest in teaching pharmacy students. He practices in a busy community pharmacy and has taken on the responsibility of building the store's medication therapy management services. With all of his new responsibility, he is nervous about how he can spend enough time with the students to provide a worthwhile learning experience.

Why It's Essential

The experiential education that is required of all pharmacy students represents a great opportunity to learn what it takes to become an effective pharmacy practitioner. By putting into practice the didactic knowledge obtained in pharmacy school, experiential education reinforces core competencies and allows students to bear the fruit of their hard work in the curriculum by improving patient satisfaction and outcomes. Unfortunately, the experiential system also represents a complicated challenge to institutions everywhere. To preserve this vital proving ground for future pharmacists, a steady stream of pharmacists must be willing to sacrifice their own time and effort to become preceptors. Making this hurdle even more difficult to overcome, the number of students that require experiential education has never been higher. Identifying, recruiting, training, and assessing pharmacy preceptors is a daunting responsibility that requires the dedication and perseverance of numerous experiential program directors and the generosity of pharmacy practitioners.

There are many reasons for becoming a preceptor. Some pharmacists feel that precepting students provides greater job satisfaction. Others feel that the simple act of teaching is a sure-fire way to maintain their own knowledge base through repetition and review of common topics. Still others choose preceptorship as a means to expand the services that they can offer and the number of patients they can reach. Regardless of the reasons it is chosen, becoming a preceptor can be considered a professional duty as it maintains the supply of well-trained pharmacists for future generations. Those that donate their energy to the cause can be certain that they will have a positive impact on their patients and their profession.

CASE QUESTION

What are some of the benefits that T.H. can reap by precepting pharmacy students in his practice? What are the benefits to the pharmacy profession?

The transition from student to preceptor often can be difficult. Many feel as though their didactic education never provided the necessary building blocks to design, implement, and assess a learning experience for pharmacy students. This chapter serves as a starting point for new pharmacists wishing to give back and will help pharmacy students understand the preparation and time commitment of their preceptors.

DESIGNING A ROTATION

The design of a rotation begins by identifying potential learning experiences. To aid in the identification of these experiences, colleges and schools of pharmacy tend to outline specific goals for their students. These goals are an excellent starting point when designing a rotation. Matching learning experiences to the goals they will address can give structure and meaning to an otherwise unorganized collection of tasks.

QUICK TIP

If the college of pharmacy does not provide goals to help structure the rotation, the evaluation rubrics used to assess students may serve a similar purpose.

Many potential preceptors spend a great deal of time trying to identify learning experiences that they deem "acceptable" for student participation. In general, however, most of the daily activities of a pharmacist can be of some value. Tasks that might seem dull and uninteresting to the typical pharmacist, such as meeting attendance, monograph write-ups, or scheduling, all require skills that must be taught to students. The key is incorporating a wide variety of experiences that allow students to appreciate the role of the pharmacist at the practice site while providing the preceptor with opportunities to assess student progress.

An objective look at one's daily schedule will allow potential preceptors to put together a rough outline of the dates and times that the students will be involved directly with the preceptor. Depending on the schedule and practice setting, the amount of time spent with students will vary. Many preceptors identify other individuals within their practice who can serve as secondary preceptors. These individuals may be pharmacists, technicians, or other healthcare providers who can provide additional experiences to students. Although the use of secondary preceptors should be minimized, an alternative point of view can be a refreshing change of pace that brings additional value to the learning experience.

CASE QUESTION

What kinds of secondary preceptors might be available to T.H. and his pharmacy students?

To fill any remaining gaps in the rotation, students may be given assignments to complete on their own time, both on-site when a preceptor is unavailable and as homework. Common assignments include journal clubs, case presentations, new drug updates, formulary monographs, and drug information questions. These assignments should be used not only as learning opportunities for students but also as ways to improve pharmacy practice for the site. Assignments should be chosen that apply to the preceptor's practice. When presentations are given, continuing education credits can be offered to other healthcare providers who attend. When true clinical controversies are identified, students can perform literature searches in an attempt to establish institutional practices. Students can be used as catalysts for change in formulary management, as cost-saving initiatives, or as the extra help needed to get a new service off the ground.

CASE QUESTION

T.H. has been tasked with establishing a new medication therapy management service for his pharmacy. In addition to the daily tasks already scheduled, how can T.H. utilize his students to build the new service?

The last component of the student schedule is the time dedicated to feedback and assessment. It is vital that students receive timely, specific feedback to improve their pharmacy practice skills. Ideally, informal feedback can be given on a daily basis. Realistically, however, this may be difficult to achieve. For this reason, preceptors should set aside some time each week to discuss student progress toward rotation goals. Although midpoint evaluations are often optional, a formal assessment midway through the rotation should also be scheduled, especially when students are not performing as expected.

WRITING A SYLLABUS

Most students find a written syllabus to be very helpful when beginning a rotation. These documents contain important information about logistical issues (parking, lockers, start times), materials to review prior to starting the rotation, and the types of activities that will make up the bulk of the rotation. Providing the students with a written syllabus before they arrive for the first day of the rotation will give them ample time to review the details contained within and be better prepared for the experience.

Contact Information

Located near the top of the document, the preceptor's name, title, and contact information should be prominently displayed. It is helpful to include a variety of methods of contact, such as e-mail, office phone, pager, and, if the preceptor is comfortable sharing it, personal or cell phone. By including various methods of contact, there is a diminished chance for missed messages and poor communication.

Logistical Concerns

The logistical issues of parking, start date, and arrival time may be addressed next. Many preceptors find it useful to include maps of their facilities to indicate ideal locations to park, preferred building entrances, and location of the desired meeting place. This section may also include a discussion of meal options for students in the area (cafeteria, local restaurants, or where to store packed lunches).

Goals and Objectives

Next, the rotation's specific goals and objectives should be clearly explained. Again, these goals may be dictated by the individual program or created by the preceptor. If supplied, they may simply be adapted from the preceptor's manual provided by the college or school of pharmacy. By including the outcomes anticipated, students have a better understanding of what to expect going into the learning experience.

Activities and Assignments

After the goals and objectives, each major activity that students will complete should be clearly described. When including activity descriptions, incorporating as much detail as possible will decrease the time spent orienting students and answering frequently asked questions. Instead of repeating yourself month after month, students can be referred back to the syllabus to obtain the required information.

Calendar

To help students understand the rotation's organization, a calendar with important dates, common activities, and assessments clearly identified may also be included in the syllabus. Regularly scheduled activities, such as rounds or topic discussions, should be included, along with intermittent activities, such as evaluations and presentations. If there are days when the preceptor will be unavailable or students will be given time off, they should also be noted on the calendar.

QUICK TIP

Many preceptors prefer an electronic calendar to a traditional paper version. As plans change and new assignments are added, all parties can collectively view and maintain the document for consistency.

Evaluation Criteria

Perhaps one of the most important components of the rotation syllabus is the evaluation criteria. In this section, preceptors outline (in very specific detail) how students will be graded. It is recommended that precise explanations of the requirements to achieve each grade be provided, especially with regard to "honors" or "A" grades. The more detailed the explanations, the less likely students will be able to contest the grades they earn.

Attendance Policy

Many colleges of pharmacy have policies established that outline the proper way to handle absences, tardiness, and days off. If these are already established, preceptors may simply adapt the policies and forms for their rotation. If they are not provided, the preceptor should create his or her own policies for how to handle these situations. Other issues that should be addressed here include inclement weather, professional activities (organization meetings and residency interviews), and emergencies.

CONDUCTING THE ROTATION

Orientation

Although the syllabus contains a wealth of information about the way the rotation will be conducted, students will still arrive requiring a certain amount of orientation to the site. Most preceptors begin orientation with a tour of the facility. Important features to point out to students include workspace for projects, the location of restrooms, and a tour of the units/floors/departments they will be frequenting over the course of the rotation. As the students are guided throughout the practice site, be sure to introduce them to the people they will be interacting with, including secretaries, other pharmacists, and the medical team.

Orientation is also the ideal time to address any requirements the Human Resource Department has for students on site. Although it will vary from site to site, students may need to complete a brief orientation session, obtain computer access, and have photographs taken for name badges. Completing these tasks in a timely manner will allow students to become autonomous more quickly, taking additional workload off of the preceptor.

After the initial tour and trip to the Human Resource Department, the syllabus should be reviewed with the students. Although it probably was supplied to students well in advance of the start date, going through each section and addressing any last-minute questions will further clarify expectations. In particular, the goals, objectives, activities, assignments, and evaluation criteria should be discussed face to face.

Each preceptor should take some time to get to know the students he or she will be precepting. Just as the preceptor's expectations are communicated to the students, it is important to learn and understand the student's expectation of the rotation. Discussions of the student's past rotations, strengths, weaknesses, and career goals can help the preceptor tailor the learning experience to better match student expectations. Possible areas for customization include assignment topics, secondary preceptors the student will shadow, duration of orientation, and degree of preceptor involvement in patient care. For students with little to no experience, longer orientation, more preceptor involvement, and extra guidance will be required compared to those familiar with the practice setting.

The Roles of the Preceptor

Once the orientation is completed, students are ready to begin assignments, take part in patient care, and achieve the goals outlined by the preceptor. How these assignments are completed will be customized slightly for each student that enters the rotation, but the role of the preceptor tends to fall somewhere along a continuum from direct instruction and modeling to coaching and facilitation.

Direct Instruction

Direct instruction is the mainstay of the didactic portion of the pharmacy curriculum. For students who are acquiring their foundational knowledge and skills, lectures, readings, and topic discussions can be very effective methods to impart new knowledge. In the experiential curriculum, direct instruction still has a role, especially when introducing students to topics that may not have been addressed previously; however, preceptors should spend a relatively small amount of time in the direct instruction role because the main function of experiential education is to apply the knowledge obtained in pharmacy school.

Modeling

Modeling, the typical preceptor role in the early portion of the rotation, allows students to see the type of behaviors and skills that are necessary to excel on the rotation and as a practicing pharmacist. Whether it is shadowing during rounds or watching a preceptor handle a difficult patient, modeling allows students to see how the didactic knowledge they possess can be translated into effective patient care. To allow students to see the thought process behind their preceptor's actions, it may also be helpful to talk through the steps that lead the preceptor to the final conclusion.

Coaching

As students become more confident in their own knowledge and abilities, the preceptor can transition into the role of a coach. Here, students begin to take over the patient care duties that the preceptor once modeled. As they try to identify drug-related problems and make therapeutic recommendations, the preceptor will be available to critique their decisions and provide the necessary guidance. Instead of the preceptor explaining his or her process, it is now the students' turn to talk through their decisions to demonstrate their growing mastery.

Facilitating

By the end of the rotation, preceptors should begin to notice the frequency of their comments and critiques begin to dwindle. This is a sign that they are transitioning into the final role of the preceptor: the facilitator. In the facilitating role, preceptors can take a back seat to the student. By now, the student has gained the ability to evaluate and correct his or her own work. To aid in perfecting their newly acquired skills, the preceptor can direct quality learning opportunities and questions toward the students and observe their handling of the challenge. In many cases, students may not achieve the level of mastery that allows preceptors to enter a facilitator's role until their final few rotations, but when it is reached, the preceptor can feel confident that he or she has helped usher a student from the classroom to practice.

CASE QUESTION

What preceptor roles should T.H. utilize for his first student arriving during the first month of APPE rotations?

STUDENT ASSESSMENT

Strong assessment skills are rarely taught in the typical pharmacy school curriculum. Many preceptors feel ill-prepared to give students vital feedback to help them improve their pharmacy practice skills. As a result, some students receive feedback that is far too infrequent, is general in nature, and provides little guidance toward improvement. Outlined below are the major types of assessments that a preceptor can provide to students and the role of each type.

Formative Assessments

Formative assessments are made up of the frequent, timely feedback that a preceptor provides through-out the course of the rotation. The goal of providing formative feedback is to improve the pharmacy student's performance in one facet of the rotation before the final assessment. Most often, formative assessments are informal, verbal critiques that are provided immediately after a student completes an assigned task. For example, reminding a student to check for any patient questions after a counseling session can be classified as formative assessment. Formative assessments may also come in the form of written evaluations. Preceptor annotations of rough drafts for case presentations, journal clubs, and drug information questions and completed rubrics assessing a student's patient care skills are tools used to provide ongoing appraisal of the student's performance. For students who are underperforming, formative assessment may take on a more formal appearance. In these cases, regular documentation of progress (or lack thereof) is vital to corroborate the final grades the student earns.

Formative assessments will be a much larger component of the pharmacy students' assessment in the first few months of the experiential curriculum. In these early rotations, students may have numerous areas in need of improvement. To keep the assessments manageable, many preceptors will focus their assessments on three areas for improvement per assessment. As students gain confidence and improve their skills, the need for corrective feedback should decrease and assessments can be used to highlight the students' strengths.

Summative Assessments

Where formative assessments focus on a single assignment or skill, summative assessments are meant to be a comprehensive evaluation of a student's progress toward achieving the goals of a rotation. They are formal and written. The most common examples of summative assessments are the midpoint and final evaluations. Midpoint evaluations are often optional but are highly recommended. Taking time halfway through a rotation to summarize the students' progress toward rotational goals can help keep them on track for success and alleviate any surprises that may come up if only a final assessment is completed, making midpoint assessments vital for underperforming students.

Each college or school of pharmacy should provide preceptors with a standardized evaluation form. To be of real value to the student, these evaluations must be completed in a timely manner, allowing the preceptor and student to discuss the documents just prior to the end of the rotation. Instead of simply assigning grades for each goal and objective, the preceptor should include constructive comments that the student can use in future rotations. In many instances, evaluations can be long, complicated documents. To keep the workload manageable for preceptors, comments may be limited to the corrective steps the student should take in areas that need improvement and descriptions of the areas in which the student has performed exceptionally well.

CASE QUESTION

T.H. has his first student on rotation and has just suggested that they take a little time to assess both prescription and nonprescription medications during each patient visit. What type of evaluation has he just completed?

Student Self-Evaluations

If not formally a part of the college of pharmacy's experiential education assessments, preceptors should strongly consider including a student self-evaluation before discussing any formative or summative assessments. Self-evaluation is an important skill that every professional must possess before practicing independently. Once their academic careers are completed, students will not have the luxury of formal assessments and graded assignments. They will need to be able to objectively judge their own performance as pharmacists. To gain this ability, students need to practice identifying their own areas of exceptional and substandard performance. These exercises should be tailored to the individual rotation and can take as many forms as the formative and summative evaluations described above: formal, informal, written, or verbal. Before the preceptor discusses each area of the self-evaluation, the student should present his or her own thoughts. When differences in opinion exist, the preceptor should take the time to clearly describe the expectations of the student and what the student can do in the future to meet those expectations. With each successive self-evaluation, the student's self-awareness will grow and the number of discrepancies between student and preceptor evaluations should fall.

LETTERS OF RECOMMENDATION

Due to their close contact with numerous students, preceptors are often asked to write letters of recommendation. Preceptors observe, firsthand, the transition from student to practitioner. Few other role models have such a prime vantage point to comment on the maturity, growth, and skills of a student.

When approached to write a letter of recommendation, preceptors should consider what type of letter they would be able to write for the requesting student. Not every request for a letter will come from an exceptional student. In situations where the preceptor does not feel he or she could write a positive recommendation, it may be wise to have a brief meeting with the student to convey the honesty that will be required if a letter is written. Other preceptors will provide a copy of the letter of recommendation to the requesting student for review prior to submission. Whatever route is chosen, it is of vital importance that any letter that is written does not artificially inflate a student's achievements or contain any false descriptions of student performance.

To be an effective recommendation writer, a thorough understanding of the student and the position or award he or she is seeking is crucial. Prior to writing a letter, preceptors may request information about a student's achievements outside of the rotation setting. Materials that may be requested include the student's curriculum vitae, transcripts, and examples of projects and assignments from other rotations or courses. If additional information is required, preceptors may request to have a meeting with the student to answer lingering questions. Along with these examples of student merit, preceptors should also collect information about the letter's destination, such as due dates, addresses, forms, and descriptions of the position or award.

Letters of recommendation can follow a number of styles and formats. One example of a letter of recommendation is provided (see **Figure 17-1**), but numerous others exist. Most letters begin with an opening statement that identifies the author of the letter, the student, and the position or award that is being sought. Next, a brief description of the nature and duration of the relationship between the preceptor and the student should be included. In addition to the length of time the student spent with the preceptor, a description of the practice setting and the student's responsibilities can also be explained. Preceptors should definitely highlight the skills displayed that exceeded expectations and may consider including any potential weaknesses discovered while on rotation. Important skills to describe include communication (patient, provider, and presentation skills), critical thinking ability, autonomy, and knowledge base. Within these descriptions, specific examples should be chosen over broad generalities. The details of the situations and events that exemplified the student's abilities are a much more effective portrayal than a positive remark.

Next, the student's academic record, awards, and leadership roles can be described. Because many of these experiences likely occurred away from the rotation site, the preceptor will need to rely on his or her interactions with the student and the student's curriculum vitae when describing these achievements. By being thorough in the collection of this information, a more complete picture of the student can be surmised from the letter. If there are any personal qualities that the student possesses that would help him or her stand out from the crowd, such as honesty, a sense of humor, or dependability, a brief description of them may also be included in the letter of recommendation.

QUICK TIP

Very short letters of recommendation can send a negative message, and lengthy letters can be a chore to read. The typical letter should be between one and two pages in length.

Lastly, each letter of recommendation should conclude with an overall impression of the student and his or her suitability for the award or position being sought. Preceptors can describe whether they would be interested in the candidate for positions at their own institution and how the student compares to other students they have had in the past. A final statement should summarize the degree of enthusiasm the preceptor has for the student and encourage the recipients to seek further contact if unanswered questions remain.

SUGGESTED READING

Cuellar LM, Ginsburg DB. *Preceptor's Handbook for Pharmacists*. 2nd ed. Bethesda, MD: American Society of Health-System Pharmacists; 2009.

Doty RE. *Getting Started as a Pharmacy Preceptor*. Washington, DC: American Pharmacists Association; 2011.

Figure 17-1. Example of a Recommendation Letter

Jason Billings, PharmD
Memorial Medical Center
Department of Pharmacy
100 Main Street
Cleveland, OH 44102

January 20, 2013

Dear Dr. Billings,

I am writing to inform you of my recommendation of Bethany Student for your PGY1 pharmacy practice residency. I had the pleasure of getting to know Bethany as her Internal Medicine preceptor over the past 2 months. Throughout that time, she demonstrated a number of important attributes that are vital to becoming a successful pharmacy resident.

While completing daily case presentations, Bethany routinely performed at a level well above her current experience. More importantly, however, she constantly strove to improve this knowledge base, working on her own time to study relevant material. Later, during one-on-one medication education rounds and large-group warfarin education sessions, she displayed strong communication skills, translating complex medical issues into language the patients could easily understand. Her interactions with patients were always professional, yet warm and friendly. During daily topic discussions she was an active participant and demonstrated an eagerness to learn advanced materials not yet covered in the curriculum. Lastly, for her final presentation, Bethany evaluated the billing and renal dosing procedures of our Catheterization Lab. Throughout the data collection and evaluation, she required little to no guidance from pharmacy staff, and the results of the project significantly impacted both patient care and the budget at our facility.

As the coadvisor to the Student Society of Health-System Pharmacists (SSHP), I have also had the chance to work closely with Bethany as this new student-pharmacist organization is built from the ground upward. She has played an integral role in the group as an active member, executive committee member, and, most recently, secretary. With the help of the other executive committee members, Bethany has expanded leadership opportunities via the addition of task forces that allow other pharmacy students to get more involved, identified qualified presenters for the speaker's series, and shaped the future course of SSHP. Despite the significant workload involved in developing a new organization, Bethany also has assumed leadership positions in the Academy of Student Pharmacists and Lambda Lambda Sigma, among other on-campus organizations.

To simply describe Bethany's involvement in these organizations by the titles she has received, however, would not accurately reflect the degree of her involvement. She has truly excelled in her ability to bring disparate groups together to organize brand new joint events, such as the Annual Golf Outing, the Pharmacy Quiz Bowl, and many other successful events. I was very impressed by her ability to both delegate responsibilities effectively to her peers and simultaneously be unafraid to jump in and accomplish what is necessary to have a successful function.

In addition to the attributes listed above, Bethany has simply been a joy to work with. She is easygoing, enthusiastic, knowledgeable, and works extremely well with her colleagues and preceptors. Had she stayed in this area, I can assure you that I would be actively recruiting her for my own residency program. If you require any additional information, please do not hesitate to contact me.

Sincerely,

John Smith, PharmD, BCPS
Clinical Pharmacist, Internal Medicine
PGY1 Residency Program Coordinator
General Medical Center
e-mail: john.smith@generalmc.org

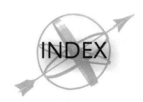

INDEX

A

abbreviations, 20-21
  to avoid, 21-22
  base solutions, 34
  diagnosis, 40-41
  drug administration, preparation, 35-36
  drug preparations or remedies, 36-37
  family history, 39
  history of present illness, 37-38
  laboratory, 40-41
  medication application methods, 37
  medications, 39-40
  past medical history, 38-39
  quantities, 34-35
  review of symptoms, 41-42
  social history, 39
  surgical history, 38-39
absolute risk reduction (ARR), 51, 52
abstracting services, 85
academic rotation
  networking, 205
  preparation, 191-192
  scholarship of teaching and learning, 205
  student performance assessment, 200-203
  teaching portfolio, 203-204
  teaching skills, 192-200
  typical day, 192
Accreditation Council for Pharmacy Education, 9, 111, 209, 260
  core IPPE domains, 112
  CPE credits 261
active learning techniques, 194, 195
adult daycare, 231-232
advanced pharmacy practice experience (APPE), 4, 111
  career stepping stone, 245-246
  first impressions, 7-8
adverse drug event books, 94
adverse drug reactions, 77, 235
alanine aminotransferase, 140
alkaline phosphatase, 140
alpha spending, 71
altruism, 5

ambulatory care rotation, 113, 209-222
  drug-related problems, 213-215
  patient visits, 218-219
  phone-based services, 219
  physical assessment skills, 216-218
  preparation, 209-211
  scope of practice, 221-222
  special populations, 220-221
  typical day, 211, 213
American College of Clinical Pharmacy, 5
American Diabetes Association, 160
American Journal of Health-System Pharmacy, 92
American Journal of Pharmaceutical Education, 205
American Pharmacists Association (APhA), 252, 259, 262
American Society of Consultant Pharmacists, 225, 240, 262
American Society of Health-System Pharmacists (ASHP), 144, 246, 252
  Midyear Meeting, 254, 255
amoxicillin, 75, 79, 85
analysis, drug information, 79
Annals of Pharmacotherapy, 92
anticoagulation, 222
antipsychotics, 240
appesartan, 51, 53
arterial blood gases, 142
aseptic technique, 149
aspartate aminotransferase, 140
aspirin, 56
assessment statement, 101
assignment-type questions, 76, 78
assisted living facility, 231
audience
  formal case presentation, 103-104
  informal case presentation, 105
  response systems, 199
audits, 188

B

background information, 76-77
  questions, 77
barium study, 130
base solutions, 34

V

vancomycin, 85
IVPB, 148-149
-vascular, 20
ventilation-perfusion (V/Q) scan, 130
veterinary medicine books, 95
video uploading/hosting, 199
visual aids, 105
-volemic, 20

W

warfarin, 53
web conferencing, 200
website, 199
wellness programs, 172
white blood cell counts, 138
wiki, 199
Wikipedia, 89
Wisneski, S. Scott, 3-17
work-life balance, 255, 257
writing test items, 201-202
written papers, 91

X

X-rays, 128